Neuroliterature
Patients, Doctors, Diseases

Literary perspectives on
disorders of the nervous system

AJ LARNER

AJ Larner MD MRCP(UK) DHMSA PhD

Consultant Neurologist, Walton Centre for Neurology and Neurosurgery, Liverpool, L9 7LJ, United Kingdom

Society of Apothecaries' Honorary Lecturer in the History of Medicine, University of Liverpool, United Kingdom.

e-mail: a.larner@thewaltoncentre.nhs.uk

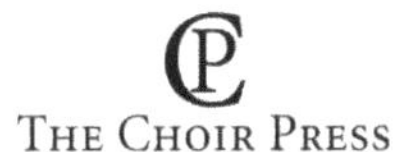

The Choir Press

First published in the United Kingdom in 2019 by
The Choir Press

ISBN 978–1–78963–056–5

Contents

Foreword

Patients, Doctors and Diseases are intricately intermingled and disease intrigues all human beings with its unhealthy and morbid interest. We are all subject to misfortunes of health at various stages of our lives and we do not know for how long we are going to continue to be part of the fraternity of live humans and therefore when we will succumb, transiently or permanently, to accident or illness. It is one of the risks of living.

We are all potential patients therefore and to read about others in the past who have suffered some disease process is highly intriguing. In the pages that follow we find descriptions of twelve persons who have either been a victim of illness or who have written about the misfortunes of another. These accounts make good reading and help explain some of the strengths and weaknesses of the characters portrayed and of their literary inventors.

Doctors too are fascinated by disease and have been accused sometimes of treating their patients as scientific preparations, bearers of disease states, problems to be solved by science, and it was as a result of this, often justified, impression that the concept of the medical humanities was developed. Humanely, we try to treat the patient as a person and not as a chemical or physical problem. However, the illnesses of doctors are also important stuff. Perhaps it is of value for doctors to suffer in order to understand more clearly what their patients are going through. Here we find essays on nineteen doctors or quasi-doctors whose lives were disturbed by illness. What effects do their illnesses have upon the writings of these medics?

And so we also come to the diseases themselves, twenty-one items discussed here, and to the effects upon our world of these infirmities. Disease is what we decide to regard as sufficiently outside our normal understanding of health and so it is a relative term and varies with the passage of time. Treatments proliferate and become, to our way of thinking, specific and more refined. The concept of Whiggishness, namely that our world gets better and better as a result of our endeavours, and this includes the "conquering" of disease, is open to debate. Each time we overcome some disease condition we tend to open up a whole new field of difficulties. The current fear that overuse of antibiotic drugs will, as in the past, lead to proliferation of organisms that are resistant has led to considerable political and economic debate and exhortations to reduce the use of such drugs in farmed animals. Thus does disease change, and our perceptions of advances in medicine with it. There is bound to be more to come with developments in technology. But let us still not forget the patient and his infirmity when here we read of some curious diseases.

Dr Larner is a prolific author in many areas of medical history and especially biography, published over a long period. Here he draws together some of his contributions which will not only fascinate us but educate us too. A second volume will be much welcomed.

Christopher Gardner-Thorpe

President of the Faculty of the History and Philosophy of Medicine and Pharmacy, Worshipful Society of Apothecaries of London

Introduction

My interest in medical history is longstanding, dating at least from Medical School days.[1–3] A period in laboratory research during my clinical training years afforded an opportunity to study for the Diploma in the History of Medicine of the Society of Apothecaries in London, one requirement for which was the writing of a dissertation, for which the African travel journals of Dr Gustav Nachtigal (1834–1885), so engagingly translated by Allan and Humphrey Fisher, provided a rich source of medical narrative.[4,5] This focus on Africa lead on, naturally enough, to Dr David Livingstone and his medical colleagues, Dr John Kirk and Dr Charles Meller.[6–8] A study of the life and work of Dr Edward Tyson (1651–1708) also dates from these years.[9]

An invitation from Dr Roger Barker and Dr Alasdair Coles to be the History of Neurology editor at the newly founded journal *Advances in Clinical Neuroscience & Rehabilitation* in 2001 was a major stimulus to engagement with medical narratives, and the publication of a number of articles ensued, many in *ACNR*. These accounts, principally of neurological disease, which form the core of this volume, are of both professional and lay origin, the latter taken from sources including novels, essays, letters and diaries (hence "Neuroliterature"). These lay narratives, as well as being of intrinsic interest, give a patient, as opposed to faculty, perspective on disorders of the nervous system and hence broaden our medical sensibility to and perception of the experiential aspects of disease, contributing to what has been termed (by Kathleen Montgomery Hunter[10]) the narrative structure of medical knowledge. Both medicine and literature are concerned with narrative, and hence are kindred subjects; a fuller account of their rich interrelationships is given elsewhere.[11]

Chapters have been grouped under the broad headings of Patients (these might be described as autopathographies[12]), Doctors, and Diseases. Some liberties have been taken, for example included in the Doctors section are non-qualified individuals who nonetheless may have made medical observations. Accounts of fictional doctors are (largely) eschewed, as other authors have covered this area.[13–15]

Since my reading has been undertaken principally for recreation and pleasure, fitted into the interstices of busy clinical practice in general neurology[16–18] with a specialist interest in cognitive neurology,[19–23] the resulting mix is eclectic but nevertheless will hopefully be both informative and entertaining for the reader.

AJ Larner

References

1. Larner AJ. Ignaz Phillip Semmelweis. *Oxford Medical School Gazette* 1985;36(2): 5–7.
2. Larner AJ. A portrait of Richard Lower. *Endeavour* 1987;11:205–208.
3. Larner AJ. Richard Lower (1631–1691): a pioneer of cardiologic research. *Am J Cardiol* 1992;69:565.
4. Larner AJ. Dr Nachtigal's casebook: medicine and illness in North Africa 1869–1874. Dissertation for the Diploma in the History of Medicine, Worshipful Society of Apothecaries of London, 1995, unpublished.
5. Larner AJ, Fisher HJ. Dr. Gustav Nachtigal (1834–1885): a contribution to the history of medicine in mid-nineteenth century Africa. *J Med Biogr* 2000;8:43–48.
6. Larner AJ. Charles Meller and the medicine of the tropics in the mid-nineteenth century: pioneer or plagiarist? *St Mary's Gazette* 1998;104(2):47–49.
7. Larner AJ. Charles Meller and John Kirk: medical practitioners and practice on Livingstone's Zambesi expedition, 1858–64. *J Med Biogr* 2002;10:129–134.
8. Larner AJ. Ophthalmological observations made during the mid-19th century European encounter with Africa. *Arch Ophthalmol* 2004;122:267–272.
9. Larner AJ. Edward Tyson and "The Anatomy of a Pygmie", 1699. *J Med Biogr* 2000;8:78–82.
10. Hunter KM. *Doctors' stories. The narrative structure of medical knowledge.* Princeton: Princeton University Press, 1991.
11. Larner AJ. Neurology and literature. *Neurosciences and History* 2017;5:47–51.
12. Farrar CB. The autopathography of C.W. Beers. *Am J Psychiatry* 1908;65:215–228.
13. Posen S. *The doctor in literature. Volume 1. Satisfaction or resentment.* Oxford: Radcliffe, 2005.
14. Posen S. *The doctor in literature. Volume 2. Private life.* Oxford: Radcliffe, 2006.
15. Surawicz B, Jacobson B. *Doctors in fiction. Lessons from literature.* Oxford: Radcliffe, 2009.
16. Larner AJ. *A dictionary of neurological signs* (4th edition). London: Springer, 2016.
17. Larner AJ, Coles AJ, Scolding NJ, Barker RA. *A-Z of neurological practice. A guide to clinical neurology* (2nd edition). London: Springer, 2011.
18. Larner AJ. *Teleneurology by internet and telephone. A study of medical self-help.* London: Springer, 2011.
19. Larner AJ. *Neuropsychological neurology: the neurocognitive impairments of neurological disorders* (2nd edition). Cambridge: Cambridge University Press, 2013.
20. Larner AJ (ed.). *Cognitive screening instruments. A practical approach* (2nd edition). London: Springer, 2017.
21. Larner AJ. *Transient global amnesia. From patient encounter to clinical neuroscience.* London: Springer, 2017.
22. Larner AJ. *Dementia in clinical practice: a neurological perspective. Pragmatic studies in the Cognitive Function Clinic* (3rd edition). London: Springer, 2018.
23. Larner AJ. *Diagnostic test accuracy studies in dementia: a pragmatic approach.* (2nd edition). London: Springer; 2019 (in press).

Patients

Antony van Leeuwenhoek (1632–1723): diaphragmatic flutter (respiratory myoclonus)

Antony van Leeuwenhoek, a draper from Delft in the Netherlands, is renowned for his pioneering work in microscopy.[1] Beginning in the 1670s, his skill in grinding lenses smaller than the head of a pin allowed him to observe, with his single lens instruments, red blood cells, the striations of muscle, spermatozoa, and "animalcules", possibly protozoa, possibly bacteria.[2] Many of his observations (116 in all) were published in the *Philosophical Transactions* of the Royal Society of London, of which he became a corresponding Fellow through his contact with Henry Oldenburg.

Towards the end of his long life (which was exactly contemporaneous with that of Sir Christopher Wren), Leeuwenhoek communicated some clinical observations to the *Philosophical Transactions.*[3] In a letter dated 19th March 1723 and entitled *De globulorum sanguineorum magnitudine* (On the size of the particles of the blood), there are two brief paragraphs in which he describes his recent state of health:

> Not long ago, after January finished, I was seized by a violent movement around that large and vital organ we call the diaphragm, so much indeed that those standing around were not a little alarmed. When the movement eased off, searching for a name for this illness, the doctor, who was there, answered it to be a palpitation of the heart. I think the doctor was in fact wrong. For although while the movement was happening I several times felt the arterial pulse with my hand, I did not feel any acceleration. Starting up again every now and then, the violent movement lasted about three days, during which time my stomach and intestine ceased to function. I thought I was at death's door.
>
> I am of the opinion an obstruction was stuck in my diaphragm, not smaller than an imperial penny.

This may not have been his first such attack. In 1716, aged 83, he wrote to Dr Abraham van Bleyswijk of Delft recording an episode in which he was very short of breath, accompanied by tightness of the chest, pain which he thought arose from the diaphragm and stomach rising to the throat. He ordered warm water, after which he vomited. This apparently occurred just before a courtesy (rather than medical) visit from Herman Boerhaave (1668–1738), but time apparently did not allow for a discussion of these symptoms with the great doctor.[2]

In a subsequent letter to the Royal Society, dated 31st May 1723, Leeuwenhoek described the histology of the diaphragm in sheep and oxen, and reiterated his belief that his illness of the previous winter was characterised by palpitations arising from the diaphragm. He persisted in this idea: after his death on 26th August 1723, the minister of Leeuwenhoek's church, the Reverend Mr Peter Gribius, wrote to inform the Royal Society of his passing, observing that:

> The notion possessed our good old man that he lay a-dying of a distemper of his diaphragm, though in fact 'twas of his lungs.[2]

Hence, Leeuwenhoek complained of episodic epigastric pulsations not in time with his pulse, shortness of breath, and thoraco-abdominal pain, possibly associated with vomiting, symptoms which he believed to be diaphragmatic rather than cardiac in origin.

These are now recognised as the characteristic clinical features of diaphragmatic flutter. This name was coined by Porter in 1936,[4] prior cases having been described as diaphragmatic tic, tremor or chorea. Nosologically it has been suggested that diaphragmatic flutter is a variant of palatal myoclonus,[5,6] although unlike the latter diaphragmatic flutter stops during sleep.[7] The pathophysiology has been shown by diaphragm electromyography to be involuntary diaphragm contraction at a frequency of 0.5–8.0 Hz.[6] A high frequency variant (9–15 Hz) has also been reported, with symptoms of hiccups, belching and retching.[8]

Subsequent reports of diaphragmatic flutter have been relatively few, and have often appeared in journals devoted to respiratory medicine or critical care medicine rather than neurology, with presentations as recalcitrant asthma, inspiratory stridor, or difficulty in weaning from mechanical ventilation. From the neurological perspective most cases are primary or idiopathic[5] although postencephalitic, postviral, and tardive forms[9] have been reported.

Phillips and Eldridge stated that Leeuwenhoek self-medicated his symptoms with port wine laced with nutmeg, apparently with initial benefit, but on symptom recurrence retrial was ineffective.[6] However, I have not been able to find a source for these statements. Though such treatment might be welcome to some patients, the evidence base is at best slim. Anecdotal efficacy has been reported with phenytoin[6] and, in the high frequency variant, carbamazepine.[8]

Leeuwenhoek's clinical observations recorded in his letter to the Royal Society of 19th March 1723 reflect his "strong allegiance to empirical observation"[10] which is manifest in his microscopical work. He had no formal training in either science or medicine. His contribution to the field of movement disorders, though previously acknowledged,[6] is not mentioned in reviews of the history of myoclonus.[11,12] Based on his account of his own symptoms, it would seem that he richly merits the eponymous renown of "Leeuwenhoek's syndrome or disease" for his description of diaphragmatic flutter or respiratory myoclonus.[13]

Acknowledgements

I thank Andrew Makower for help with Latin translation; any remaining errors are my own.

Adapted from: Larner AJ. Antony van Leeuwenhoek and the description of diaphragmatic flutter (respiratory myoclonus). *Mov Disord* 2005;20:917–918.

References

1. Reiser SJ. *Medicine and the reign of technology*. Cambridge: Cambridge University Press, 1978:69–90 [at 71–72].
2. Dobell C. *Antony van Leeuwenhoek and his "little animals", being some account of the father of protozoology and bacteriology and his multifarious discoveries in these disciplines collected, translated and edited, from his printed works, unpublished manuscripts, and contemporary records.* London: John Bale, Sons and Danielsson, 1932 [at 83–86,90–91,95].
3. Leeuwenhoek A. De globulorum sanguineorum magnitudine. *Phil Trans Roy Soc Lond* 1723;32:341–343 [at 342].
4. Porter WB. Diaphragmatic flutter with symptoms of angina pectoris. *JAMA* 1936;106:992–994.
5. Iliceto G, Thompson PD, Day BL, Rothwell JC, Lees AJ, Marsden CD. Diaphragmatic flutter, the moving umbilicus syndrome, and "belly dancers" dyskinesia. *Mov Disord* 1990;5:15–22.
6. Phillips JR, Eldridge FL. Respiratory myoclonus (Leeuwenhoek's disease). *N Engl J Med* 1973;289:1390–1395.
7. Walton D, Bonello M, Steiger M. Diaphragmatic flutter. *Pract Neurol* 2018;18:224–226.
8. Vantrappen G, Decramer M, Harlet R. High-frequency diaphragmatic flutter: symptoms and treatment by carbamazepine. *Lancet* 1992;339:265–267.
9. Burn DJ, Coulthard A, Connolly S, Cartlidge NF. Tardive diaphragmatic flutter. *Mov Disord* 1998;13:190–192.
10. Cook HJ. Anton van Leeuwenhoek. In: Black J, Porter R (eds.). *A dictionary of eighteenth-century world history*. Oxford: Blackwell, 1994:404.
11. Marsden CD, Hallett M, Fahn S. The nosology and pathophysiology of myoclonus. In: Marsden CD, Fahn S (eds.). *Movement Disorders*. London: Butterworth, 1982: 196–248.
12. Goetz CG, Chmura TA, Lanska DJ. History of myoclonus: Part 8 of the

MDS-sponsored history of movement disorders exhibit, Barcelona, June 2000. *Mov Disord* 2001;16:545–547.

13. Barker RA, Scolding NJ, Rowe D, Larner AJ. *The A-Z of neurological practice. A guide to clinical neurology*. Cambridge: Cambridge University Press, 2005:481.

Elizabeth Gaskell (1810–1865): "a habit of headaches"

To the old adage, variously ascribed to either Benjamin Franklin (1706–1790) or Daniel Defoe (ca. 1660–1731), to the effect that nothing is certain in life except death and taxes, it might be appropriate to add a third trial, namely headache. The reasons for suggesting this are both historical and epidemiological.

The written historical record indicates headache troubled our ancestors in Mesopotamia some 6000 years ago,[1] and it is possible, though not amenable to confirmation or refutation, that the practice of trepanation or trephination of the skull, dating to prehistoric times, might have been undertaken, at least in some instances, for the relief of headache.[2]

Modern epidemiological surveys suggest a lifetime prevalence of headache of between 70% and 90%,[3] meaning that only a minority of individuals go through a lifetime without experiencing at least one headache (and as a minority might therefore be deemed abnormal). Most headaches are borne without soliciting professional medical assistance, but nevertheless at least 20–25% of the outpatient workload of a hospital specialist in neurology is made up of patients complaining of headache.[4] According to the World Health Organisation, headache disorders rank in the top ten of the most disabling conditions globally.[5]

The ubiquity of headache may therefore render the finding of accounts of headache in literary texts hardly worthy of comment, even mundane. However, the old advice to potential authors to "write what you know" may prompt the curious neurologist to wonder whether such usages might reflect an underlying headache disorder in the author. Such an analysis has been undertaken, for example, with Jane Austen (1775–1817), based on the characters in her novels with headache and the author's extant correspondence.[6] Since many characters in the novels and shorter fiction of Elizabeth Gaskell are reported to have headaches, it may be worth enquiring whether she too was a sufferer.

Many references to medical issues, their impact, and treatment, may be found in the two volumes of Mrs Gaskell's correspondence (covering the period 1832–1865)[7] and in the brief fragment of diary which she kept (1835–1838).[8] Of these, references to headache form a very significant part yet, to my knowledge, no extended analysis of the headaches suffered by Mrs Gaskell, her family and friends, has been presented hitherto, although mentioned in passing in biographical work.[9]

The neurological assessment of a complaint of headache will encompass various factors, including but not necessarily limited to, age at onset, duration of headache disorder, headache characteristics, provoking and relieving factors, family history of headache, and treatments used and their efficacy. Headache is not a uniform syndrome, with many different types being recognised in modern classification systems based on differences in these various factors. However, most headaches are deemed "primary" (i.e. no specific cause identified: most commonly migraine), in distinction from "secondary" or symptomatic headaches which have an identifiable underlying cause (e.g. brain tumour, albeit an extremely infrequent cause).[10] Some details on all of these various factors may be extracted from a reading of Elizabeth Gaskell's correspondence.

The clinical record

The first definite report from Gaskell's pen that she has suffered from a headache is in her letter to Charles Dickens, provisionally dated 12th January 1850, when she reports "My head & eyes ache so, with crying over the loss of three dear little cousins, who have died of S[carlet]. Fever since I last wrote ….".[11] However, the onset of her headache disorder certainly predates this. A letter from Meta Gaskell to her former governess, Miss Fergusson, with postmark 23rd April 1848, states that "Mama has got a bad headache, & did not get up this morning".[12] In August 1849 Mrs Gaskell reports to Catherine Winkworth that she and her husband William have been invited to a dance "but I'm going to have a headache", possibly suggesting a familiarity with the effects of headache.[13] An even earlier reference is found in one of Gaskell's earliest extant letters, addressed to Harriet Carr and dated August 1832, in which she commiserates with Harriet about the latter's headaches and suggests a possible remedy, sal volatile, from which Gaskell has "'derived great benefit myself" and which she claims to have been suggested by "an M.D. in the shape of Dr Holland", presumably Henry Holland, son of her Uncle Peter Holland.[14] Uglow states that "her letters to Harriet are full of remedies for the headaches that plagued them both".[15] This may put the onset of Gaskell's headaches back to her early twenties or even late teenage years. Of possible relevance here, if it be the case that art truly imitates life, is the headache suffered by Molly Gibson when aged 11 or 12 years old in the novel *Wives and Daughters*.[16] Gaskell's daughter Julia may have suffered from headaches from as early as the age of 5 years.[17]

The tendency to intermittent headaches evidently continued throughout Gaskell's life. Definite or possible reports of headache are mentioned in correspondence dated definitely or provisionally to 1852,[18] 1853,[19] 1854,[20] 1855,[21] 1856,[22] 1857,[23] 1858,[24] 1860,[25] and 1865.

That the propensity was lifelong is indicated in a letter to Madame Scherer dated 11th April 1865 in which Gaskell states "I am really afraid of being completely incapacitated for writing my story unless I take care of my precious and troublesome head; which begins to ache so very easily".[26] The last report of headache is in a letter to George Smith, provisionally dated 23rd August 1865,[27] less than 3 months before Gaskell's death. The duration of headache disorder may therefore be confirmed as decades, encompassing most or all of her adult life.

Most of Gaskell's references to headache are incidental, rather than detailed accounts of headache characteristics such as a clinician would wish to elicit. Nonetheless, she does give some descriptions of headache and her responses to them, including "atrocious", "felling", "very stupid with repeated headaches", "so ill", "too much blinded with head-ache to read", "deadly", and "stupefied".[28] One "*dreadful* headache" (Gaskell's italics) leaves her "utterly Kilt & incapable", kilt being a dialect word apparently meaning exhausted.[29]

The term "migraine" is used by Gaskell on only one occasion: visiting a confectioner's shop whilst in Germany, she reported to the girl that she had a "migraine affreuse".[30] A different terminology is employed in a letter to Bentley of 1853, perhaps the longest account devoted to her pain, when, echoing her correspondent, she speaks of "tic & neuralgia; from which I have suffered most acutely for years".[31] The terms migraine, tic and neuralgia are not necessarily mutually exclusive in this discourse, since they do not necessarily carry the same technical meanings with which a modern clinician would use them. Writing in the 1870s, Francis Kilvert described his symptoms interchangeably as headache, face ache, and neuralgia.[32]

Gaskell's headaches clearly affected both her social and occupational functions. For example, she "could not go to the Examination of the Schools at Swinton", has "been stopping at home", and has to "come home in the middle of the festivities".[33] Headache "would incapacitate me for work" and "makes me write confusedly".[34] Taking writing to be Gaskell's occupational function, headaches clearly impinged on the writing of *North and South*, on the proof corrections of the *Life of Charlotte Brontë*, and on the writing of *Wives and Daughters* which is described as "behindhand".[35]

A question asked by practically every headache patient is what causes their headaches, and many speculations may be advanced to answer this. Provoking factors suggested by Mrs Gaskell include "heat & sun", "misty foggy Manchester", "the air of Manchester" (her claim that she hardly ever has headaches anywhere else than Manchester is not substantiated by the letters), "thunder yesterday", and "glare and heat".[36] Ambient conditions might also be implicated by "going .. to the theatre" the day before; on another theatre visit "We sat right under the very much raised stage, on the front row, & I think I got

Braidized for I had such a headache with looking up", Braidized suggesting a form of hypnotism.[37] Her daughter Julia's "constant feeling of sickness & headache" prompts the plan to "have the drains up in the yard & see if anything is wrong there".[38] The absence of emotional or psychic factors as headache precipitants in the correspondence, rather than physical or sensory factors, is striking (and contrasts with Gaskell's fiction[39]), although Uglow states that Elizabeth's "migraines and neuralgia … were often the results of stress".[40]

Certain headache types, particularly migraine, have a tendency to run in families, suggesting genetic contributions to aetiology. From a reading of the correspondence it is evident that the Gaskell family history was positive for headache. Others afflicted were her daughters Marianne,[41] Meta,[42] and Julia,[43] with Florence the only one seemingly spared. Other Gaskell correspondents noted to have headaches are Eliza Fox, Charlotte Brontë, Mrs Shadwell, Selina, Ellen Larghe, Harriet Carr, and Harriet Anderson (possibly *née* Carr).[44]

Little is said about headache treatment, presumably because the options, other than bed rest,[45] were limited to grin and bear it. Recovery from headache was associated with a "weak happy state of easy exhaustion, which follows on the cessation of extreme pain" which permitted letter writing and driving.[46] Resort to medication is infrequently reported. In the German confectioner's shop, "*rum & peppermint*!! .. *was* wonderful for the headache" (Gaskell's italics). The headache provoked by thunder prompts "my prussic acid medicine made up" (efficacy not stated), and in correspondence with a fellow sufferer of "tic & neuralgia" rubbing the affected part with viratria ointment is recommended as a remedy which Gaskell has found curative, based in part on the recommendation of her cousin Sir Henry Holland. His authority is also claimed for sal volatile (i.e. ammonium carbonate smelling salts, also known as hartshorn, which give off ammonia on exposure to air) which Gaskell recommended to Harriet Carr, reporting that she herself had "derived great benefit" from this treatment.[47] For Julia's headaches, Gaskell recommends "opening medicine", specifically stewed rhubarb.[48]

Discussion

It is recognised that the existing correspondence of Mrs Gaskell, though forming a "treasure hoard[,] can distort, since its record is inevitably incomplete".[49] Nonetheless, it would seem from this record that, just as "[s]he certainly suffered all her life from periods of low spirits and exhaustion",[50] Elizabeth Gaskell also was subject to headaches throughout her adult life, covering at least the period 1850 to 1865, and very possibly from before 1832. Evidence has been adduced to support a diagnosis of headache disorder in other authors based on their extant correspondence (e.g. Charlotte Brontë[51]) or diaries (e.g. Francis Kilvert,[32] Sofia Tolstoy[52]).

Gaskell's headaches were often sufficiently severe to interfere with her daily occupations, as well as her writing. Three of her four daughters also are reported to have had headaches. Retrospective diagnosis is risky, but the features described in the correspondence combine to suggest a diagnosis of migraine.

Perhaps more important than any retrospective diagnosis is the question as to whether Gaskell's headaches informed her fictional writing. The frequency of characters with headache, extending throughout her writing career (see Table) suggests that this may have been the case. Correspondences between life and fiction may be noted, for example Gaskell's recommendation of sal volatile as a treatment, and its use by Mrs Carson in *Mary Barton*.[53] However, as with other authors, such as Jane Austen, Gaskell also used headache as a convenient literary device with gendered meanings, such as a metaphor for other difficulties (emotional, domestic) or as an excuse or avoidance strategy.[54] Hence headache may be a further example of Gaskell's use of illness to transform realism to romanticism, as argued by Angus Easson, illness being a "marker of crisis not just in the body but also in the mind and the psyche; symptoms and diagnosis are not so important as the significance of sickness".[55]

Acknowledgement

Adapted from: Larner AJ. "A habit of headaches": the neurological case of Elizabeth Gaskell. *Gaskell Journal* 2011;25:97–103.

References

1. Rose FC. The history of migraine from Mesopotamian to Medieval times. *Cephalalgia* 1995;15 Suppl15:1–3.
2. Arnott R, Finger S, Smith CUM (eds.). *Trepanation. History, Discovery, Theory.* Lisse: Swets & Zeitlinger, 2003.
3. Rasmussen BK, Jensen R, Schroll M, Olesen J. Epidemiology of headache in a general population – a prevalence study. *J Clin Epidemiol* 1991;44:1147–1157; Torelli P, Abrignami G, Berzieri L et al. Population-based pace study: lifetime and past-year prevalence of headache in adults. *Neurol Sci* 2010;31 Suppl1:S145–S147.
4. Larner AJ. NHS Direct for headache. *J Neurol Neurosurg Psychiatry* 2003;74:1698; Larner AJ. Trigeminal autonomic cephalalgias: frequency in a general neurology clinic setting. *J Headache Pain* 2008;9:325–326.
5. Stovner LJ, Hagen K, Jensen R et al. The global burden of headache: a

documentation of headache prevalence and disability worldwide. *Cephalalgia* 2007;27:193–210.
6. Larner AJ. "A transcript of actual life": headache in the novels of Jane Austen. *Headache* 2010;50:692–695; Larner AJ. Jane Austen's (1775–1817) references to headache: fact and fiction. *J Med Biogr* 2010;18:211–215.
7. Chapple JAV, Pollard A (eds.). *The letters of Mrs Gaskell.* Manchester: Manchester University Press, [1966] 1997 (henceforward *Letters*); Chapple J, Shelston A (eds.). *Further letters of Mrs Gaskell.* Manchester: Manchester University Press, 2000 (henceforward *Further Letters*).
8. Chapple JAV, Wilson A (eds.). *Private voices: The diaries of Elizabeth Gaskell and Sophia Holland.* Keele: Keele University Press, 1996.
9. Uglow J. *Elizabeth Gaskell: a habit of stories.* London: Faber & Faber, 1993:73 (re Mrs Carsons in *Mary Barton*),77 266,299,359,367,419,452,524 (re Hester Rose in *Sylvia's Lovers*),564 (Meta Gaskell),565 (account of Mme Mohl).
10. Goadsby P. Headache. In: Clarke C, Howard R, Rossor M, Shorvon S (eds.). *Neurology: a Queen Square textbook.* Chichester: Wiley-Blackwell, 2009:449–464.
11. *Letters*, 100 (no.62).
12. *Further Letters*, 298.
13. *Letters*, 83 (no.49).
14. *Further Letters*, 19,20.
15 Uglow, *Elizabeth Gaskell*, 77.
16. Elizabeth Gaskell, *Wives and Daughters* (London: Penguin Classics, [1866] 2003): chapter 2 (15,17,18); chapter 9 (103).
17. *Letters*, 174 (no.109).
18. *Letters*, 191 (no.126), 200 (no.133), 848 (no.118a), 854 (no.144a); *Further Letters*, 64,74.
19. *Letters*, 858 (no.156a).
20. *Letters*, 274 (no.185), 294 (no.200), 325 (no.222).
21. *Letters*, 871 (no.267).
22. *Further Letters*, 153.
23. *Letters*, 435 (no.330), 447 (no.346), 464 (no.366), 466 (no.368), 491 (no.384).
24. *Letters*, 502 (no.393), 512 (no.401), 519 (no.405); *Further Letters*, 191.
25. *Letters*, 597 (no.453), 607 (no.461), 614 (no.465), 912 (no.472+).
26. *Further Letters*, 273.
27. *Letters*, 766 (no.576).
28. Respectively *Letters*, 274 (no.185), 325 (no.222), 464 (no.366), 466 (no.368), 502 (no.393), and *Further Letters*, 153,191.
29. *Letters*, 614 (no.465).
30. *Letters*, 519 (no.405).
31. *Letters*, 250 (no.167).
32. Larner AJ. Francis Kilvert (1840–1879): an early self-report of cluster headache? *Cephalalgia* 2008;28:763–766.
33. Respectively, *Letters*, 200 (no.133), 512 (no.401), 912 (no.472+).

34. Respectively, *Further Letters*, 153,191.
35. Respectively, *Letters*, 294 (no.200) and 325 (no.222; also noted by Uglow, *Elizabeth Gaskell*, 359,367); 464 (no.366), 766 (no.576).
36. Respectively, *Letters*, 519 (no.405), 597 (no.453), 607 (no.461), 912 (no.472+); *Further Letters*, 273.
37. Respectively, *Letters*, 614 (no.465); *Further Letters*, 64. Mesmerism was possibly a subject of interest to Gaskell, see Hilton C. Elizabeth Gaskell and mesmerism: an unpublished letter. *Med Hist* 1995;39:219–235.
38. *Letters*, 937 (no.575a).
39. Larner AJ. Headache in the writings of Elizabeth Gaskell (1810–65). *J Med Biogr* 2015;23:191–196.
40. Uglow, *Elizabeth Gaskell*, 266.
41. *Letters*, 212 (no.141), 530 (no.414, apparently after a head injury), 769 (no.580), 847 (no.116a), 911 (no.472+); *Further Letters*, 296.
42. *Letters*, 605 (no.460, in the context of a bad cold), 736 (no.553, "the old headaches, and tendency to fainting"), 744 (no.560, "bewildering whirling headache").
43. *Letters*, 174 (no.109), 602–603 (no.457), 937 (no.575a, "sickness & headache").
44. Respectively, *Letters*, 109 (no.69), 127 (no.76), 653 (no.487), 790 (no.602), 795 (no.611); *Further Letters*, 19,20;155.
45. *Letters*, 491 (no.384).
46. *Letters*, 512 (no.401), 447 (no.346).
47. Respectively, *Letters*, 519 (no.405, also noted by Uglow, *Elizabeth Gaskell*, 452), 912 (no.472+), 250–251 (no.167a); *Further Letters*, 19. For Henry Holland, see Hill B. "More fashionable than scientific". Sir Henry Holland, Bt, M.D., F.R.C.P., F.R.S. (1788–1873). *Practitioner* 1973;211:548–552.
48. *Letters*, 602–603 (no.457).
49. Shelston A. *Brief lives: Elizabeth Gaskell.* London: Hesperus, 2010:19.
50. Ibid., 24.
51. Larner AJ. Charlotte Brontë (1816–1855): migraineur? *Eur J Neurol* 2009;16 Suppl3:329.
52. Larner AJ. "Neurological literature": headache (part 8). *Adv Clin Neurosci Rehabil* 2011;11(2):21.
53. Elizabeth Gaskell, *Mary Barton: A tale of Manchester life* (London: Penguin Classics, [1848] 2003):201–202.
54. Kempner J. A sociologic perspective on migraine in women. In: Loder E, Marcus DA (eds.). *Migraine in Women.* Hamilton: Decker, 2004:166.
55. Easson A. Introduction. In: Elizabeth Gaskell, *Ruth* (London: Penguin Classics, [1853] 2004):xiv-xv.

Some characters afflicted with headache in the works of Elizabeth Gaskell

Mary Barton (1848)	Mrs Carson, Mary Barton
The Moorland Cottage (1850)	Mrs Browne
Mr Harrison's Confessions (1851)	Caroline Tomkinson
Ruth (1853)	Ruth Hilton, Henry Bellingham, Jemima Bradshaw
Cranford (1853)	Matilda Jenkyns, Miss Pole
North and South (1855)	Margaret Hale, Mrs Hale, Mrs Thornton, Fanny Thornton, Mr Thornton, Bessy Higgins
Half a life-time ago (1855)	William Dixon, Susan Dixon
The Manchester Marriage (1858)	Norah Kennedy
The Grey Woman (1861)	Madame the Baroness de Roeder
Sylvia's Lovers (1863)	Sylvia Robson, Hester Rose
A Dark Night's Work (1863)	Ellinor Wilkins, Mr Wilkins, Miss Monro
Cousin Phillis (1864)	Cousin Holman
Wives and Daughters (1866)	Molly Gibson, Miss (Sally) Browning, Mrs Goodenough

David Livingstone (1813–1873): uvulectomy

In April 1852, in Cape Town, South Africa, Dr David Livingstone, then 39 years of age and yet to commence the explorations of Africa which would bring him to public attention, underwent the surgical procedure of uvulectomy. This article reviews the history of Livingstone's uvulectomy, its indications and outcome, as documented by his own writings. The practice of uvulectomy in indigenous African societies, and some contemporary ideas about uvulectomy, are also considered in order to try to ascertain why Livingstone elected to undergo this procedure.

Introduction

Surgery of the uvula has become familiar in recent times, in isolation or, more commonly, as a component of uvulopalatopharyngoplasty, in the treatment of snoring, and of obstructive sleep apnoea syndrome when nasal continuous positive pressure ventilation cannot be tolerated.[1, 2] The procedure of uvulectomy, also known as uvulotomy, cionectomy, kionectomy (kion = Greek for uvula), or staphylectomy, was known to the ancients, being described in the works of Hippocrates and Galen, among others, and also in Hindu medicine.[3,4] However, although long practised, the operation has not always met with approval. For example, writing in 1911 in the *Preface on Doctors* published alongside the play *The Doctor's Dilemma*, George Bernard Shaw (1856–1950) stated:

> The surgeon need not take off the rich man's (or woman's) leg or arm: he can remove the appendix or the uvula, and leave the patient none the worse after a fortnight or so in bed . . .[5]

Speaking of "Fashions and Epidemics" Shaw writes:

> Tonsils, vermiform appendices, uvulas, even ovaries are sacrificed because it is the fashion to get them cut out, and because the operations are highly profitable.[6]

Thus it is reasonable to inquire into the indications and beliefs that prompted Dr David Livingstone (1813–1873) to undergo uvulectomy in the mid-nineteenth century.

Livingstone's uvulectomy

Although several of Livingstone's biographers mention his uvulectomy,[7–10] no article specifically devoted to the subject has been located by the author.

The first mention in Livingstone's papers of a problem with the uvula dates from 9th January 1850 in a letter addressed to JJ Freeman of the London Missionary Society, then Livingstone's employers:

> I have wished for a long time to have the uvula excised, and thank you heartily for your kind invitation to accompany you for the purpose.[11]

The exact date of onset of these symptoms is not recorded but presumably postdates his arrival in Africa since he had not apparently sought treatment in Glasgow or London. Within a month (5th February 1850), Livingstone wrote similarly to his sister, Agnes:

> We had a pleasant visit from Mr Freeman ... He wished me to go with him down to the [Cape] Colony in order to get my uvula excised, but I could not go. It plagues me much in speaking, having become too long.[12]

Later in the same year (31st July), Livingstone wrote to his father-in-law and fellow missionary, Dr Robert Moffat:

> I must go somewhere for surgical aid, perhaps the Cape for the best. If in London I should get Sir Benjamin Brodie for nothing.[13]

Why Livingstone thought he would be able to secure the services of such a distinguished surgeon gratis is not clear.

On 24th August 1850 he wrote again to JJ Freeman:

> If I go down to the Colony to get my uvula excised ... [14]

Then to Robert Moffat on 17th October 1850 he confides:

> I feel very unsettled in reference to our Cape journey. We need supplies, and my throat needs doctoring.[15]

Nothing further was done at this time, and one year later (1st October 1851) Livingstone wrote to A Tidman, also of the London Missionary Society:

> I shall be obliged to go southwards, perhaps to the Cape, in order to have my uvula excised and my arm mended ... [16]

One possible reason for the delay is mentioned in a further letter to Tidman (17th October 1851):

> After our return last year . . . I postponed my own wants, & did not proceed to the Cape in order to have my uvula excised, in order to allow her [Mrs Livingstone] rest.[17]

According to Blaikie, Livingstone's first biographer, at that time:

> Dr Livingstone had a strong desire to go to the Cape for the excision of his uvula, which had long been troublesome. But, with characteristic self-denial, he put his own case out of view, staying with his wife, that she might have the rest and attention she needed. He tried to persuade his father-in-law to perform the operation, and, under his direction, Dr Moffat went so far as to make a pair of scissors for the purpose; but his courage, so well tried in other fields, was not equal to the performance of such a surgical operation.[18]

As this biography was prepared at the request of the "venerable Dr Moffat",[19] among others, there seems no reason to doubt this account.

The operation

Livingstone and his family finally reached Cape Town on 16th March 1852. At this time the city boasted a powerful professional medical elite.[20] While preparing for the departure of his family for England, Livingstone also was preparing to have his uvula dealt with, as he informed Robert Moffat (2nd April 1852):

> I am in poor spirits. My throat became worse in [*sic*] the way down. My opinion is that it ought to be operated on immediately, but Dr Abercrombie thought it might be benefitted by the daily application of a strong solution of lunar caustic. He rubs it every morning. I sometimes think it is a little better, but at other times I feel it decidedly worse. The caustic being on it daily makes it feel raw, yet the gowks here will have me to speak or lecture or I don't know what. I don't like to break away from Dr Abercrombie, as he seems anxious to try, but as soon as I can do so I will, and get the operation performed, & then away.[21]

Livingstone's speaking difficulties, alluded to in this extract, were perhaps also attested to by the appearance of a publication entitled "Notes of a Tour to the River Sesheke, in the Region North of Lake Ngami, by Dr Livingston [*sic*]" in the *South African Commercial Advertiser* of 7th April 1852, in the introduction to which it is stated that Livingstone consents to publication "only in consequence of the urgent wishes of friends whom I cannot otherwise favour, being incapacitated by a disease in the throat for public speaking".[22]

Dr James Abercrombie (1797–1871) was a prominent Cape Town physician, surgeon and accoucheur. Born in Edinburgh, he gained the LRCS of Edinburgh in 1816, moved to the Cape in 1817 and was licensed there in 1819. He became well known in both medical and religious circles, as reflected in his obituary which described him as "an accomplished physician and a generous, big-hearted and Christian gentleman".[23] It is not recorded where Livingstone consulted him, but his residence at 27 Loop Street, where he lived from 1827 to 1862,[24] seems likely.

Livingstone must have applied his persuasive powers in favour of surgery, for his private journal subsequently notes tersely (paraphrasing St Paul's Epistle to the Ephesians, 3:8):

> Got my uvula excised, which I hope will enable me more fully to preach unto the gentiles the unsearchable riches of Christ.[25]

The precise date of the operation is not mentioned. Livingstone was more forthcoming about the procedure in a further letter to Robert Moffat, dated 26th April 1852:

> I got my uvula cut off, and have had all the back part of the throat smeared almost daily with a strong solution of lunar caustic. The uvula is now quite small, but the parts around are still swollen. The tongue feels as if it needed oiling. I made my first attempt at speaking in English last night in Union Chapel, and feel much the worse for it. The Dr [presumably Abercrombie] is displeased with the attempt, and certainly I have no reason to be pleased with it. I felt dreadfully at a loss for words in English, while ideas came up in barrowfuls. I became quite hoarse in about ten minutes after I began. I imagined I was recovered from the attack on the Karoo about which I informed you, but am now painfully conscious of being much worse than when I passed through Kuruman. Yet I have hopes of being ultimately well. The breath suffers no obstruction as it did before the uvula was cut. The piece taken off was about this size [illustration *ca.* 2 cm x 1 cm]. It sometimes fell down on the opening of the windpipe in sleep & made me start up as if suffocating. I shall certainly not speak in public again ... What a little thing is sufficient to bring down to old-wifishness such a tough tyke as I consider myself. Poor proud human nature is a great fool after all.[26]

Livingstone reported the outcome of his surgery in a letter of 12th October 1852:

> The throat, I am sorry to say, is not so much benefitted as I expected.[27]

Writing to his parents on 30th September 1853, nearly 18 months post-surgery, Livingstone states that:

> My throat became well during the long silence of travelling across the desert. It plagues again now that I am preaching in a moist climate.[28]

During his return to Great Britain on furlough in 1856–1858, when he was often called upon to speak in public, contemporaries noted Livingstone to have "broken hesitating speech".[29]

The uvula problem was also mentioned, in passing, in Livingstone's first 'best seller', *Missionary travels and researches in South Africa*, published in 1857. Speaking of his missionary work, he states:

> Our services having necessarily been all in the open air, where it is most difficult to address large bodies of people, prevented my recovering so entirely from the effects of clergyman's sore throat as I expected, when my uvula was excised at the Cape.[30]

Some further 'follow-up' information is also given:

> I gave many public addresses to the people of Sesheke ... They often amounted to between five and six hundred souls, and required an exertion of voice which brought back the complaint for which I had got the uvula excised at the Cape.[31]

Later he wrote:

> "Clergyman's sore throat" ... partially disabled me from the work.[32]

Thereafter, nothing further about the uvula has been discovered in Livingstone's voluminous output. Not least perhaps, this was because of preoccupation with other, more pressing, health problems, most particularly the African fever, probably malaria.[33, 34] Livingstone writes that the first attack "seized" him on 30th May 1853;[35] a little over two years later (June 1855) he reported his twenty-seventh attack.[36] Livingstone's writings also contain incidental and informative comments on other health issues.[37]

Uvulectomy in indigenous African societies

Uvulectomy performed by traditional healers has been reported from many indigenous African societies, within the borders of modern day Nigeria,[38–42] Cameroon,[43] Niger,[44] Tanzania,[45–47] Ethiopia,[48,49] Sudan,[48,50] Egypt[51,52] and Morocco,[53] as well as from Jordan and Arabia.[48,54]

Although these areas coincide largely with the distribution of Islam, the procedure may not necessarily have religious origins; certainly it is not related to the rites enjoined in the Koran.[55, 56] Wind suggests independent origins maintained by cultural mechanisms.[55] The procedure has both ritual and therapeutic purposes,[56] the former connected with the naming ceremony of children. In recent times a study in Niamey, the capital of Niger, found that around 20% of children had undergone uvulectomy by the age of five years; the frequency differed in different ethnic groups but was commonest in some subgroups of the Hausa where it formed part of the ritual naming of the child and was stated to prevent death due to "swelling of the uvula".[44] Hausa barber surgeons also perform the operation in Nigeria.[38,39]

That the procedure has been practised at least since the time of Livingstone's travels, if not long before in all probability, is indicated by travel narratives of Europeans in the nineteenth century. For example, the German medical traveller Dr Gustav Nachtigal (1834–1885), who visited Saharan Africa between 1869 and 1874,[57] observed childhood uvulectomy in several locations including Fezzan (modern day Libya), Borno (Nigeria), Tibesti and Borku (both in Chad).[58] For example, he reports that amputation of the uvula is:

> ... an operation which I have found in general use as a prophylactic measure against many kinds of illness in all the Muslim Negro countries visited by me ... [59]

Moreover, in Borku:

> ... in their new homeland the Arabs had also adopted the custom of the Negroes and half-Negroes of cutting off the uvula of children with scissors as a presumed protection against a whole series of diseases ... [60]

This observation seems to corroborate the suggestion that the practice did not originate with Islam.[55]

Why did Livingstone chose uvulectomy?

Why Livingstone should have thought the uvula was the cause of his preaching difficulties, and that uvulectomy was the desired solution, is a challenging question. One speculation might be to suggest that Livingstone's desire for uvulectomy stemmed from his observation of the procedure performed by indigenous medical practitioners during his years in Africa. This seems highly unlikely, if not impossible. Livingstone did not visit the aforementioned territories wherein uvulectomy was prevalent, with the exception of Tanzania, and his visit there did not occur until more than a decade after his uvulectomy had been performed.[61] He spent his early years in Africa, up to 1852, with the Bechuana people (now known as Tswana), also called Bakuena or Bakwains. He reported diseases encountered among these people and the practices of their healers, noting that "The surgical knowledge of the native doctors is rather at a low ebb",[62] and he also described Bechauna rituals including circumcision[63] but uvulectomy is not mentioned.

Another possibility is that Livingstone's belief in uvulectomy might have its origins in his medical education. Although some details of his medical training and career are known,[64] Livingstone's own writings say very little about this aspect of his life.[65] It seems likely that his knowledge of diseases of the throat was minimal (as for diseases of the eye[37]). His training occurred sometime before the widespread use of the laryngoscope[66] although he was familiar with the stethoscope.[65] However, Livingstone may have been aware of the work of the surgeon James Yearsley (1805–1869), perhaps best known for his 'artificial tympanum'[67] but also noted for tonsillotomy and uvulectomy.[56,68–70] Yearsley popularised a "cure for stammering … by making, as I excise the tonsils or uvula, an aperture in the valvular obstruction", as reported in the *Lancet* in 1841.[71] (Of possible note, this journal formed part of Livingstone's reading, as reported in Blaikie's account of his activities *circa* 1845.)[72] Yearsley's claims did occasion controversy, fully aired in the *Lancet*,[73,74] including a financial claim against him for a failed procedure,[75] although Yearsley himself noted that just over 20% (65/300) of his patients did not benefit from surgery.[74] Although Livingstone never mentions stammering per se, he may nonetheless have been impressed with the reported efficacy of the operation on others with speech impediment.

Conclusion

It is well recognised that a patient's belief in a medical procedure may contribute to its apparent efficacy, irrespective of whether or not it does in fact 'work'. Livingstone clearly believed that uvulectomy was the solution to his difficulties in public speaking, and clearly was disappointed with the apparent failure of the operation. With the benefit of hindsight, we are perhaps not surprised by this outcome but, before indulging in what the historian EP Thompson (1924–1993) has graphically called "the condescension of posterity", it is worth reflecting on the possibility, if not likelihood, that many of the procedures currently undertaken may excite similar feelings in future generations. Studies of efficacy utilising, where possible, the methodology of the randomised double-blind placebo-controlled clinical trial may reduce this risk.[76]

Acknowledgments

I thank Dr Humphrey Fisher for helpful comments on this article. Adapted from: Larner AJ. David Livingstone's uvulectomy. *J Med Biogr* 2006; 14:104–108.

References

1. Coleman J, Rathfoot C. Oropharyngeal surgery in the management of upper airway obstruction during sleep. *Otolaryngol Clin N Am* 1999;32:263–276.
2. Davies RJO, Bates G, Stradling JR. The surgical treatment of snoring and obstructive sleep apnoea. In: Morris PJ, Wood WC (eds.). *Oxford textbook of surgery* (2nd edition). Oxford: Oxford University Press, 2000:2991–2995.
3. Wright J. *A history of laryngology and otology* (2nd edition). Philadelphia & New York: Lea & Febiger, 1914 [at 52, 80, 31 respectively].
4. Stevenson RS, Guthrie D. *A history of oto-laryngology.* Edinburgh: E & S Livingstone, 1949 [at 14 (Hippocrates), 10 (Hindu)].
5. Shaw GB. *The doctor's dilemma. A tragedy.* Harmondsworth: Penguin, 1982:10.
6. *Ibid.*, 68–69; also mentioned in the play itself [at 101].
7. Blaikie WG. *Personal life of David Livingstone.* London: John Murray, 1880:89,99,108,126,132.
8. Seaver G. *David Livingstone: his life and letters.* London: Lutterworth, 1957:147.
9. Ransford O. *David Livingstone: the dark interior.* London: John Murray, 1978:69.
10. Mitchison A. *Who was . . . ? David Livingstone. The legendary explorer.* London: Short Books, 2003:18,52–53.
11. Schapera I (ed.). *Livingstone's missionary correspondence 1841–1856.* London: Chatto & Windus, 1961:142.
12. Schapera I (ed.). *David Livingstone: family letters 1841–1856.* London: Chatto & Windus, 1959 (2 volumes):II.74.
13. *bid.* II.89.
14. Schapera (*op. cit.* ref. 11):152.
15. Schapera (*op. cit.* ref. 12):II.109.

16. Schapera (*op. cit.* ref. 11):177; also Blaikie (*op. cit.* ref. 7):99.
17. Schapera (*op. cit.* ref. 11):188–189.
18. Blaikie (*op. cit.* ref. 7):89.
19. *Ibid.* iv.
20. Deacon H. Cape Town and "country" doctors in the Cape Colony during the first half of the nineteenth century. *Soc Hist Med* 1997;10:25–52.
21. Schapera (*op. cit.* ref. 12):II.169.
22. Schapera I (ed.). *Livingstone's private journals 1851–1853.* London: Chatto & Windus, 1960:80n4. The text of the article appears, with minor alterations, in *Journal of the Royal Geographical Society* 1852;22:163–173.
23. Burrows EH. *A history of medicine in South Africa up to the end of the nineteenth century.* Cape Town & Amsterdam: AA Balkema, 1958:110–111.
24. Laidler PW, Gelfand M. *South Africa. Its medical history 1652–1898. A medical and social study.* Cape Town: C Struik (Pty) Ltd, 1971:170n104.
25. Schapera (*op. cit.* ref. 22):80.
26. Schapera (*op. cit.* ref. 12):II.177–178; also Blaikie (*op. cit.* ref. 7):126.
27. Schapera (*op. cit.* ref. 11):227–228.
28. Schapera (*op. cit.* ref. 12):II.229.
29. Ransford (*op. cit.* ref. 9):119–120.
30. Livingstone D. *Missionary travels and researches in South Africa; including a sketch of sixteen years' residence in the interior of Africa, etc.* London: John Murray, 1857:164.
31. *Ibid.* 205.
32. *Ibid.* 578.
33. Cook GC. Doctor David Livingstone FRS (1813–1873): "the fever" and other medical problems of mid-nineteenth century Africa. *J Med Biogr* 1994;2:33–43.
34. Larner AJ. Charles Meller and John Kirk: medical practitioners and practice on Livingstone's Zambesi expedition, 1858–64. *J Med Biogr* 2002;10:129–134.
35. Livingstone (*op. cit.* ref. 30):169–170; see also 146.
36. *Ibid.* 404.
37. Larner AJ. Ophthalmological observations made during the mid-19th century European encounter with Africa. *Arch Ophthalmol* 2004;122:267–272.
38. Maclean U. *Magical medicine: a Nigerian case- study.* London: Allen Lane The Penguin Press, 1971:65–66.
39. Fleischer K. Uvula-Exzision in Afrika. Ein traditioneller Brauch – auch heute noch lebendig. *Curare* 1980;3:19–22.
40. Ijaduola GTA. Uvulectomy in Nigeria. *J Laryngol Otol* 1981;95:1127–1133.
41. Ijaduola GTA. Hazards of traditional uvulectomy in Nigeria. *East Afr Med J* 1982;59:771–774.
42. Oyelami OA. Traditional uvulectomy among preschool children in the far north eastern Nigeria. *J Trop Pediatr* 1993;39:314–315.
43. Einterz EM, Einterz RM, Bates ME. Traditional uvulectomy in northern Cameroon. *Lancet* 1994;343:1644.

44. Prual A, Gamatie Y, Djakounda M, Huguet D. Traditional uvulectomy in Niger: a public health problem? *Soc Sci Med* 1994;39:1077–1082.
45. Jarvis JF, Mivathi SN. Uvulotomy among East African tribes. *J Laryngol* 1959;73:436–438.
46. Haddock DR, Chiduo AD. Uvulectomy in coastal Tanzania. *Central African Medical Journal* 1965;11:331–334.
47. Manni JJ. Uvulectomy, a traditional surgical procedure in Tanzania. *Ann Trop Med Parasitol* 1984;78:49–53.
48. Sarnelli T. Resection of uvula in native medicine of Arabia, Kordofan, and Ethiopia. *Revue de Medecine Tropical* 1940;1:288–293.
49. Bonnlander BH. Uvulectomy. *JAMA* 1980;243:515.
50. Arkell AJ. Removal of the uvula in Darfur. *Sudan Notes and Records* 1936;19:322–323.
51. Rubinstein A. Absence of uvula in south Sinai Bedouins. *JAMA* 1979;242:323.
52. Nathan H. Mutilation of the uvula among Bedouins of the south Sinai. *Isr J Med Sci* 1982;18:774–778.
53. Apffel CA. Uvulectomy, ethnic mutilation or prophylactic surgery? An Oriental tale. *JAMA* 1965;193:164–165.
54. Nalin DR. Death of a child submitted to uvulectomy for diarrhoea. *Lancet* 1985;1:643.
55. Wind J. Cross-cultural and anthropobiological reflections on African uvulectomy. *Lancet* 1984;2:1267–1268.
56. Hunter L. Uvulectomy – the making of a ritual. *S Afr Med J* 1995;85:901–902.
57. Larner AJ, Fisher HJ. Dr. Gustav Nachtigal (1834–1885): a contribution to the history of medicine in mid-nineteenth century Africa. *J Med Biogr* 2000;8:43–48.
58. Nachtigal G. *Sahara and Sudan* (transl. AGB Fisher, HJ Fisher; 4 volumes). London: Christopher Hurst, 1971–1987:I.135,393; II.376,419,449; III.201.
59. *Ibid.* I.393.
60. *Ibid.* II.376.
61. Shepperson G (ed.). *David Livingstone and the Rovuma.* Edinburgh: Edinburgh University Press, 1965.
62. Livingstone (*op. cit.* ref. 30):112–116.
63. *Ibid.* 128–131.
64. Morris DE. The medical career of Dr David Livingstone. *Scott Med J* 1984;29:183–186.
65. Livingstone (*op. cit.* ref. 30):4–6.
66. Reiser SJ. *Medicine and the reign of technology.* Cambridge: Cambridge University Press, 1978:51–55.
67. Kerr AG. James Yearsley: reflections of an otologist. *J Laryngol Otol* 1991;105:249–251.
68. Yearsley J. *Stammering and other imperfections of speech, treated by surgical operations on the throat.* London: Churchill, 1841.
69. Yearsley J. *Treatise on the enlarged tonsil and elongated uvula. In connexion with*

defects of voice, speech, and hearing, difficult deglutition, susceptibility to sore throat, impeded respiration, disturbed sleep, throat-cough, nasal obstruction, and the imperfect development of health and strength in youth. London: J Churchill, 1842.

70. Obituary. James Yearsley MD MRCS Eng. *Lancet* 1869;2:108.
71. Yearsley J. Operations for stammering. *Lancet* 1840–1;1:884–885.
72. Blaikie (*op. cit.* ref . 7):68.
73. Poett J. Operations for stammering. *Lancet* 1840–1;2:414–416.
74. On the cure of stammering by the removal of the uvula and tonsils. *Lancet* 1840–1;2:587–593.
75. Symonds JF. Ten guineas for clipping the uvula. *Lancet* 1840–1;2:594.
76. Matthews JR. *Quantification and the quest for medical certainty*. Princeton: Princeton University Press, 1995.

Charlotte Brontë (1816–1855): migraineur

There has been much interest in the health of the Brontë siblings, perhaps unsurprisingly in view of their early deaths and, in the cases of Charlotte, Emily, and Anne, the premature truncation of their genius. Pulmonary tuberculosis was undoubtedly the most likely cause of death of Maria, Elizabeth, Emily and Anne, whilst Branwell's health was undermined by his use of opium.[1] Charlotte's demise may well have been due to hyperemesis gravidarum (excessive vomiting in pregnancy) although other possibilities have been advanced, including tuberculosis with secondary Addison's disease (failure of the adrenal glands) and an infectious diarrhoeal illness, perhaps typhoid.[2] It has also been suggested that Charlotte suffered depression.[3] However, little has been said on the subject of her headaches.[4]

Epidemiological studies suggest that headache is a ubiquitous symptom, globally ranking in the top ten of the most disabling conditions (according to the World Health Organisation).[5] For that reason, a writer's allusions to headache may be thought hardly worthy of additional comment. However, patient, as opposed to professional, accounts of disease and its treatment are increasingly valued by historians of medicine since they present the perspective of the recipients, rather than the deliverers, of medical care, and hence are hopefully free of the whiggish tendencies which may permeate reports emanating from the medical faculty. Furthermore, it is well-recognised that headaches have the capacity to interfere with daily activities, including social and occupational functions, and hence might be anticipated to influence a writer prone to their effects. A number of examples of writers afflicted with headache and who include characters with headache in their major novels may be adduced from the literary canon, including Elizabeth Gaskell and (possibly) Jane Austen.[6]

The aim of this paper is to collate and analyse accounts of headache found in the extant letters of Charlotte Brontë and in the novels written by the Brontë sisters. The three volumes of Charlotte Brontë's extant letters, edited by Margaret Smith,[7] were examined, as were two biographies, by Elizabeth Gaskell[8] and by Juliet Barker,[9] as well as the seven completed novels by the Brontë sisters. All references to headache, pain in the head, migraine, and bilious attacks were noted. This methodology was used previously when examining the works of Jane Austen and of Elizabeth Gaskell.[6]

The search for specific terms was also informed by a reading of T.J. Graham's *Modern Domestic Medicine*, Patrick Brontë's (1826) edition of which was heavily annotated. Graham lists four chief species "Of Head-ache", namely: sick or bilious; nervous; rheumatic or chronic; and hemicranias; but acknowledges that "All these species ... are closely connected and apt to run into each other".[10] Likewise, although modern headache classification systems recognise many different types of headache, these may broadly be divided into "primary" (i.e. no specific cause identified; most commonly migraine), and "secondary" or symptomatic headaches which have an identifiable underlying cause (e.g. intracranial infection, inflammation, tumour).[11]

The neurological assessment of a patient complaining of headache typically aims to establish various facts, including the age at headache onset, duration of headache disorder, headache characteristics, provoking and relieving factors, family history of headache, and treatments used and their efficacy, all of which may help with specific headache diagnosis.[12] Information relating to many of these factors may be extracted from a reading of Charlotte Brontë's correspondence.

Charlotte Brontë's headaches: facts

The first definite report from Brontë's pen that she has suffered from a headache dates from June 1843, when she was aged 27. In a letter to Ellen Nussey sent from Brussels she states:

> Today the weather is gloomy and I am stupefied with a bad cold and a headache[13]

It was to be the first of many such accounts over the ensuing 12 years of her life, many addressed to Ellen Nussey: references have been identified in her letters from every succeeding year with the exceptions of 1847 and 1855. The last mention, in a letter to Miss Wooler of 15th November 1854, states that "it is long since I have known such comparative immunity from headache, sickness and indigestion, as during the last three months", a coincidence with the early months of marriage that is perhaps significant, Barker opining that the "happiness of married life transformed her health".[14] Nonetheless it is clear that the duration of the headache disorder encompassed most of Charlotte's adult life.

Contemporaneous witness accounts of Charlotte Brontë's headaches are provided by her father, Patrick, and by her friend and biographer Elizabeth Gaskell. Patrick Brontë reported to Ellen Nussey on 12th July 1850 that his daughter was "labouring under one of her usual bilious attacks".[15] Elizabeth Gaskell, writing to an unknown correspondent (provisionally dated 25th August 1850), recounts personally witnessing one of Charlotte's headaches:

> I then saw how severely her nerves were taxed by the effort of going amongst strangers. We knew beforehand that the number of the party would not exceed twelve; but she suffered the whole day from an acute headache brought on by apprehension of the evening.[16]

What was the nature of this headache disorder? Evidently it was intermittent or episodic, with attacks lasting anything from 3 hours to a week or more.[17] Headache descriptors used in the correspondence include thundering, nervous, neuralgic and obnoxious.[18] Gastrointestinal symptoms were frequent and prominent accompaniments of headache, variously described as sickness, poor appetite, indigestion, bilious attacks, and dyspepsia.[19] In March 1852, "frequent head-aches" were accompanied by "a swelled face and tic in the cheek bone", and attacks of "Tic Douloureux" were reported by Patrick Brontë when writing to Mrs Gaskell to cancel a proposed visit to Haworth in June 1853.[20] No mention of the words "migraine" or "hemicrania", or of symptoms suggestive of the sensory disturbances frequently encountered in migraine, such as photophobia, phonophobia, and osmophobia,[21] have been found.

What impact did these headaches have? It is clear that they affected both social and occupational functions. Headaches left Charlotte "incapacitated [...] from occupation", "quite weak and washy", in low spirits and a poor companion.[22] Letter writing was difficult and sometimes curtailed because of headaches.[23] As for writing novels, there is mention of difficulty in completing volume three of *Villette* in November 1852:

> ... it would speedily be finished – could I but ward off certain obnoxious headaches which [...] are apt to seize and prostrate me.[24]

As mentioned, a visit from Mrs Gaskell had to be cancelled because of "frequent sharp attacks of 'Tic Douloureux', 'in the head,' which have rendered her utterly unable to entertain you as she could wish".[25] Undoubtedly Charlotte's experience of headache allowed her to sympathize with Mrs Gaskell over her daughter Julia's headache.[26]

What were the causes of these headaches? Clinical experience indicates that almost without exception headache sufferers try to identify a cause or causes for their headaches, and Charlotte Brontë was no exception, advancing a number of possible explanations. Of these, physical or sensory factors appear to predominate over emotional or psychic precipitants. The weather is commonly inculpated, including the east wind or cold wind, Autumn, fog, closeness and oppression of air, and change of temperature.[27] Close work or "sitting too closely to my writing" may perhaps relate to Charlotte's visual difficulties, and another of her bodily explanations states that headache "proceeds from the stomach".[28] Visits and visitors might also be associated with headache. Examples of the former are the anticipation of an evening meeting with Thomas Arnold at Fox How in August 1850, and a visit to Mrs Gaskell on 22nd April 1853 when an unexpected guest was also in attendance.[29] Examples of the latter are the departure of Joe Taylor and of the Bishop of Ripon. Elizabeth Gaskell speaks of Charlotte's "nervous dread of encountering strangers".[30]

Travel, particularly going away from home, often seems to have been associated with headache, so much so that its absence is notable: in June 1850, Charlotte reports that she "performed the journey [to Brookroyd] with less inconvenience from headache ... than I ever remember". Despite these experiences of headache associated with or exacerbated by movement, Charlotte states that headaches "often haunt sedentary people".[31] A combination of travel and the anticipation of encountering strangers, with sleep deprivation thrown in for good measure, may perhaps explain the headaches attending her first meeting with the publisher George Smith in London in September 1848:

> I paid for the excitement of the interview by a thundering head-ache and harassing sickness.[32]

Emotional or psychic factors may also have contributed to the collapse of health featuring headaches following Branwell's death in September 1848.[33]

What medical opinions were sought and what treatments were given for these headaches? Incidentally, a doctor's diagnosis of "bilious fever" is mentioned around the time of Branwell's death.[34] Notoriously, William Ruddock, called in to attend to Charlotte in December 1851, prescribed mercury and succeeded in poisoning his patient. With hindsight, this was a situation in which Charlotte might have heeded Emily's refusal of any "poisoning doctor",[35] although to be fair to Ruddock the use of mercury was commonplace, Graham's *Modern domestic medicine* mentioning a "mercurial alterative every other night" as a headache treatment. Nothing deterred, Ruddock went on in January 1852 to try quinine, evidently against Charlotte's inclination.[36] Charlotte herself mentions the use of sal volatile ("roused me a little"), hop tea, and blistering ("seems to have done [...] some good but I am yet weak and bewildered").[37] Change of air, for example sea air, might be deemed a logical, if difficult to arrange, approach if ambient weather conditions were deemed culpable, but generally taking to bed was the only realistic manoeuvre.[38] There is no mention of the use of opiates for headache, in keeping with Charlotte's denial to Mrs Gaskell that she had ever taken opium, and despite the description of its effects in *Villette*.[39]

Brontë headaches: fiction

Despite this evidence from the correspondence for her headache disorder, and despite the recognition that she was at her best as a novelist when drawing on personal experience,[40] Charlotte Brontë's fictional works contain few and only passing references to characters suffering from headaches.

David Perkin has identified a reference to headache in the juvenile work *Caroline Vernon* (1839).[41] In *Jane Eyre*, confined to the Red Room at Gateshead Hall, Jane's "head still ached and bled with the blow and fall" she had received from John Reed.[42] In *Shirley*, Miss Keeldar:

> went to Mr Helstone and expressed herself with so much energy, that that gentleman was at last obliged, however unwillingly, to admit the idea that his niece was ill of something more than a migraine.

Later, Mr Helstone "gave himself headaches, with stooping to pick up gloves, handkerchiefs, and other loose property" for Shirley when he imagines her marrying Sir Philip Nunnely. Following the ejection of Mr Sympson, Shirley states "My head aches and I am tired" before laying her head on a cushion and falling asleep.[43] In *Villette*, Miss Marchmont tells Lucy "My head aches now with talking too much" after narrating until two in the morning the story of her lover's death. At the "Pensionnat de demoiselles", "one or two of the *pensionnaires* complained of headache" and are attended by Dr John, originally summoned by Madame Beck to attend her feverish daughter, Georgette. Blanche and Angélique then "had the migraine. Dr John had written a prescription; voila tout!". Reflecting on her secret love for Monsieur Paul, Lucy realises "What I now suffered was called illness – a headache".[44] I find no references to headache-related terms in *The Professor*.

Considering the other Brontë novels, in *Wuthering Heights* Catherine reports in her manuscript that "My head aches, till I cannot keep it on the pillow". Master Linton wonders that Heathcliff's long elegant locks of hair "don't make his head ache. It's like a colt's mane over his eyes!". Mrs Linton tells Ellen that Edgar "either for a head-ache or a pang of envy, began to cry" following her "few sentences of commendation to Heathcliff". On the third night of regaining Ellen's company after her illness, Catherine "complained [to Ellen] of a head-ache, and left me". Another possible reference is Catherine's report to Nelly that a "thousand smiths' hammers are beating in my head".[45]

In *Agnes Grey*, the eponymous governess finds that travelling to church crushed in the corner of the carriage "invariably made me sick" leading to "a feeling of languor and sickliness, and the tormenting fear of its becoming worse; and a depressing head-ache was generally my companion throughout the day".[46] In *The Tenant of Wildfell Hall*, Helen Graham tells Gilbert that "my head aches terribly" and, pressing her hand to her forehead, that "I must have some repose". Her diary account tells "how my head ached and how internally wretched I felt", perhaps in part because of "sleeping and eating so little" for a day or two. Another possible reference is to Helen's aching temples. When she ceases to write in the night "I find my head aches terribly". Answering Annabella briefly and coldly, Helen wonders whether "perhaps she thought I had a headache and could not bear to talk". Lady Lowborough explains her husband's immediate departure to "unpleasant intelligence from home [...] and that he had suffered it so to bother his mind that it had brought on a bilious headache".[47]

Discussion: headache diagnosis and its implications

Charlotte Brontë's extant letters contain more than 50 personal references to headache. It is evident from these that she suffered from intermittent headaches through much of her adult life, at least from 1843 to 1854 (aged 27-38 years). Correspondence, by the intermittent nature of its composition and the opportunistic nature of its survival, can never give a full clinical picture sufficient to satisfy a neurological examination. Nevertheless, it is clear from the available material that Charlotte's headaches were severe, often associated with feelings of sickness, interrupted social and occupational activities, may have been triggered by travel, sleep deprivation, overwork, and by cessation of mental and physical activity (clinically referred to as "let down", as seen in the phenomenon of "weekend migraine"). The sum of these characteristics suggests a tentative (and retrospective) syndromic diagnosis of migraine, specifically migraine without aura.[11] Headache may have contributed to her depression,[3] or vice versa, since concurrence of chronic headache and affective disorder is commonly noted in clinical practice. Evidence supporting a diagnosis of headache disorder has previously been presented for other authors based on their extant correspondence (e.g. Elizabeth Gaskell[6]) or on surviving diaries (e.g. Francis Kilvert, Sofia Tolstoy[48]).

In the current classification of headache, the two major categories of "primary" headache are migraine and tension-type headaches.[11] Tension-type headaches were originally called tension headaches, based on the erroneous belief that they were caused by undue tension in the musculature of the scalp. Tension-type headaches are deemed rather featureless, in contradistinction from migraine, often manifesting as a tight band-like painful sensation around the head, of variable severity, which may last for hours, days or even weeks. The exact relationship between migraine and tension-type headaches remains uncertain with one possibility being that they are in fact different manifestations of similar pathophysiological mechanisms. Co-existence of more than one primary headache type in the same person is certainly not unusual, and so it might be suggested that some of Charlotte's headaches, for example those lasting for days,[17] might have been categorised as tension-type. However, prolonged headaches are reported less frequently in her correspondence than the more evidently migrainous events. Whether this was because they were less frequent or because they were deemed not worthy of mention cannot be known.

Despite her experience of probable migraine, Charlotte Brontë seldom referred to headaches in her major novels, even in *Jane Eyre* (1847), a work subtitled "An Autobiography" (although this subtitle may have been at the suggestion of her publishers Smith, Elder[49]). This omission may perhaps be contrasted with her short-sightedness which probably served (as did her values[50]) as a model for the character of William Crimsworth in *The Professor*. Hence Charlotte Brontë's absence from a list of authors who are claimed to have used their own experience of migraine in their writings, which includes *inter alia* William Shakespeare, John Dryden, Cervantes, Alexander Pope, Jonathan Swift, Lewis Carroll, Anthony Trollope, GK Chesterton, Rudyard Kipling, and Arthur Ransome,[51] would seem to be justified. Interestingly, it is Anne Brontë's novelistic accounts of headache, particularly in *Agnes Grey*, which seem clinically the most accurate account of migraine. Migraine often runs in families,[52] so Anne herself may have been afflicted; alternatively, it is well-recognised that headaches have effects on family members other than the sufferer, so Anne may have been familiar with Charlotte's headaches (there may be an analogy here with Anne's portrayal of the alcoholism of Arthur Huntingdon in *The Tenant of Wildfell Hall* drawn from observation of Branwell's problems[53]).

Accounts of neurological disease written by authors of fiction, including but not limited to headache, are of value, since they open perspectives which are not necessarily available in contemporaneous medical texts.[54] Fictional representations of illness are recognised to operate within larger cultural frameworks.[55] In this context, it is interesting to note similarities between Elizabeth Gaskell's and Charlotte Brontë's accounts of their headaches (e.g. their perceived relationship to weather conditions, their treatment with sal volatile), suggesting shared cultural norms. However, whereas Elizabeth Gaskell frequently used characters with headache as an authorial device,[56] as did Jane Austen,[6] Charlotte Brontë did not, despite her personal experience. One may only speculate as to why this might be so. Lois Keith has pointed out, in the context of fictional portrayals of childhood paraplegia, that "linking otherwise inexplicable medical conditions to inner states of turmoil and distress was popular with the medical profession long before Freud and psychoanalytic thinking",[57] a linkage which may also hold true for novelists: most of Jane

Austen's and Elizabeth Gaskell's female headache sufferers face some form of emotional, often amatory, distress or conflict at the time that their headaches are alluded to.[6,56] It is possible Charlotte Brontë had other ways to express the internal psychic states of her characters without needing to resort to metaphorical representations of illness.

Acknowledgment

Adapted from: Larner AJ. Charlotte Brontë's headaches: fact and fiction. *Brontë Studies* 2012;37:208–215.

References

1. Rhodes P. A medical appraisal of the Brontës. *Brontë Society Transactions* 1972;16:101–109; Helm WH. Tuberculosis and the Brontë family. *Brontë Studies* 2002;27:157–167; Alexander C. Smith M (eds.). *The Oxford Companion to the Brontës.* Oxford: Oxford University Press, 2006:243–244.
2. Gallagher HW. Charlotte Brontë: a surgeon's assessment. *Brontë Society Transactions* 1985;18:363–370; Fitzgerald JA. Death of elderly primigravida in early pregnancy. Charlotte Brontë. *NY State J Med* 1979;79:796–799. For tuberculosis with secondary Addison's disease, see Weiss G. The death of Charlotte Brontë. *Obstet Gynecol* 1991;78:705–708. For typhoid, see Gordon L. *Charlotte Bronte. A passionate life.* London: Virago, 2008:356–358 (henceforward *Gordon*).
3. Todd J, Dewhurst K. The periodic depression of Charlotte Brontë. *Perspect Biol Med* 1968;11:208–216.
4. A brief account of CB's headaches is given in Larner AJ. Charlotte Brontë (1816–1855): migraineur? *Eur J Neurol* 2009;16 Suppl3:329. A reading of CB's letters also informs Larner AJ. Kilvert and cholera. *Journal of the Kilvert Society* 2009;Issue 28:22–23.
5. Stovner LJ, Hagen K, Jensen R et al. The global burden of headache: a documentation of headache prevalence and disability worldwide. *Cephalalgia* 2007;27:193–210.
6. For Elizabeth Gaskell, see Larner AJ. "A habit of headaches": the neurological case of Mrs Elizabeth Gaskell. *Gaskell Journal* 2011;25:97–103; for Jane Austen, see Larner AJ. "A transcript of actual life": headache in the novels of Jane Austen. *Headache* 2010;50:692–695; Larner AJ. Jane Austen's (1775–1817) references to headache: fact and fiction. *J Med Biogr* 2010;18:211–215.
7. Smith M (ed.). *The Letters of Charlotte Brontë* (3 volumes). Oxford: Clarendon Press, 1995–2004 (henceforward *Letters*).
8. Easson A (ed.). *Elizabeth Gaskell. The Life of Charlotte Brontë.* Oxford: Oxford World's Classics, 1996 (henceforward *Gaskell*).
9. Barker J. *The Brontës.* London: Phoenix, 1995 (henceforward *Barker*).

10. Graham TJ. *Modern Domestic Medicine: A popular treatise, illustrating the symptoms, cause, distinction, and current treatment of the diseases incident to the human frame; embracing the modern improvements in medicine. Etc.* London: Simpkin & Marshall, 1844 (9th edition):478–482 (henceforward *Graham*).
11. International Headache Society Classification Subcommittee. The international classification of headache disorders, second edition. *Cephalalgia* 2004;24 Suppl1:1–160.
12. Lipton RB, Scher AI, Silberstein SD, Bigal ME. Migraine diagnosis and comorbidity. In: Silberstein SD, Lipton RB, Dodick DW (eds.). *Wolff's headache and other head pain.* Oxford: Oxford University Press, 2008 (8th edition):153–175; Larner AJ, Coles AJ, Scolding NJ, Barker RA. *A-Z of Neurological Practice. A Guide to Clinical Neurology.* London: Springer, 2011 (2nd edition):315–317.
13. *Letters*, I:325; *Barker*, 422.
14. *Letters*, III:301; *Barker*, 765
15. *Letters*, II:423.
16. Chapple JAV, Pollard A (eds.). *The Letters of Mrs Gaskell.* Manchester: Mandolin, 1997:127 (no. 76); *Gaskell*, 431.
17. *Letters*, II:395 (3 hours); II:126 (one week); III:175 (ten days).
18. *Letters*, II:113 (thundering); II:639 (nervous); II:710 (neuralgic); III:78 (obnoxious).
19. *Letters*, I:382; II:113,126,268,336,513,541,620,635,643; III:57,114 (sick or sickness); II:126 (poor appetite); II:285; III:24 (indigestion); II:249; III:129 (bilious attacks); III:233 (dyspepsia).
20. *Letters*, III:25,173.
21. For the technical (neurological) meaning of these terms, see Larner AJ. *A Dictionary of Neurological Signs.* New York: Springer, 2011 (3rd edition): 279,278,258 respectively.
22. Respectively, *Letters*, III:174; II:635; I:373,382.
23. For example, *Letters*, I:390,466; III:58,183,236. *Gaskell*, 436.
24. *Letters*, III:78.
25. *Letters*, III:173; *Gaskell*, 436.
26. *Letters*, II:15 and n6. Chapple JAV, Pollard A (eds.). *The Letters of Mrs Gaskell.* Manchester: Mandolin, 1997:174 (no. 109).
27. *Letters*, I:390; III:52 (wind); II:512 (Autumn); II:513 (fog); II:636 (closeness and oppression of air); II:729 (change of temperature).
28. *Letters*, II:241,249 (close work); II:621 (stomach).
29. *Gaskell*, 353; *Barker*, 652 (visit to Thomas Arnold); *Letters*, III:158n1; *Barker*, 726 (visit to Gaskell).
30. *Letters*, II:395 (visit of Joe Taylor); III:129; *Barker*, 725 (Bishop of Ripon). 30. Quote, along with another example of anticipatory headache, is from *Gaskell*, 431.
31. *Letters*, I:373,382; II:113–114,635,636,639,643,675; III:16,55 (travel); II:421 (journey [to Brookroyd]); III:221 (sedentary).

32. *Letters*, II:113–114; *Barker*, 559–560. *Gordon*, 417, points out that this is the only letter from CB to Mary Taylor which survives.
33. *Letters*, II:126; *Barker*, 569.
34. *Letters*, II:127.
35. *Letters*, II:152; *Barker*, 575.
36. *Letters*, II:734; III:4,9,19,25. For William Ruddock, see Mackay R. *Dr William Ruddock (1814–1860): a brief memoir*, reviewed in *Brontë Studies* 2002;27:76–78; *Barker*, 690. *Graham*, 479.
37. *Letters*, II:113 (sal volatile); II:19 (hop tea); III:175 (blistering).
38. *Letters*, II:218,621 (air); II:126 (bed).
39. *Gaskell*, 441, but see also 565n for possible evidence to the contrary; *Gordon*, 256, states that Mrs Gaskell "tended to give in to stress with migraines, neuralgia, and spells of lassitude, propped by opiates" but I find no evidence based on Gaskell's correspondence for her using opiates for her headaches; Larner AJ. "A habit of headaches": the neurological case of Mrs Elizabeth Gaskell. *Gaskell Journal* 2011;25:97–103. In *Villette* (London: Penguin Classics, 2004), ch. 38, 496, opiates were administered to Lucy shortly after her illness has been called a headache. In *Shirley* (London: Penguin Classics, 2006), ch. 28, 479, Shirley asks Louis to administer a strong narcotic, laudanum, if the bite of the rabid dog Phoebe leads to hydrophobia.
40. *Barker*, 500.
41. Perkin GD. Headache. *J Neurol Neurosurg Psychiatry* 1995;59:632.
42. Charlotte Brontë. *Jane Eyre*. London: Penguin Classics, 2006: ch. 2, 18.
43. Charlotte Brontë. *Shirley*. London: Penguin Classics, 2006: ch. 24, 395; ch. 27, 444; ch. 31, 522.
44. Charlotte Brontë. *Villette*. London: Penguin Classics, 2004: ch. 4, 46; ch. 11, 110,111; ch. 38, 496.
45. Emily Brontë. *Wuthering Heights*. London: Penguin Classics, 2003: Vol. 1, ch. 3, 22; ch.7, 59; ch. 10, 98; Vol. 2, ch. 10, 245; Vol. 1, ch. 11, 116. In Torgerson BE. *Reading the Brontë Body: Disease, Desire, and the Constraints of Culture*. Basingstoke: Palgrave Macmillan, 2005:117 it is claimed that Catherine Linton feigns headache in her discussion with Ellen. For ill-health in *Wuthering Heights*, see also Lemon C. Sickness and health in *Wuthering Heights*. *Brontë Society Transactions* 1963:14:23–25.
46. Anne Brontë. *Agnes Grey*. London: Penguin Classics, 2004: ch. 7, 126–127.
47. Anne Brontë. *The Tenant of Wildfell Hall*. London: Penguin Classics, 1996: ch. 12, 103; ch.19, 164; ch. 31, 273; ch. 33, 307; ch. 34, 309; ch. 38, 345.
48. For Kilvert, see Larner AJ. Francis Kilvert (1840–1879): an early self-report of cluster headache? *Cephalalgia* 2008;28:763–766. For Sofia Tolstoy, see Larner AJ. "Neurological literature": headache (part 8). *Adv Clin Neurosci Rehabil* 2011;11(2):21.
49. *Letters*, I:540.
50. *Gordon*, 149.
51. Blau JN. *Understanding headaches and migraines. A practical guide to avoiding*

and coping with all forms of headache. London: Consumers' Association/ Hodder & Stoughton, 1991:97, reportedly based on writings of EMR Critchley but no citation given. For a different diagnostic formulation on the nature of Arthur Ransome's headaches (viz. cluster headache), see Larner AJ. Arthur Ransome's headache disorder. *Mixed Moss* [The Journal of the Arthur Ransome Society] 2006:3–9.

52. *Barker*, 198, reports that Emily Brontë had "severe bilious attacks" following a dog bite in 1833. This event was the origin for the episode in *Shirley* (see note 39) when the heroine fears the possibility of rabies following a dog bite: *Shirley*. London: Penguin Classics, 2006:650n8.
53. *Gordon*, 193.
54. For an example of an author's account of personally experienced epilepsy, see Larner AJ. "A ray of darkness": Margiad Evans's account of her epilepsy (1952). *Clin Med* 2009;9:193–194; Larner AJ. Margiad Evans (1909–1958): a history of epilepsy in a creative writer. *Epilepsy Behav* 2009;16:596–598.
55. For examples of fictional representations of illness in the Brontës' novels, see Torgerson BE. *Reading the Brontë Body: Disease, Desire, and the Constraints of Culture*. Basingstoke: Palgrave Macmillan, 2005.
56. Larner AJ. Headache in the writings of Elizabeth Gaskell (1810–65). *J Med Biogr* 2015;23:191–196.
57. Keith L. *Take up thy bed and walk: death, disability and cure in classic fiction for girls*. London: Routledge, 2001:28. See also Larner AJ. Some literary accounts of possible childhood paraplegia and neurorehabilitation. *Dev Neurorehabil* 2009;12:248–252.

Fyodor Dostoevsky (1821–1881): epilepsy

Although their influence did not reach western Europe until some years after his death, the works of the Russian novelist Fyodor Mikhailovich Dostoevsky (1821–1881) have intrigued writers, philosophers and theologians ever since. For example, Dostoevsky is "a significant presence in the margins of much that has been written" in the Archbishop of Canterbury's 2005 Clark Lectures delivered at Trinity College, Cambridge.[1] Likewise, neurologists have taken Dostoevsky as a subject for study, because of his epilepsy, and that ascribed to a number of his characters.

Perhaps the first neurologist to write on Dosteovsky's epilepsy was Sigmund Freud (1856–1939). Freud had briefly received some training under Charcot (1825–1893) in Paris before turning to psychiatry. In an article entitled *Dostoevsky and parricide*, first published in 1928, Freud stated that:

> Dostoevsky called himself an epileptic. . . . it is highly probable that this so-called epilepsy was only a symptom of his neurosis and must accordingly be classified as hystero-epilepsy – that is, as severe hysteria.

Freud's reasoning for thinking Dostoevsky's seizures psychogenic was based on the timing of their inception:

> The most probable assumption is that the attacks went back far into his childhood, that their place was taken to begin with by milder symptoms and that they did not assume an epileptic form until after the shattering experience of his eighteenth year – the murder of his father. It would be very much to the point if it could be established that they ceased completely during his exile in Siberia . . . [2]

In the biography by Dostoevsky's daughter, it was "according to family traditions" that the onset of epilepsy occurred on learning of the death of his father, Mikhail Andreyevich (sometime head physician at the Malinsky Hospital for the Poor in Moscow), but Dostoevsky's own letters contradict this.

Ingenious though Freud's psychoanalytical formulation was, it was vigorously challenged shortly after its translation into English (in the *Realist* of July 1929) by the historian EH Carr (1892–1982), then preparing a biography of Dostoevsky[3] (and some years away from commencing his monumental fourteen-volume *History of Soviet Russia* for which he is chiefly remembered). His analysis of the extant sources suggested that, quite contrary to Freud's belief,

Dostoevsky's seizures did not start until during his imprisonment in exile in Omsk, i.e. not earlier than 1849, some years after his father's death in 1839, and indeed was not unequivocally diagnosed as epilepsy until 1857, shortly after his first marriage.[4]

If not pseudoseizures, or non-epileptic seizures, then from what type of epilepsy did Dostoevsky suffer? A number of authors, including neurologists, have examined the issue, as well as delineating epileptic characters in Dostoevsky's works.[5–14] Alajouanine, one of the successors to Charcot's chair, believed Dostoevsky had partial and secondarily generalised seizures with ecstatic auras,[5] but Gastaut initially plumped for idiopathic generalised seizures.[6] Voskuil felt that the seizures began in 1846 (Carr had examined, and discounted, the evidence for this[4]) and suggested complex partial seizures with secondarily generalised nocturnal seizures and ecstatic auras.[7] Gastaut, returning to the subject, acknowledged the possibility of a silent temporal lesion but such as permitted "almost immediately secondary generalization to each seizure".[8] DeToledo suggested, on the basis of Smerdyakov's admission of feigning a seizure to provide himself with an alibi for the murder of his father Old Karamazov in Dostoevsky's 1879–80 novel *The Brothers Karamazov* (an episode perhaps recapitulating Dostoevsky's experience of his own father's death), that Dostoevsky was well acquainted with the possible secondary gain of seizures, but he stopped short of bringing the historical wheel full circle back to Freud by suggesting that Dostoevsky had pseudoseizures.[9] Rosetti and Bogousslavsky suggested seizure onset in 1846 and that Dostoevsky's father was not in fact murdered, *en route* to their conclusion that Dostoevsky suffered from temporal lobe epilepsy, most likely left mesiotemporal (this lateralisation based on Dostoevsky's postictal aphasia, since ecstatic auras are thought to be non-lateralising), with complex partial and secondarily generalized seizures, with a relatively benign course.[10] Mesial temporal lobe epilepsy is also the diagnosis favoured by Baumann et al.[11]

Whatever its particular nature, what impact did this seizure disorder have on Dostoevsky's art? Siegel and Dorn[15] have traced six characters with epilepsy in Dostoevsky's oeuvre, of which the most notable are Prince Myshkin in *The Idiot* (1868) and Smerdyakov in *The Brothers Karamazov*. Certainly the former has an experience of mystical ecstasy akin to Dostoevsky's ecstatic auras, whereas Smerdyakov's epilepsy, as related above, is according to Carr "a piece of machinery necessary to the plot, and appears to have no other artistic or spiritual significance".[4]

Ecstatic auras, a feeling of absolute harmony and happiness, a sense of spiritual exaltation and triumph, a feeling of power to transcend the limits of the material world, comparable with Mahomet's vision of Paradise, were first recorded by Dostoevsky in 1865. Such ecstatic auras have sometimes been labelled as "Dostoyevsky's epilepsy," although this terminology does not appear in the various ILAE classifications of seizures; such auras have been associated with focal right temporal abnormalities.[16,17] In one case, ecstatic auras have been reported to be induced by watching television – not as implausible as it may at first appear, since such episodes were independent of the content of the television programme – but these were associated with generalised rather than focal epileptiform activity.[18]

Acknowledgment

Adapted from: Larner AJ. Dostoevsky and epilepsy. *Adv Clin Neurosci Rehabil* 2006;6(1):26.

References

1. Williams R. *Grace and necessity. Reflections on art and love.* London: Morehouse/Continuum, 2005:170.
2. Freud S. Dostoevsky and parricide. In: Dickson A (ed.). *Penguin Freud Library volume 14: Art and Literature.* London: Penguin, 1985:441–460.
3. Carr EH. *Dostoevsky (1821–1881). A new biography.* London: George Allen & Unwin, 1931.
4. Carr EH. Was Dostoevsky an epileptic? *Slavonic and East European Review* 1930;December:424–431.
5. Alajouanine T. Dostoiewski's epilepsy. *Brain* 1963;86:209–218.
6. Gastaut H. Fyodor Mikhailovitch Dostoevsky's involuntary contribution to the symptomatology and prognosis of epilepsy. *Epilepsia* 1978;19:186–201.
7. Voskuil PHA. The epilepsy of Fyodor Michailovitch Dostoevsky (1821–1881). *Epilepsia* 1983;24:658–667.
8. Gastaut H. New comments on the epilepsy of Fyodor Dostoevsky. *Epilepsia* 1984;25:408–411.
9. DeToledo JC. The epilepsy of Fyodor Dostoyevsky: insights from Smerdyakov Karamazov's use of a malingered seizure as an alibi. *Arch Neurol* 2001;58:1305–1306.
10. Rosetti AO, Bogousslavsky J. Dostoevsky and epilepsy: an attempt to look through the frame. In: Bogousslavsky J, Boller F (eds.). *Neurological disorders in famous artists* (Frontiers of Neurology and Neuroscience Volume 19). Basel: Karger, 2005:65–75.
11. Baumann CR, Novikov VP, Regard M, Siegel AM. Did Fyodor Mikhailovich Dostoevsky suffer from mesial temporal lobe epilepsy? *Seizure* 2005;14:324–330.
12. Hughes JR. The idiosyncratic aspects of the epilepsy of Fyodor Dostoevsky. *Epilepsy Behav* 2005;7:531–538.
13. Seneviratne U. Fyodor Dostoevsky and his falling sickness: a critical analysis of seizure semiology. *Epilepsy Behav* 2010;18:424–430.

14. Iniesta I. Epilepsy in the process of artistic creation of Dostoevsky. *Neurologia* 2014;29:371–378.
15. Siegel AM, Dorn T. Dostojewskijs Leben im Wechselspiel zwischen Epilepsie und Literatur. *Nervenarzt* 2001;72:466–474.
16. Cirignotta F. Todesco CV, Lugaresi E. Temporal lobe epilepsy with ecstatic seizures (so-called Dostoevsky epilepsy). *Epilepsia* 1980;21:705–710.
17. Morgan H. Dostoevsky's epilepsy: a case report and comparison. *Surg Neurol* 1990;33:413–416.
18. Cabrera-Valdivia F, Jimenez-Jimenez FJ, Tejeiro J, Ayuso-Peralta L, Vaquero A, Garcia-Albea E. Dostoevsky's epilepsy induced by television. *J Neurol Neurosurg Psychiatry* 1996;61:653.

Phineas Gage (1823–1860): the beginnings of neuropsychology

1848 was a year of political revolutions in Europe. In the same year, in the field of neuroscience, a freak occurrence would also prove to have a revolutionary impact. Few neurologists will be unfamiliar with the name of Phineas P Gage, nor with the extraordinary work-related accident which befell him on the afternoon of 13th September 1848 in Burlington, Vermont, USA.[1,2] Excavating rock with blasting powder, in his capacity as a railroad foreman, an accidental ignition caused a tamping iron approximately 1.1 m (43 inches) long, 3 cm thick at its widest point, and weighing 13 pounds, to smash through the left side of Gage's face, entering just below the cheekbone, and emerge from the top of his skull, landing some 25–30 yards away, smeared with brain. Gage was thrown back, a few convulsive movements of the extremities were observed, but he was able to speak within a few minutes.

Fewer neurologists may be familiar with Dr John Martin Harlow, the railway physician who attended Gage within two hours of the accident. Harlow continued to treat Gage in the following days when death from infection seemed imminent. He then continued to observe the changes in Gage's personality, up to the time of his death from status epilepticus in 1860. Moreover, it was Harlow who persuaded the family to permit exhumation of Gage's skull five years after his death (no post mortem was performed). Harlow published his findings in two papers,[3,4] without which record Gage might not be remembered at all.

Gage's skull was subsequently donated to the Warren Anatomical Museum at Harvard University School of Medicine. Modern neuroimaging techniques have been used to study Gage's skull and reconstruct the probable path of injury caused by the tamping iron.[5] This has permitted more precise definition of the lesion location, and suggests that both left and right prefrontal cortices were injured.

As Harlow's account records in detail the behavioural changes manifested by Gage after the accident,[4] and is still regarded as one of the best accounts of behavioural disorder following prefrontal damage, clinical-anatomical correlation is possible. From an efficient and capable work foreman, Gage became irreverent, capricious, profane and irresponsible, and showed defects in rational decision making and the processing of emotion, such that his employers refused to return him to his former position. Harlow argued that the frontal lobe lesion had caused a loss of planning skills.[4] These neurobehavioural changes, sometimes labelled "pseudopsychopathic" or "sociopathic", are now regarded as typical of orbitofrontal injury, having been observed in other patients with selective lesions of this area.[6]

However, other case histories indicate the need to differentiate this clinical picture from that following injury to other parts of the frontal lobes. For example, a more recent account of a patient with frontal lobe injury due to an iron bar penetrating the skull, with prolonged follow up, reported prominent apathy, difficulties with planning, and lack of drive, yet stability of function within the domestic, professional and social setting (*cf.* Gage), associated with bilateral dorsolateral prefrontal injury.[7] Disinhibited, apathetic, and akinetic types of frontal lobe syndrome are described, associated respectively with orbitofrontal, frontal convexity and medial frontal lesions. Long term recovery from unilateral brain injury from a penetrating iron bar has been described with little in the way of functional neuropsychological compromise.[8]

Although we accept the landmark status of Gage in the development of ideas relating to cortical localisation,[2] the contemporary response to Harlow's reports was, to say the least, muted.[1] However, the account did appear at a propitious time. Broca was publishing his observations correlating aphasic syndromes with focal brain injury (1861), and Fritsch & Hitzig's electrical stimulation studies of the exposed cortex were soon to follow (1870). Ferrier's experimental observations in monkeys (1878) largely confirmed Harlow's clinical findings in Gage.

Gage is unquestionably one of the most famous patients in neurological history, a fixture in neurological textbooks and the subject of many papers. (Regrettably these often err in their assertions about him, principally because they neglect the original Harlow reports.[9]) A cursory study of the history of medicine indicates that it is unusual for the names of patients, rather than their doctors, to be recorded for posterity (one eponymous exception which immediately springs to mind is Christmas disease). Why should it be, then, that Gage is remembered, and not Harlow? Many speculations might be advanced: perhaps the extraordinary nature of the accident he suffered, the very fact that he survived, his memorable name, the fact that he was written up. More significant, however, may be the possibility, evident with the benefit of hindsight, that this case represents part of a paradigm shift, a "natural experiment" which demonstrated the possibilities of correlating particular personality and behavioural changes with focal injury to the brain, and hence the correlation of function with location. This practice continues in modern neuropsychology, where detailed case histories may be compared with structural and functional neuroimaging findings to help elucidate the workings of the brain.[10]

Acknowledgment

Adapted from: Larner AJ, Leach JP. Phineas Gage and the beginnings of neuropsychology. *Adv Clin Neurosci Rehabil* 2002;2(3):26.

References

1. O'Driscoll K, Leach JP. "No longer Gage": an iron bar through the head. *BMJ* 1998;317:1673–1674.
2. Haas LF. Phineas Gage and the science of brain localisation. *J Neurol Neurosurg Psychiatry* 2001;71:761.
3. Harlow JM. Passage of an iron bar through the head. *Boston Med Surg J* 1848;13:389–393.
4. Harlow JM. Recovery from the passage of an iron bar through the head. *Publications Mass Med Soc* 1868;2:327/9–346 (3:1–21) [reprinted in *Hist Psychiatry* 1993;4:271–281].
5. Damasio H, Grabowski T, Frank R, Galaburda AM, Damasio AR. The return of Phineas Gage: clues about the brain from the skull of a famous patient. *Science* 1994;264:1102–1105.
6. Eslinger PJ, Damasio AR. Severe disturbance of higher cognition after bilateral frontal lobe ablation: patient ENR. *Neurology* 1985;35:1731–1741.
7. Mataró M, Jurado MA, García-Sánchez C, Barraquer L, Costa-Jussà FR, Junque C. Long-term effects of bilateral frontal brain lesion: 60 years after injury with an iron bar. *Arch Neurol* 2001;58:1139–1142.
8. Aji BM, Ghadiali EJ, Jacob A, Larner AJ. Passage of an iron bar through the head: 50–year follow-up. *J Neurol* 2012;259:1247–1248.
9. Macmillan M. Restoring Phineas Gage: a 150th retrospective. *J Hist Neurosci* 2000;9:46–66.
10. Shallice T. *From neuropsychology to mental structure.* Cambridge: Cambridge University Press, 1988.

Louisa May Alcott (1832–1888): headache in fiction and fact

Introduction

The American author Louisa May Alcott (1832–1888) is mostly remembered for her novel, *Little Women, or Meg, Jo, Beth and Amy* (1868), although she was a prolific author with many other works to her name. Such was the popularity of this one book, detailing the exploits of the March sisters (loosely based on the author's own siblings), that a sequel quickly emerged, *Little Women, or Meg, Jo, Beth and Amy, Part Second* (1869; this book is sometimes published under the title of *Good Wives*, presumably to distinguish it from the original *Little Women*). The March family, and in particular Jo March (based on Alcott herself), also form the axis around which revolve the characters in two later books, *Little Men: Life at Plumfield with Jo's boys* (1871) and *Jo's boys, and how they turned out* (1886).

To the neurological eye, the trilogy (or tetralogy, depending on how you count *Part Second*) permits an analysis of headache disorders seen in one family over a period of about 20 years (all subsequent page references are to the Library of America edition[1]). A brief account of the headaches in *Little Women* (1868) has previously been offered.[2] At the outset Meg is 16, Jo15, Beth 13, and Amy the youngest is probably 12 (p.10,155).

The Little Women

Meg, aged 16, attends a party, following which she was "glad when it was all over, and she was quiet in her bed, where she could think and wonder and fume till her head ached" (p.98). At a subsequent party, the girls' neighbour, Laurie, warns Meg of the possibility of "a splitting headache tomorrow" if she drinks too much champagne (p.106). Many years later, Meg's daughter, Daisy, has headache when her paramour is about to depart to Europe (p.884).

At age 15, Jo gets "raging headaches by reading too long" (p.121) when her usual daily routine of looking after a trying elderly relative, Aunt March, comes to an end and the "experiment" of not working is tried. Aged 19, she undertakes "to be as lively and amiable as an ... aching head ... would allow" when preparing for visits to the house from Amy's superior friends (p.276). An entrée into literary society subjects Jo to philosophical discussions, "and the only thing 'evolved from her inner consciousness', was a bad headache after it was all over" (p.374); at this time she may be 20 or 21 (since Beth is between the ages of 18 (p.341) and 19 (p.397)).

At the age of around 25, Jo, meeting her suitor, Mr Bhaer, reports herself "so tired" when she "discovered that ... her head ached". Five years later, aged 30, she is now married ("Mrs Bhaer"), has 2 children, and helps with the teaching and care of the pupils at Plumfield, bequeathed to her by Aunt March. One pupil, Nan, a girl of perhaps 10, reports "Didn't my sage tea make Mother Bhaer's headache go away?" (p.712). Sage Tea or infusion of Sage, *Salvia officinalis*, has been claimed to relieve nervous headache. Sage was officially listed in the United States Pharmacopoeia from 1840 to 1900.

We hear of no further headaches in the subsequent 10 years of Jo's life, despite her pupils being involved in various vicissitudes, including shipwreck and imprisonment, although some of her pupils are occasionally afflicted: George Cole ("Stuffy": p.788, 1000, ascribed to overeating); Nat (p.888, "took his head in both hands as if it ached"); and Dan (p.1048, allegedly being read to too fast).

Beth, aged 13, has headaches which force her to lie on the sofa and cuddle her cats (p.42). Later she develops headaches at the onset of a febrile illness, which she self-diagnoses as scarlet fever based on her reading of her mother's book, and from which she nearly dies (p.186,187).

Amy, the youngest of the March sisters, seems unaffected by headache throughout the saga.

Louisa Alcott

Alcott herself certainly suffered from headaches (subsequent references are from Harriet Reisen's biography of Alcott,[3] unless otherwise stated), for example in 1843, after harvesting at her father's ill-fated utopian farm, Fruitlands (p.79). During her work as a nurse (entirely without training) in a Washington DC hospital during the American Civil War in 1863, she suffered a febrile illness with headache, forcing her to return home.[4]

Problems with headache were particularly notably in the early months of 1867 when, according to her journal, Alcott "Did nothing all month but sit in a dark room & ache. Head and eyes full of neuralgia." (p.205). She frequently used opiates to treat these headaches (p.210,223,242,250). In 1869 she complained that headaches kept her from working as she once could "fourteen hours a day" (p.221), and also suffered from headaches and other symptoms (rheumatism, laryngitis) when writing later in that year (p.223). Whether the headaches were part of, or entirely separate from, a multisystem disorder characterised by later diagnosticians as lupus[5] is not entirely clear, but certainly in 1869 they occurred with other symptoms possibly indicative of a multi-system disease (p.223).

Conclusion

Louisa May Alcott may be included in the cadre of nineteenth century female novelists who wrote of and suffered from headaches, such as Charlotte Brontë,[6] Elizabeth Gaskell,[7,8] and (probably) Jane Austen.[9,10]

Acknowledgment

Adapted from: Larner AJ. Louisa May Alcott and headache. *Adv Clin Neurosci Rehabil* 2014;14(2):20.

References

1. Alcott LM. *Little Women. Little Men. Jo's Boys.* New York: Library of America, 2005.
2. Larner AJ. "Neurological literature": headache (part 2). *Adv Clin Neurosci Rehabil* 2006;6(2):37–38.
3. Reisen H. *Louisa May Alcott. The woman behind Little Women.* New York: Henry Holt & Co., 2009:79,205,210,221,223,228,242,250.
4. Alcott LM. *Civil War hospital sketches.* Mineola, New York: Dover Publications, 2006 [1863]:54.
5. Hirschhorn N, Greaves IA. Louisa May Alcott: her mysterious illness. *Perspect Biol Med* 2007;50:243–259.
6. Larner AJ. Charlotte Brontë's headaches: fact and fiction. *Brontë Studies* 2012;37:208–215.
7. Larner AJ. "A habit of headaches": the neurological case of Elizabeth Gaskell. *Gaskell Journal* 2011;25:97–103.
8. Larner AJ. Headache in the writings of Elizabeth Gaskell (1810–65). *J Med Biogr* 2015;23:191–196.
9. Larner AJ. "A transcript of actual life": headache in the novels of Jane Austen. *Headache* 2010;50:692–695.
10. Larner AJ. Jane Austen's (1775–1817) references to headache: fact and fiction. *J Med Biogr* 2010;18:211–215.

Francis Kilvert (1840–1879): a diarist's account of cluster headache?

Francis Kilvert (1840–1879) was an Anglican clergyman of the mid-Victorian age who worked in rural parishes in the Welsh border country and in southern England. He would probably be unknown to posterity were it not for the fact that he kept a diary for the last 10 years of his life (1870–1879), selections from which were published many years later (1938–1940) to public acclaim. The diary has become acknowledged as one of the most notable in the English language, principally as a social documentary of rural life in an era long past. In addition to these features of historical interest, Kilvert's diary may also be of note to neurologists since it shows that he suffered from headaches and facial pain.[1] This article collates all Kilvert's references to headache and facial pains, the nature of which suggests a possible diagnosis of cluster headache.

Methods

The three volumes of selections from Kilvert's diary, made by William Plomer and originally published between 1938–1940, which cover the periods 1st January 1870 to 19th August 1871, 23rd August 1871 to 13th May 1874, and 14th May 1874 to 13th March 1879 respectively (henceforward referred to as I, II, and III), were read and all references to headache, face-ache, face pain or neuralgia were systematically recorded. A selection of more recent commentaries on the diarist and his works were also consulted.[2–5] There are no detailed contemporaneous records of Kilvert other than his diary.

Results

In the approximately 1300 published pages of the diary, twenty-three references were found to Kilvert's headaches (seven), face-ache or facial pain (eleven), and neuralgia (five). Only ten of these references survive the cut for Plomer's 1944 selection from his original selections. Kilvert mentions these symptoms in six of the nine years of the diary for which any substantial amount of material remains. Of these ailments, the index appended to the 1961 reprint of the diary includes only face-ache (six references).

Seven other individuals with these symptoms are also mentioned in the diary, each on only one occasion: Mrs Crichton "upstairs with neuralgia"

(I:28); "old Jones in bed who complained of a headache" (I:55); Baskerville who "rode down with neuralgia" (I:333); Dora, Kilvert's sister, who "had a headache" (II:27); his father, suffering from severe cold and face ache (II:110); Emma Griffiths suffering from face-ache (II:163); and Mrs Lewis "ill with neuralgia" (III:390). Kilvert's own headache disorder may have made him more acute in noting these problems in others.

Whether the different terms used by Kilvert represent different entities, or are different ways of describing the same symptoms, is not entirely clear. Headache and face-ache seem to occur simultaneously in February 1871, and in December 1871 as exemplified by the following quotes:

> Monday 4th December 1871: Knocked all to pieces today with face ache, feeling miserable, stiff, sick and nohow (II:93).
>
> Tuesday 5th December 1871: Shattered with face ache and want of sleep, weak and miserable. Everything seemed unreal and grotesque (II:93).
>
> Wednesday 6th December 1871: A wretched groaning night, sleepless except for some feverish grotesque bad dreams about daybreak. Gnawing face pain and a splitting bursting headache from the heat of the room and the vile gas (II:94).
>
> Sunday 10th December 1871: . . . home by the upper road crazy with face ache, weak and wretched, and the road never seemed to be so long (II:96).

It seems possible that the "bad headache" with "fresh cold and greater tightness of chest" of March 1878 (III:384) may have been distinct from earlier episodes of face-ache and neuralgia. Clearly Kilvert may have used these words in a sense different from their current medical usage. For example, at one point he reports himself "miserable all day with an attack of cholera and diarrhoea" (II:99), but the diagnosis of cholera as currently understood is untenable.[6]

The character of Kilvert's headache symptoms is severe, for example:

> Wednesday 1st March 1871: . . . all night and all today I have been groaning with a bursting raging splitting sick headache (I:307).

Other headache descriptors used by Kilvert include splitting (I:38), crushing (I:301), racking (I:325), and bursting (II:94). Of note, however, nowhere are the words "throbbing" or "pulsating" used to describe the headache.

Face-ache is similarly severe (see quotes above, II:93,94,96), and sleep disturbance is a frequent accompaniment (I:306; II:93,94,232,234). Feelings of restlessness are also mentioned, both in association with face-ache ("awake all night walking about the room . . . unable to rest anywhere"; II:232) and in relative isolation:

> Thursday 14th March 1872: After dinner today I was seized with a strange fit of nervous restlessness ... with it came a twinge of neuralgia and toothache (II:149–150).

Neuralgia is often mentioned just as the single word, but it may also render Kilvert "prostrate" (III:89) and cause sleep disturbance (III:391). A sudden cessation of face-ache, ascribed by Kilvert to an abscess breaking, occurs on one occasion (II:234).

The date of symptom onset is unknown, but the first mention comes in only the second month of the diary (I:38) and the tone of the written entry does not suggest that this is a new or unfamiliar occurrence, so onset prior to the age of 29 years may be assumed.

The frequency of symptoms is of particular note, specifically the clustering of attacks: in late February/early March 1871 headache and face-ache are mentioned three times in five days. This pattern is replicated in later entries: face-ache, face pain and headache are mentioned four times in seven days in December 1871; face-ache and "mouth ... so bad" four times in four days in July 1872; neuralgia is mentioned twice in two days in October 1874; and neuralgia is reported to have been "very troublesome all the week" in April 1878. The duration of bouts would therefore seem to be a few days at most, with long intervals between bouts, the longest apparently being October 1874 to March 1878 (although only one day of the diary for 1877 survives). The duration of individual attacks is not specified, although the impression is that they can last several hours (I:38,140,306,307; II:94,232,234; III:391,447).

Possible symptom triggers are identified by Kilvert. Alcohol is suggested on one occasion ("Drank too much port after dinner . . . last night and a splitting headache all today in revenge"; I:38). The bout of December 1871 follows immediately after a dinner in honour of his birthday (3rd December) at which champagne is consumed, although a later exposure to champagne (II:288) is not followed by any report of ill effects. Heat, from a crowded public gathering (I:301) or from a poorly ventilated gas-heated room (II:94), is blamed, as is cold ("from sitting on a tombstone in the Churchyard"; II:232).

As regards treatment, there seems little that can be done other than to wait until symptoms pass off. Though mentioned as a possible trigger, alcohol is also tried for symptom relief: "after dinner and four glasses of port I felt better" (II:96), sometimes in conjunction with laudanum (I:140). Sal volatile is mentioned on one occasion (II:232). Improvement of symptoms after sleep also occurs (II:149–150).

Medical intervention does not seem to have been sought, even when Kilvert saw the local practitioner, Dr Clouston, in town on the same day that he was having symptoms (II:94). In the July 1872 bout, Kilvert wrote a note asking Clouston to come, and after a sleepless night changed the wording "begging the doctor to come as soon as possible" but as he gave the note to the postboy the "abscess broke" and the pain resolved, and the note was not sent (II:234).[7,8] Kilvert was a regular visitor to his dentist, Gaine, a train journey away in Bath (I:328,376; II:100,446; III:114–115,229,325,357,428), and on occasion had teeth "stopped". One such procedure (23rd December 1871) occurred shortly after a bout of face ache. The tooth was "so sensitive that it could only be stopped temporarily and it was necessary to destroy the nerve" (II:100). However, there is no explicit linkage made between this and the prior symptoms to suggest that Kilvert thought these were of dental origin.

Discussion

Kilvert's published diary is a fragment of the whole work. Following his death, his widow destroyed parts of it relating to herself and possible other of Kilvert's amatory relationships, and of the 22 notebooks originally delivered to William Plomer perhaps only a third of the material was selected as worthy of publication, this at a time of marked paper shortage. Only two of the original notebooks are known to survive, and the original typescript of all 22 notebooks was also, amazingly enough, destroyed. It is therefore unlikely that much, if any, new material will come to light. It is possible that the full text of the diary may have included additional references. For example, in an extract from one of the extant notebooks not selected for inclusion in the published diary by Plomer, but subsequently published by Grice (153), another individual with headache is mentioned: "Helen had a sad headache from the fierce glare of the sun".[4]

Previous Kilvert commentators[2–5] have made occasional note of their subject's headaches but to my knowledge there has been no prior systematic analysis of all references. Le Quesne,[2] who may have shared with Kilvert a headache disorder (p.1), suggests that "the pain in his eyes that frequently troubled him" may have been migraine (p.45). However, my reading of the diary finds no mention of pain in the eyes, although to be sure Kilvert several times mentions problems with his eyesight (I:37; II:52–53,88; III:45,75,358,431,443), especially when trying to read services in dim church interiors, and wonders what one young lady will think of his "poor disfigured eyes" (II:37). None of these reports coincides with episodes of headache or face pain. Lockwood[3] states (p.146) that "Some think he [Kilvert] had a squint. If that is so, and it is not unlikely, it would account for his attacks of neuralgia and headaches. They could easily stem from strain in trying to overcome the deficiency in his vision". Whilst refractive errors are a recognised cause of headache,[9] and headache ascribed to "eye strain" prompting a visit to an optician is a frequent route followed by patients with primary headache disorders,[10] it would seem unlikely to account for Kilvert's severe and periodic symptoms. Glaucoma may present with acute and systemic symptoms, but the aforementioned lack of symptom association with low light environments argues against acute angle closure.

Grice refers to neuralgia and headache in the last years of Kilvert's life as components of his "failing health", accepts "eating and drinking too much and sitting in an overheated room" as causes for the headaches, and opines that his neuralgia and face ache were "probably both the same". He also cites a letter of Lois Lang-Sims which states: "[Kilvert] was occasionally overwhelmed by psychic invasions. Evidently he suffered from a severe form of migraine, a common accompaniment of psychic sensitivity".[4] Toman mentions Kilvert's headaches and face-ache only in passing, when illustrating the burdens placed on him by the absence of his Vicar, even when Kilvert was in ill-health.[5]

The information vouchsafed to us from the diary suggests Kilvert had a syndrome of severe headache and facial pain, occurring periodically, associated with sleep disturbance and restlessness. Although detail is insufficient to fulfil current diagnostic criteria,[9] the symptom pattern, especially the periodicity and the accompanying restlessness, would seem to fit better with a diagnosis of cluster headache than with migraine without aura. Against this formulation, there is no convincing account of autonomic symptoms, and the bouts are apparently of short duration, although such "minibouts" have been described as part of the cluster headache cycle.[11] The absence of any mention of unilaterality of symptoms is odd, although this absence has also been noted in the account of another writer, Arthur Ransome (1884–1967), whose letters and autobiography might otherwise suggest a diagnosis of cluster headache.[12] Although a recognised cause of facial pain, there is no strong evidence to suggest dental problems were the cause of Kilvert's symptoms, although there is a long history of dental treatment being undertaken inappropriately in primary headache disorders.[13,14] Atypical facial pain, a diagnosis of exclusion, must also enter the differential diagnosis.

Should the formulation of cluster headache be accepted, Kilvert's diary may be one of the earliest accounts of this syndrome. Wilfred Harris published his seminal monograph which introduced the term "periodic migrainous neuralgia" in 1926,[15] which was acknowledged by later authors as the first record of cluster headache in the English medical literature,[16,17] although it postdated a possible account by Romberg ("ciliary neuralgia", 1851/3). Other possible, and earlier, accounts have been suggested in the works of Nicolaas Tulp dating from1641,[18] Thomas Willis from the late seventeenth century,[19] Gerhard van Swieten in 1745,[20] Giovanni Battista Morgagni in 1761, the Scotsman Robert Whytt in 1764, and Marshall Hall in 1836.[21] These accounts were all by medical practitioners, so Kilvert may still retain the laurel for the first patient self-report. Other authors who may have suffered from cluster headache include Franz Kafka (1883–1924)[22] and Arthur Ransome.[12]

Acknowledgments

Adapted from: Larner A. Headache, face-ache and neuralgia. The neurological case of the Reverend Francis Kilvert. *Journal of the Kilvert Society* 2008; Issue 26:18–19; and Larner AJ. Francis Kilvert (1840–1879): an early self-report of cluster headache? *Cephalalgia* 2008;28:763–766

References

1. Larner AJ. Neurological literature: headache (part 3). *Adv Clin Neurosci Rehabil* 2007;7(1):27–28.
2. Le Quesne AL. *After Kilvert.* Oxford: Oxford University Press, 1978:45,199.
3. Lockwood D. *Francis Kilvert.* Bridgend: Seren Books, 1990:146–148.
4. Grice F. *Francis Kilvert and his world.* Horsham: Caliban Books, n.d. [1983]:127,130,199.
5. Toman J. *Kilvert: the homeless heart.* Almeley: Logaston Press, 2001:145,146.
6. Larner AJ. Kilvert and cholera. *Journal of the Kilvert Society* 2009;Issue 28:22–23.
7. Larner AJ. Kilvert and the medical profession. *Journal of the Kilvert Society* 2010;Issue 31:53
8. Larner AJ. Hay's "universally acclaimed" junior doctor. *Journal of the Kilvert Society* 2012;Issue 35:187–188
9. International Headache Society Classification Subcommittee. The international classification of headache disorders, second edition. *Cephalalgia* 2004;24(suppl1):1–160.
10. Larner AJ. What role do optometrists currently play in the management of headache? A hospital-based perspective. *Optometry in Practice* 2005;6:173–174.
11. Sjaastad O, de Souza Carvalho D, Fragoso YD, Zhao JM. Cluster headache: on the significance of so-called minibouts. *Cephalalgia* 1988;8:285–291.
12. Larner AJ. Arthur Ransome's headache disorder. *Mixed Moss* [The Journal of the Arthur Ransome Society] 2006:3–9.
13. Larner AJ. Unnecessary extractions. *Br Dent J* 2007;203:442.
14. Larner AJ. "A transcript of actual life": headache in the novels of Jane Austen. *Headache* 2010;50:692–695.
15. Harris W. *Neuritis and neuralgia.* London: Oxford University Press, 1926:301–313.

16. Symonds CP. A particular variety of headache. *Brain* 1956;79:217–232.
17. Boes CJ, Capobianco DJ, Matharu MS, Goadsby PJ. Wilfred Harris' early description of cluster headache. *Cephalalgia* 2002;22:320–326.
18. Koehler PJ. Prevalence of headache in Tulp's Observationes Medicae (1641) with a description of cluster headache. *Cephalalgia* 1993;13:318–320.
19. Pearce JMS. Cluster headache and its variants. *Headache Quarterly Curr Treat Res* 1991;2:187–191.
20. Isler H. Episodic cluster headache from a textbook of 1745: van Swieten's classic description. *Cephalalgia* 1993;13:172–174.
21. Eadie MJ. Two mid-18th century descriptions of probable cluster headache. *J Hist Neurosci* 1992;1:125–130.
22. Ekbom T, Ekbom K. Did Franz Kafka suffer from cluster headache? *Cephalalgia* 2004;24:309–311.

Arthur Ransome (1884–1967): headache disorder

Arthur Ransome is best known as the author of the *Swallows and Amazons* series of twelve children's books published between 1930 and 1947, although prior to this he also worked as a journalist and observed the early years of the Russian Revolution first hand.[1,2]

In *We didn't mean to go to sea* (1937), as the Swallows are making their way across the North Sea, Arthur Ransome gives us this account of Able Seaman Titty Walker:

> ... Titty suddenly clutched the coaming of the cockpit and leant over it.
>
> "She's being sick," said Roger ...
>
> "Leave me alone," said Titty, "... It's only one of my heads. I'll be all right if I lie down for a bit."
>
> ... Down in the fore-cabin Titty scrambled into her bunk. Something was hammering in her head as if to burst it.[3]

To a practising neurologist with an interest in headache disorders, this sounds like childhood migraine without aura, apparently induced by seasickness or at least by the motion of the sea. The question which such a passage immediately provokes, at least for this neurologist, is whether the author himself suffered from headaches and was drawing on his own experience in writing this. Other examples of "literary headaches" which reflect the authors' own experience have been documented, including Mikhail Bulgakov[4] and, possibly, Lewis Carroll.[5,6]

To investigate whether Arthur Ransome did suffer from headaches, I have consulted as primary sources his autobiography, edited by Rupert Hart-Davis (henceforward A),[7] and the selected letters which have been published, edited by Hugh Brogan (henceforward B).[8] As the definitive secondary source I have used Hugh Brogan's biography, (henceforward C).[1] As a brief perusal of the index of Brogan's biography will show (C:451), throughout his life Ransome suffered from an "anthology of ailments" (C:419); a detailed pathography of Ransome could fill many pages. However, headache is not specifically mentioned in Brogan's index, and to my knowledge has not been examined hitherto.

Symptoms

The autobiography first mentions "violent headaches" during Ransome's visit to France in 1907 at the age of 23:

> I was troubled at that time with violent headaches, for which I found walking the best though a painful cure. I used to set out from my studio half-blind with pain and, stumbling resolutely on, would find the pain lessening and at last gone altogether. (A:124)
>
> I have never learned to draw, but at this time I always carried a sketch-book in my pocket and, on the long walk that resulted from that fortunate headache, I did a number of drawings of gargoyles. (A:126)

There is no mention of headache in Ransome's *Bohemia in London*, published in 1907, a great part of which work was, according to Rupert Hart-Davis, autobiographical.[9] Nor are headaches mentioned during the stressful time of the Douglas legal case, in 1912–13, when Ransome was also experiencing difficulties with his first wife, Ivy, from whom he was estranged and eventually divorced.

The next mention of headaches occurs when Ransome was in Russia, in 1915, aged 31. He reports:

> ... I was growing rapidly more and more ill, losing much too much blood [from the bowel] and at the same time being unable to throw off a succession of violent headaches that made work all but impossible. This neuritis was not improved by letters from Wiltshire [from his wife, Ivy] which ... led me to believe that my daughter was dangerously ill. (A:179)

This problem is also mentioned in a letter to his mother, Edith (27th July 1915):

> ... it's sickening being unable to work, and also unable to keep still, and waking every day with a most frantic headache which only clears off for a few hours in the middle of the day. (B:25)

Interestingly, it was around this time that Ransome was preparing his book *Old Peter's Russian Tales* for publication ("I was ... putting in all free hours on the book of Russian folk-stories"; A:179), which included the story of *Little Master Misery* whose head ached early in the morning, and also *The Three Men of Power*, two of whom suffer headaches after being beaten by the little man a yard high.[10] However, in retrospect this was a happy time:

> I forget the ... wild headaches one after another (A:182)

Around this time Ransome was also troubled with haemorrhaging from the bowel which eventually required surgery. It was in the immediate postoperative period that he wrote his first telegram to the *Daily News* newspaper, standing in for their usual correspondent who was also ill:

> I had a violent headache that evening and another next day when I wrote my second telegram. For some weeks the headaches and the telegrams seemed inseparable . . . (A:184)

Whilst still convalescing following his operation which was performed on 9th August 1915, he wrote to his mother (2nd September 1915):

> I get headaches at once if I try to work. . . . however, after telegraphing I lie down, and the headache goes as soon as my blood is evenly distributed (C:105)

Recuperating in England (September-October 1915):

> I did some quiet fishing in Wiltshire and at Coniston, though suffering, in spite of writing only a couple of articles and no telegrams, a further lot of frantic headaches. (A:185)

However, Brogan reports of this period that:

> His journey home, and sojourn there, were uneventful, except that the strain of living with Ivy brought on a recurrence of his headaches, which had previously gone away (C:106)

As he began the return journey to Russia:

> I was still in a pretty poor way, what with anaemia and those continual headaches (A:186)

Back in Russia, in February 1916:

> I was having one headache after another (A:190)

Likewise, following a further home visit, returning to Russia again in December 1916:

> I reached Petrograd on December 11, after a journey spoilt by violent headaches (A:205)

Brogan states that:

> Arthur started back to Russia on 2 December [1916], suffering once more from violent headaches, caused by a brief but thoroughly unsatisfactory visit to Ivy (C:114)

Writing to his mother (6th July 1917):

> ... when I get a headache so rotten that work is an impossibility I bolt to the suburbs of Petrograd and get sunburnt and catch, actually catch, roach (B:45–46)

The final mention of headache in the autobiography occurs in 1928, when Ransome was aged 44 (i.e. more than 10 years after the previous report):

> I left for Moscow and got there on February 3 with a raging headache and feeling most unwell generally (A:329)

Writing to his mother, enumerating fish caught (4th July 1930):

> ... have so far not got my usual after fishing headache (B:173)

But the headaches had not gone away, since, writing to his mother after arrival in Aleppo, Syria, to visit his friends the Altounyan family (3rd February 1932):

> I got through the journey pretty well, only ending up with rather a bad go of pains and headache, which, however, seems to have lifted again this morning (B:202)

In 1936 Ransome "was frequently prostrated with headaches or duodenal pains or both" (C:346). This was shortly after the idea came to him for the novel *We didn't mean to go to sea*, wherein came the one mention of headache in his *Swallows and Amazons* fiction.[3]

The final mention of headache I have found came when Ransome was writing to the Renolds (13th February 1941, aged 58):

> My old brain is truly bust and wore out ... it can run headaches but not yarns. (B:281)

Not quite worn out, though, since there were still three *Swallows and Amazons* books to be published, not to mention all the other writing and editing of his later years.

Diagnostic formulation

Clearly then Ransome suffered from headaches for many years. References in all three key sources cover periods of over 20 years (A: age 23–44 years; B: 31–58 years; C: 31–52 years). But what type of headache, or headaches, did he suffer from? The internationally agreed classification of headaches provides a rich typology[11] which may assist diagnosis (admittedly these criteria were formulated well after Ransome's death, so what follows is to indulge in retrospective diagnosis, a potentially misleading undertaking).

Some of Ransome's reported headaches are clearly secondary to an obvious precipitating factor. For example, in Bucharest in 1916, he happened to be only a few yards from where a bomb dropped:

> I was quite unhurt except that I did get a bit of a headache (A:202)

In Aleppo in 1932, he wrote to his mother (21st February 1932):

> I am today feeling pretty sick and sorry for myself after my first inoculation for typhoid. . . . I feel sick, headachy, and bone-achy, with a swelled up arm (B:203; also C:324)

However these are the exceptions rather than the rule. Moreover, whilst it may be understandable to blame the difficulties with Ivy for some of the headaches (C:106,114), this cannot be the whole explanation for so long-lasting a disorder.

Unfortunately, the information vouchsafed in the various sources is not sufficient to permit a definitive diagnosis to be made. The questions a neurologist would like to ask in a clinical encounter are not involuntarily answered by the author. However, some characteristics are at least suggested.

Firstly, the character of the headaches: they are variously described in such a way ("half-blind with pain"; "neuritis"; "violent"; "frantic"; "wild"; "raging") as to suggest extreme severity. These were not the "normal" headaches which everyone battles through occasionally, being sufficiently intrusive to prevent work, and being associated with systemic upset ("feeling most unwell generally").

Details of headache timing are sparse, although it is mentioned on one occasion that Ransome is "waking every day with a most frantic headache". The relationship to fishing is also intriguing: is this in any way a consequence of the early morning start required ("got up today at 1.30 a.m."; B:173), hence sleep deprivation? The later description of the headaches as "continual" is a little problematic: it is not clear whether this means that they are present all the time (continuous, every minute of every day) or that they are recurring every day though not present for all of the day. The report of "one headache after another" would perhaps be more consistent with the latter interpretation. One might also infer, from Ransome's silence on the subject, that there were periods of headache remission; clearly matters were very bad in 1915, 1916, and possibly 1917, but then there are no reports of headache until the late 1920s.

Although lying down is the response to headache in one passage (C:105), more striking are the allusions to a preference for movement ("walking the best though a painful cure"; "unable to keep still"; "bolt to the suburbs"). This would be an unusual response to migraine headaches, wherein headache is exacerbated by usual physical activities, and a desire to remain still or to lie down is the norm.

Movement is a more usual response to the entity variously known as cluster headache, Harris's syndrome, migrainous neuralgia, or trigeminal autonomic cephalalgia. This is an episodic, stereotyped, strictly unilateral, primary headache syndrome of extreme severity, much commoner in men than women, most often beginning in the third or fourth decade of life, with typical periodicity with respect both to time of day and over months or years. Headaches may occur daily, often at the same time, for weeks or months (a "cluster"), then remit for weeks or months, only to recur at a later time with similar periodicity.[12] Smoking is reported to be a risk factor for cluster headache, in which connection Ransome's predilection for strong tobacco may be significant. The suggestion of headache periodicity from the published sources would be in keeping with the diagnosis. However, the strict unilaterality of cluster headaches is not mentioned in any of the sources I have consulted. Whether the unpublished letters or other sources might provide the key to this medical detective work remains to be explored. Chambers, Ransome's most recent biographer,[2] mentions his subject's headache and/or neuralgia on seven occasions, most (6) occurring between June 1914 and late 1917, the exception being 1928 (p.85,100,108,124,148,158,342).

Another possible explanation for the passage quoted from *We didn't mean to go to sea* is that it might possibly be drawn from the human model for Titty, Mavis Altounyan. (I am not aware of any account of Captain Flint suffering headaches.) In Taqui Altounyan's memoir of her childhood, *In Aleppo Once*,[13] which mentions "Uncle Arthur" (p.153, 160–3, 175, 181), but not the aforementioned complications of his inoculation, she comments that on receipt of *Swallows and Amazons* the family judged the portrayal of Titty to be "very true to life" (p.163). Interestingly, Titty/Mavis is the only one of the Altounyan children reported by Taqui to suffer from a headache (p.101–102), admittedly in the context of a cough and a fever; she is also sick when rounding a series of corkscrew bends as the family travel up into the mountains, possibly indicating sensitivity to movement (p.123). Suggestive evidence, but not compelling. Moreover, as has been rightly said, "the tempting game of pinning real people to the characters cannot be taken too far".[14]

Acknowledgment

Adapted from: Larner AJ. Arthur Ransome's headache disorder. *Mixed Moss* [The Journal of the Arthur Ransome Society] 2006:3–9

References

1. Brogan H. *The life of Arthur Ransome.* London: Cape, 1984.
2. Chambers R. *The last Englishman. The double life of Arthur Ransome.* London: Faber and Faber, 2009.
3. Ransome A. *We didn't mean to go to sea.* Harmondsworth: Puffin, 1969 [1937]:135.
4. Zayas V. Sympathy for Pontius Pilate. Hemicrania in M.A. Bulgakov's "The Master and Margarita". *Eur J Neurol* 2005;12(suppl2):296 (abstract P2506).
5. Larner AJ. "Neurological literature": headache. *Adv Clin Neurosci Rehabil* 2006;5(6):23–24.
6. Larner AJ. "Neurological literature": headache (part 2). *Adv Clin Neurosci Rehabil* 2006;6(2):37–38.
7. Hart-Davis R (ed.). *The autobiography of Arthur Ransome.* London: Cape, 1976.
8. Brogan H (ed.). *Signalling from Mars: the letters of Arthur Ransome.* London: Cape, 1997.
9. Ransome A. *Bohemia in London.* Oxford: Oxford University Press, 1984 [1907]:xii.
10. Ransome A. *Old Peter's Russian Tales.* London: Jane Nissen, 2003 [1916]:135,137,204,205,207.
11. International Headache Society Classification Subcommittee. The international classification of headache disorders, second edition. *Cephalalgia* 2004;24(suppl1):1–160,
12. Barker R, Scolding NJ, Rowe D, Larner AJ. *The A-Z of neurological practice. A guide to clinical neurology.* Cambridge: Cambridge University Press, 2005:187–189.
13. Altounyan T. *In Aleppo Once.* London: John Murray, 1969.
14. Hardyment C. *Arthur Ransome and Captain Flint's trunk.* London: Cape, 1984:42.

Jean Langlais (1907–1991): stroke-induced aphasia and Braille alexia without amusia

Introduction

Language is a symbolic code used for communication. Though typically spoken and written, language may also be gestured or signed in the visual domain, or represented in the tactile domain as raised dots (Braille). As early as 1878 John Hughlings Jackson (1835–1911) predicted that a deaf-mute might be deprived of the system of sign language by a cerebral lesion, a supposition amply confirmed by observations of "aphasia" for sign-language in the deaf, which usually indicates left hemisphere damage.[1] In an analogous manner, Macdonald Critchley (1900–1997) predicted that blind Braille readers might well lose their tactuo-linguistic skill as a result of brain damage,[2] a prediction which has also been confirmed by reports of Braille alexia, albeit rare.[3]

One of these cases of Braille alexia, reported in French, concerned a blind organist, designated in the paper as "M. J.L. (84097) né le 15 février 1907".[4] This patient has been identified as Jean Langlais (1907–1991), whose artistic and clinical history is presented here. A brief account of his stroke and its consequences may be found in his biography.[5]

Background

Jean Langlais was born on 15th February 1907 in the village of La Fontenelle in Brittany. He lost his sight around the age of 2 or 3 years; the cause was never ascertained, but it may possibly have been as a consequence of congenital glaucoma and/or eye infection. He first learned to read Braille around the age of 10 years when he entered, in 1917, the Institut National des Jeunes Aveugles in Paris, the institution where Louis Braille (1809–1852) had spent most of his life. As Langlais was interested in music, initially the piano and violin, he also mastered Braille for music, which utilizes the same constellations of raised dots as for language, such that the same patterns may, depending on context, represent letters or musical notation. The Institut had a long tradition of teaching music and supplied blind organists to many churches from the 1820s onward, hence after the age of 16 Langlais devoted himself to the organ. One of his teachers at the Institut was André Marchal (1894–1980), an organist who was blind from birth. Langlais entered the Conservatoire de Paris in 1927, where his teachers included the celebrated organists Marcel Dupré (1886–1971) and Charles Arnould Tournemire (1870–1939) for organ studies, and Paul Dukas (1865–1935) for composition. Langlais won the first prize at the Conservatoire in 1930 and his first compositions were published in 1932. In 1945 he was appointed the organist at St Clotilde in Paris, a position previously held by Cesar Franck (1822–1890), and which Langlais was to hold until 1988.[6]

Contemporary with not only Marchal and Dupré but also a number of other noted organists working in Paris, including Maurice Duruflé (1902–1986) and Olivier Messiaen (1908–1992), the latter a personal friend, Langlais was noted for a large output of organ music, some based on Gregorian themes enhanced by polymodal harmonies, including three concertos with orchestra as well as several liturgical choral works. One vocal piece was entitled *Hommage à Louis Braille* (1951). Langlais was also known for his recitals and was a renowned improviser, as well as being a teacher. A number of his works feature "name motifs", in which notes are used to correspond to letters through the double (musical/verbal) meaning of Braille notation, so that names and complete sentences may be written in the form of a musical theme.[7] Currently, little of Langlais' oeuvre is easily available on disc,[8] but his work remains in the repertoire of many cathedral organists and choirs.

Case Report[9]

On 1st July 1984, aged 77, Langlais suffered a stroke affecting the territory of the left middle cerebral artery. Symptom onset occurred whilst he was playing at a mass in the cathedral of Dol-de-Bretagne. Initially he had right hemiplegia and, since he was right-handed, was unable to speak. He was hospitalised in Saint-Malo for one week, and in fifteen days was able to walk and use his right arm and hand. Thereafter, he was seen at the Hôpital de la Salpêtrière in Paris, initial assessment occurring 10 weeks after the acute event, and continuing at the patient's home over the subsequent two months. Neurological examination of the motor system and sensation was normal by this time. Structural brain imaging with CT scan showed extensive hypodensity in the left temporal lobe affecting Wernicke's area in particular.

There were marked difficulties with spoken language. Output was fluent with normal articulation and intonation, but blockages, *conduit d'approche*, rare phonemic paraphasias and neologisms were evident; discourse was empty with jargon aphasia. Comprehension of simple questions and orders concerning daily life were preserved, allowing satisfactory communication, but more complex orders proved impossible to carry out. Familiar voices were easily identified. Naming to tactile confrontation of 7 common objects was preserved but to verbal description was impaired. Repetition was impaired for monosyllabic words and simple phrases. Repetition of musical notes given verbally was possible if the repetition was by singing, but impossible if the patient was required to verbalise the notes without singing.

Concerning the written word in Braille, reading aloud was almost impossible, with 50% errors for letters, 70% for simple syllables. Errors were more frequent for long words than for short words. Comprehension of simple phrases was impossible even if certain words were identified. However, these difficulties were not due to tactile agnosia: identification of each Braille sign was perfect. Writing Braille, with a tablet and a punch, the patient retained great manual dexterity and could copy letters, syllables and common words not exceeding five letters, but paragraphias were evident when writing spontaneously or to dictation.

In contrast to the aphasia, the patient was able to hum a tune or sing a melody without error, but notes could not be named without singing them.

In summary, there was a Wernicke type aphasia, consistent with structural imaging findings (left temporoparietal infarct), and with concordant alexia and agraphia for Braille, but without amusia. For reading and writing, the difficulty was interpreted as a failure of integration of signs ("tactemes", as opposed to the graphemes of written language) confined to the domain of linguistic ability with sparing of musical ability, suggesting different cerebral localisation for these faculties.

Progress

Six weeks after the cererbal infarct, Langlais was able to play a Bach chorale, considered an easy piece. At eleven weeks, he was able, at the request of his doctors, to play Franck's Pastorale, a performance which was considered by musical listeners as exemplary, without technical fault and showing qualities of interpretation and sensibility perhaps superior to those evinced in his recording of the piece in 1975. He resumed concerts at the organ of St Clotilde in October 1984 (3 months post-stroke), and on 24th October recorded for French television a series of improvisations on themes of Franck which were unanimously judged exemplary and brilliant. From November 1984, Langlais resumed giving lessons on playing and improvisation, judged by his pupils to be of the same quality as before his stroke, though his aphasia necessarily reduced the verbal exchanges. His wife, also an organist, noted that his musical "grammar" (scales, modulation, transposition) was executed without error, and pieces could be identified and continued after hearing the first few bars although verbal naming was impossible. Musical Braille notation could be decoded and played perfectly, and music could be written in Braille, despite continuing verbal alexia and agraphia for Braille. Musical composition was resumed in 1985. Consulting the chronological list of his works, there was no obvious decline in output in subsequent years, post-stroke pieces including sixteen works for organ, three hymns, two choral works, and a variety of instrumental pieces. Included are works dedicated to his doctors, Signoret and van Eeckhout. "Name motifs" also occur in post-stroke pieces.[10]

Discussion

The French encyclopaedist Denis Diderot (1713–1784) opined that in "a blind person the theatre of the soul is to be found within the finger-tips".[11] This statement may be particularly true of an artist like Langlais, whose music was both read and played not by sight but by touch. This may be a reflection of the extraordinary augmentation of perceptual abilities associated with sensory deprivation in other modalities, including tactile faculties in the blind, the phenomenon known as hyperpilaphesie.[12]

The findings in Jean Langlais may be summarised as a striking ability to read and write music in Braille notation but an inability to read and write verbal language in the same Braille notation. Such a double dissociation, used in cognitive neuropsychology as one of the cornerstones for making inferences about mental structure,[13] suggests functional and anatomical independence of the mental processes subserving linguistic and musical abilities, at least in this patient (note that he had both "invested" heavily in the development of musical skills and been blind from a young age, i.e. "early blind"). Since the tactile elements of Braille are identical for both musical and linguistic notation, the selective deficit in Langlais implies a disorder of higher order, integrative rather than perceptual, processing, which would accord with an associative type of agnosia.[14] Indeed the pattern of Braille alexia in Langlais corresponds perfectly to the explanation emphasized by Critchley, that "the loss of skill is not . . . the result of any loss of the peripheral sense of touch, but is a high-level disorder of linguistic interpretation".[15] However, other mechanisms may operate in other patients with Braille alexia, with at least one case reported with apparent tactile sensory impairments indicative of an apperceptive, rather than associative, agnosia.[16]

Acknowledgments

Adapted from: Fisher CAH, Larner AJ. Jean Langlais (1907–91): an historical case of a blind organist with stroke-induced aphasia and Braille alexia but without amusia. *J Med Biogr* 2008;16:232–234; and Larner AJ, Fisher CAH. Amazing brains: Questions arising from the neurological histories of two blind organists. *Organists' Review*2009;November:38–39.

References

1. For discussion of sign language and its deficits, see: Critchley M. *Aphasiology.* London: Edward Arnold, 1970:325–347; Kimura D. Neural mechanisms in manual signing. *Sign Language Studies* 1981;33:291–312; Ellis AW, Young AW. *Human cognitive neuropsychology. A textbook with readings.* Hove: Psychology Press, 1996:262–265; Rönnberg J, Söderfeldt B, Risberg J. The cognitive neuroscience of signed language. *Acta Psychol Amst* 2000;105:237–254; and Gordon N. The neurology of sign language. *Brain Dev* 2004;26:146–150. Classic accounts of patients with sign aphasia include: Douglass E, Richardson JC. Aphasia in a congenital deaf mute. *Brain* 1959;82:68–80; Sarno JE, Swisher LP, Sarno MT. Aphasia in a congenitally deaf man. *Cortex* 1969;5:398–414; Kimura D, Battison R, Lubert B. Impairment of nonlinguistic hand movements in a deaf aphasic. *Brain Lang* 1976;3:566–571; Chiarello C, Knight R, Mandel M. Aphasia in a prelingually deaf woman. *Brain* 1982;105:29–52; Bellugi U, Poizner H, Klima ES. Brain organization for language: clues from sign aphasia. *Human Neurobiology* 1983;2:155–170; and Poizner H, Bellugi U, Iragui V. Apraxia and aphasia for a visual-gestural language. *Am J Physiol* 1984;246:R868–R883.
2. Critchley M. *The divine banquet of the brain and other essays.* New York: Raven Press, 1979:90.
3. For reports of Braille alexia see: Gloning I, Gloning K, Weingarten K, Berner P. Uber einen Fall mit Alexie der Brailleschrift. *Wien Z Nervenheilkd Grenzgeb* 1954;10:260–273; Birchmeier AK. Aphasic dyslexia of Braille in a congenitally blind man. *Neuropsychologia* 1985;23:177–193; Signoret J-L, van Eeckhout P, Poncet M, Castaigne P. Aphasie sans amusie chez un organiste aveugle. *Rev Neurol Paris* 1987;143:172–181; Perrier D, Belin C, Larmande P. Trouble de la lecture du Braille par lésion droite chez une patiente devenue aveugle. *Neuropsychologia* 1988;26:179–185; Hamilton R, Keenan JP, Catala M, Pascual-Leone A. Alexia for Braille following bilateral occipital stroke in an early blind woman. *Neuroreport* 2000;11:237–240; Maeda K, Yasuda H, Haneda M, Kashiwagi A. Braille alexia during visual hallucination in a blind man with selective calcarine atrophy. *Psychiatry Clin Neurosci* 2003;57:227–9; and Larner AJ. Braille alexia: an apperceptive tactile agnosia? *J Neurol Neurosurg Psychiatry* 2007;78:907–908.
4. Signoret *et al.* 1987, *op. cit.* ref 3:173.
5. Labounsky A. *Jean Langlais. The man and his music.* Portland, Oregon: Amadeus Press, 2000: 314–316; this briefly alludes to the Signoret *et al.* 1987 paper.
6. The definitive biography is Labounsky 2000 (*op. cit.* ref 5). Langlais's second

wife, Marie-Louise Langlais, also wrote a biography, *Ombre et lumière* (Paris: Combre, 1995). For brief biographical details, see also Signoret *et al.* 1987, *op. cit.* ref 3:173; Sadie S (ed.). *The Grove concise dictionary of music.* London: Macmillan, 1988:446; and Latham A (ed.). *The Oxford companion to music.* Oxford: Oxford University Press, 2002:671. Websites with useful information about Langlais are: www.musimem.com/langlais.htm and http://perso.orange.fr/langlais/index.htm.

7. Examples may be found in Labounsky 2000, *op. cit.* ref 5:156, 164, 190, 192, 252, 256, 260, 265–6, 267, 271, 273, 283, 288, 289, 298, 305, 319, 326.
8. Labounsky has recorded the complete organ works (1979–2003) in 24 CDs for the Musical Heritage Society.
9. Based on a translation by the CAH Fisher and AJ Larner from the French of Signoret *et al.* 1987, *op. cit.* ref 3, supplemented by the account in Labounsky 2000 (*op. cit.* ref 5:314–316).
10. Labounsky 2000, *op. cit.* ref 5:342–363; 318; 319; 319 and 326, respectively.
11. Cited in Critchley 1979, *op. cit.* ref 2:265.
12. For a further example of a blind organist with apparently extraordinary perceptual skills, possibly colour-touch synaesthesia, see Larner AJ. A possible account of synaesthesia dating from the seventeenth century. *J Hist Neurosci* 2006;15:245–249. A different interpretation of these faculties, namely dermo-optical perception, is suggested by Brugger P, Weiss PH. Dermo-optical perception: the non-synesthetic "palpability of colors" a comment on Larner (2006). *J Hist Neurosci* 2008;17:253–255.
13. Shallice T. *From neuropsychology to mental structure.* Cambridge: Cambridge University Press, 1988
14. Larner AJ. *A dictionary of neurological signs* (2nd edition). New York: Springer, 2006:8–9.
15. Critchley M. *The citadel of the senses and other essays.* New York: Raven Press, 1986:198.
16. Larner 2007, *op. cit.* ref 3.

Margiad Evans (1909–1958): epilepsy in a creative writer

Margiad Evans was the pseudonym used by Peggy Eileen Whistler (1909–1958) as the author of a series of acclaimed novels in the 1930s and 1940s, such as *Country Dance* (1932), *The Wooden Doctor* (1933), *Turf or Stone* (1934), *Creed* (1936), and *Autobiography* (1943). She also wrote short stories, poems, reviews and radio broadcasts up to the 1950s. Although perhaps little known today, contemporary critics compared her with writers such as James Joyce and T.S. Eliot.[1–3]

Margiad Evans was diagnosed with epilepsy in her early forties. Her first major seizure occurred on the evening of 11th May 1950 whilst she was alone in her cottage, the Black House, in the village of Elkstone in Gloucestershire, and is described thus in her published account of her epilepsy, *A Ray of Darkness*:[4]

> [I] looked up at the clock … saw that it was ten minutes past eleven. The next thing I was still looking up at the clock and the hands stood at five and twenty minutes past midnight. I had fallen through Time, Continuity and Being.
>
> I felt a cold dampness and it came on me stunningly, terrifyingly, that my clothes were wet. My urine had escaped me then. Horrifyingly, in one moment, I realized the incredible, impossible, and ghastly truth – I had neither fainted nor been asleep: I had had an epileptic fit! … A horrible, perhaps incurable illness lay before me.

In the immediate aftermath, recalled later, her brain "worked … like an engine misfiring and unsteered". The seizure "was total blackness, a hole in the self" and a "separation from the will".

Relatives later suggested to her that the attack was simply a faint but in her rebuttal Margiad showed a clear ability to differentiate her symptoms from those of syncope:

> I had been close enough to it to be absolutely sure that one did not faint as I had fallen. There was a sinking away, a sick feeling, and a remembrance of it afterwards.

On 12th May 1950, the day following the seizure, Margiad was seen by her general practitioner, who prescribed Luminal (phenobarbital) and arranged a referral to “Professor T … a man of international reputation” at the “Neurological Institute outside Clystowe”, in fact Professor Frederick Golla (1878–1968) at the Burden Neurological Institute, then located outside Bristol. The published history of “The Burden” notes that “Golla’s reputation and interest in the subject [epilepsy] and the availability of brain recordings [EEG] attracted a great number of referrals”.[5] Golla saw Margiad on 8th June 1950, and following an EEG he confirmed the diagnosis of epilepsy which he thought might be due to “a slight scar on the brain from an old injury”. Margiad’s response to this diagnosis was unsparing:

> I walked out of the Institute as a person harbouring epilepsy, it was true, but free of false hopes and quite clearly defined as myself.

Epilepsy defined

The brain may be conceptualized physiologically as an electrical organ. Epileptic seizures result from abnormal electrical activity within the brain. In pathological states, brain cells (neurones) discharge in highly rhythmic and coordinated (hypersynchronous) patterns which override normal physiological brain activity and function to produce the phenomena which are witnessed and/or experienced as epileptic seizures. Many types of epileptic seizure may be delineated, according to either seizure characteristics, known as the seizure semiology, or underlying mechanism. Seizures may include motor, sensory, autonomic (relating to the automatic homeostatic mechanisms of the body, for example control of blood pressure, breathing, sweating), or psychic phenomena.

Broadly epileptic seizures may be classified according to either aetiology (i.e. cause) or neurophysiology (i.e. mechanism). Aetiologically, seizures may be either *idiopathic/primary* (i.e. cause unknown) or *symptomatic/secondary* (cause identified, e.g. brain tumour, infection, neurodegeneration such as Alzheimer’s disease). Neurophysiologically, seizures may be either *generalized* (abnormal electrical activity throughout the brain at seizure onset) or *partial/localization-related* (focal abnormal electrical activity at seizure onset, which may remain localized or spread to other brain areas, sometimes becoming generalized and resulting in a secondarily generalized seizure). Generalized seizures may take various forms such as grand mal (or generalized tonic-clonic seizures) and petit mal, and partial seizures may be *simple* if consciousness is preserved or *complex* if consciousness is impaired.[6]

A distinction may be drawn between epileptic seizures and epilepsy. Epilepsy may be canonically defined as an enduring predisposition of the brain to generate epileptic seizures, a definition which may be operationalised to mean the occurrence of two or more unprovoked seizures.[7] Margiad Evans gave a graphic account of her second seizure in *A Ray of Darkness*:

> One morning in our cottage [the Black House, Elkstone, Gloucestershire] I got up fairly early out of bed and went down stairs to make tea. I carried the tray upstairs, put it down by the bed and the next moment it seemed heard my husband saying to me as my head lay on the pillow: "How do you feel, dearie?".
>
> Astonished, I answered drowsily that I felt very well, why? "Because you have just had another attack," he said. With those words an amazement entered into me which has never left me. Ever since I have been incredulous of all things firm and material. The light has held patches of invisible blackness, Time has become as rotten as worm-eaten wood, the earth under me is full of trap-doors and the sense of being, which is life and all that surrounds and creates it, a thing taken and given irresponsibly and without warning as children snatch at a toy. Sight, hearing, touch, consciousness, torn from one like a nest from a bird!
>
> Of course it was only slowly I realized the truth as my eyes discovered a blood-stained pillow-case, my senses a tongue bitten through at the edge, for it seemed he had had as little warning as myself. It had been a swift performance. One kick, he said, as I lay down, and he cried "What are you doing?" and turned and saw. It had lasted twenty minutes. He had changed the pillow-case under my head. Twenty minutes! and less than a blink to me, for this time, as I had been lying in bed and was not hurt apart from my tongue, I felt no illness afterwards. In fact the tea was still hot and we drank it quite as usual. This was my second major or total attack of epilepsy.

This seizure probably occurred at some time in late July or early August of 1950, when Margiad was 41 years of age. It was her first witnessed seizure, since her husband, Michael Williams, had been away from home at the time of the first event. By the time of this second attack, Margiad was two to three months pregnant, a situation known to lower the threshold in some symptomatic epilepsies, probably due to the hormonal changes of pregnancy.[8]

Irrespective of professional clinical definitions of epilepsy, the second seizure was, according to her written account, a watershed for Margiad: "my security was gone". She had already acknowledged herself to be an epileptic. The "adventure of body and mind" which was to prompt the writing of "the story of my epilepsy" had begun, a journey which was to produce two accounts of epilepsy, *A Ray of Darkness* and the unpublished *The Nightingale Silenced*, which together constitute one of the earliest patient accounts of the disease. Although she evidently experienced other neurological phenomena distinct from epileptic seizures,[9,10] it is the latter which form the subject of this account, as well as a consideration of the effect of epilepsy on Margiad Evans as a creative writer.

Epilepsy in literature

Shakespeare used the word 'epilepsy' only once in his plays. In *Othello* (IV;i:50–51), the Moor collapses as Iago goads him into believing Desdemona is unfaithful:

> My lord is fallen into an epilepsy;
> This is his second fit; he had one yesterday.

Othello's rapid recovery and the circumstances of the attack suggest (to this clinician) that this was not an epileptic seizure,[11] as some commentators have seemed willing to accept,[12–14] but syncope or a vasovagal attack (in lay parlance, a faint), a much more frequent cause of loss of consciousness. This is a common, and often challenging, differential diagnosis in clinical practice even today, based on the clinical history and often requiring an eyewitness account of the episode, rather than any sophisticated diagnostic testing.[15] Indeed, Margiad Evans was able to rebut from her own experience the suggestion of her relatives that her first attack was simply a faint, evidently aware of the difference between the two. Of course there is a least one definite account of epilepsy in Shakespeare, although it is not named as such, in *Julius Caesar* (I;iii:253–256) when Casca and Brutus discuss Caesar falling in the market place and foaming at the mouth, diagnosed by Brutus as the 'falling sickness'.[16] Elizabethan 'falling sickness' almost certainly equates to modern epilepsy.

Such seizures were familiar in ancient medical literature, the earliest treatise devoted to the subject probably being that of Hippocrates of Cos, *On the Sacred Disease*, dating from the fourth century BCE. Hippocrates was clear that this was not a supernatural phenomenon:

> It is thus with regard to the disease called Sacred: it appears to me to be nowise more divine nor more sacred than other diseases, but has a natural cause . . . like other affections.

The term epilepsy derived ultimately from ancient Greek, meaning to be seized upon or attacked. However, the Oxford English Dictionary lists only one usage of 'Epilepsie' prior to that of Shakespeare (1604), dating from 1578, in the *Niewe herball or historie of plantes* by Henry Lyte (1529?-1607), a botanist and antiquary, this being a translation of the Flemish physician and botanist

Rembert Dodoens' (1516/17–1585) *Cruydeboek* of 1554, an extensive herbal which became a standard in English through Lyte's translation, and which had a dedication to Queen Elizabeth. A familiarity with botany was at that time a key element of medical training and practice.[17]

A definitive literary history of epilepsy has, to my knowledge, yet to be written, but a few examples of literary accounts of seizures may be given here. The plot of *Silas Marner, the weaver of Raveloe* (1861) by George Eliot (another Evans, this time by birth rather than pseudonym) hinges upon a theft occurring during the protagonist's fit, later described thus:

> ... he saw that Marner's eyes were set like a dead man's, and he spoke to him, and shook him, and his limbs were stiff ... just as he had made up his mind that the weaver was dead, he came all right again ... and said "Goodnight", and walked off.

This has features compatible with a complex partial seizure.[16] Fyodor Dostoevsky (1821–1881), himself an epileptic, described seizures in many of his works, notably as a key plot device in *The Brothers Karamazov* (1879–80). Freud suggested that Dostoevsky's seizures were hysterical in origin, but the evidence is against this, as first pointed out by EH Carr, for example in his 1931 biography of Dostoevsky. Dostoevsky's own experience of epilepsy may have directly informed the portrayal of seizures experienced by Prince Myshkin in *The Idiot* (1868).[18,19] Examples of epileptic seizures may also be noted in films, many focusing on 'possession' as the cause of convulsions.[20,21]

Despite these artistic presentations of seizures, first hand accounts of the experience of epilepsy were few prior to Margiad Evans's *A Ray of Darkness*, which gives insights into one woman's consciousness of the phenomenality of epilepsy.

Margiad Evans's epilepsy: personal and professional accounts

Margiad Evans's epilepsy has necessarily been described in biographical works focusing on her as a writer, albeit in passing,[1–3] and also by neurologists who were personally involved in her clinical care in the 1950s, specifically Frederick Golla[22] and William Lennox (1884–1960).[23] However, her illness and its effect on her as a writer has attracted relatively little clinical interest until recently.[24,25]

What was the nature of her epilepsy? Clinical clues may be drawn from *A Ray of Darkness* (1952) and from the unpublished manuscript of *The Nightingale Silenced* (1954–55).[26] Since the latter is addressed specifically to medical professionals, it behoves us to examine this work critically.

Whereas the first two epileptic attacks Evans suffered occurred without any appreciable warning (see above for the descriptions of these attacks), in later episodes there was a ghastly awareness of fading consciousness, associated with overwhelming psychic phenomena. Indeed many later seizures comprised solely the latter: some "convulsions were confined to mental sensations only", in which fear was the predominant and overriding feeling. Without such feelings ("panic without cause"), the seizures may not have troubled her greatly: "could fear … be wiped away, the seizures would not matter very much". But when attacks occurred these sensations were overwhelming:

> I was … incapable of controlling the sudden panic … every object became impregnated with terror. … The term "restless horror" is nearer to an approximation of the utterly evil, utterly causeless, panic I was in … There was not the slightest outward sign of an epileptic state … except this causeless fear and a certain blurring of the consciousness as though the brain had been wiped over with a dirty wet rag.
>
> An appalling terror amounting to panic seemed to emanate from every piece of furniture, every book, every saucepan. These things might have been dangerous animals, only I knew that they did not want my body: it was my mind they wanted to destroy.
>
> As soon as the attacks began to subside the panic disappeared.

This change in the nature of the seizures is clearly reported following the initiation of anti-epileptic drug therapy. Firstly treated with Luminal (phenobarbital), Evans also subsequently received Epanutin (phenytoin) and, when the seizures were particularly frequent, Mysoline (primidone). Although effective for the suppression of seizures, all these medications have unwanted adverse effects and none would be considered as first line anti-epileptic drug treatments today.

Some epileptic attacks were also accompanied by motor phenomena, always affecting the left side of her body: she reports a "strange stiffening of the left side of my body", and after a severe fit "I was very slightly paralysed in the left side and hand". Speech difficulty was also noted on occasion: "I was silent … for nearly two minutes". Of particular note to a writer, she could not write during attacks: "to continue to write is impossible even though I am right handed and the right hand is not usually disabled". Possible autonomic features were also mentioned: "it was as though a ghost walked through me chilling every chamber of my body"; "I feel as if the hair on my head was whitening … and my body withering".

The subjective phenomena so graphically described by Margiad Evans (although she was fully aware of the difficulties of rendering these phenomena intelligible to others: "My task is to be the very difficult one of giving an outside inside story") would suggest to a clinician that her seizures were of partial rather than generalized onset, and hence possibly associated with focal brain pathology. The motor phenomena (left-sided) are clearly lateralising, suggesting a right-sided brain lesion, whereas the psychic phenomenon of ictal fear (i.e. fear as part of an epileptic attack), although also of focal onset, does not permit clear lateralization.[27] Speech arrest is also recognized as an ictal phenomenon, typically associated with pathology in the left frontal lobe of the brain.[28]

Hence the seizure semiology is suggestive of focal, rather than generalized, seizures, with the possibility of multifocal onset of seizures. Today, such an account of epileptic seizures would mandate structural brain imaging, preferably with the technique of magnetic resonance imaging. Such technology lay over 30 years in the future at the time of Evans's presentation, with electroencephalography (EEG; 'brainwaves') being the only non-invasive investigative technique readily available at the time.[29] Hence no criticism can be levelled at Golla's original diagnostic formulation. It was only with the passage of time (an important investigation in many neurological conditions), and the evident progression of disease, that more invasive investigation, namely surgical exploration, was undertaken, no doubt after very careful consideration and with some misgivings. In his textbook, Lennox states of Margiad Evans that "a gliomatous brain tumour ... lay behind both seizures and, after a dozen years [*sic*, in fact eight], death. The temporal lobe was not involved".[23] The exploratory surgical intervention which allowed this diagnosis rendered Margiad Evans partially paralysed on her left side.

As previously mentioned, Margiad Evans was pregnant by the time of her epilepsy diagnosis. Her observations on this subject, in *A Ray of Darkness*, retain a resonance for women today:

> Epilepsy and pregnancy. The shock of waking every morning to such a grim problem of life.

Although there was no family history of epilepsy, Margiad was concerned, understandably, that the condition might be hereditary, and evidently contemplated abortion, still illegal at that time:

> People who could help me have written to me and asked me why not have it quietly removed and I have replied that since the second fit that is my wish and that if they knew of any one who would do it, please help me.

Her general practitioner, "Dr Y", however, maintained all would be well, visiting Margiad to read:

> ... a passage from *Nervous Diseases* by the Professor of Neurology at London University [neither book nor author identified], which he said was

the last and most up-to-date work on epilepsy. . . . there was in reality only the very slightest danger of its being hereditary.

The child was born uneventfully, but after a post partum fit concerns about safety meant that Margiad "was never again able to feed my child".

Epilepsy and creativity: is there a link?

Margiad Evans's epilepsy raises a number of questions and dilemmas which continue to challenge epilepsy management today, not least the issue of pregnancy and epilepsy mentioned above. However, for scholars of literature, possible links between epilepsy and creativity may be of more interest. The neural substrates of creativity remain a subject of mystery, although new techniques in neuroscientific research may help to uncover some of them.[30] There is increasing interest amongst the faculty regarding the effects of neurological disorders in famous artists.[31–33]

Whether brain disorders such as epilepsy may enhance or diminish creative faculties has also been a subject of interest for many years. In the visual arts, Vincent van Gogh (1853–1890) was at one time thought to have suffered from temporal lobe epilepsy, but in recent times there has been a move away from this idea to suggestions of borderline personality disorder and bipolar affective disorder.[16] Other examples of visual artists thought to have epilepsy and whose art may have been influenced by seizure activity include Kyffin Williams, Edward Lear, Charles Altamont Doyle (father of Arthur Conan Doyle), and Giorgio de Chirico.[34] In the verbal arts, Caesar wrote (in the third person) his histories of *The Gallic War* and *The Civil War*, epilepsy notwithstanding. Dostoevsky not only transcended his epilepsy but capitalised on it as a device in his fiction. Could it be possible that inspiration itself is 'some unknown form of epilepsy'?[35]

Frederick Golla may have thought so:

> . . . where writers of genius have been sufferers [of epilepsy], it is fascinating to trace how greatly their sensibility and creative activity have been enhanced by the liability of their nervous system to respond as a whole. . . . [T]he expression of her [Margiad Evans] total personality has been facilitated by the malady'.[22]

He may well have had Dostoevsky in mind, since according to *A Ray of Darkness* he suggested to Margiad Evans that she read the works of 'Dostoëffsky', presumably because he was another author with epilepsy, who had managed to incorporate his knowledge of epilepsy into several of his novels. Evans apparently declined Golla's suggestion, at least initially, although Dostoevsky is mentioned in both *A Ray of Darkness* and *The Nightingale Silenced*, being described in the latter as "the greatest descriptive writer of epilepsy". Of her own writing, Evans mentions "an older incomplete fragment of a novel about an epileptic man". This has not been identified, although there is a passage in *Turf and Stone* (1934) in which a character has episodes from childhood in which "Something like a telephone rings in my head, and then my neck seems to go numb … I have walked quite a long way and come to myself and wondered how I did it, for I couldn't remember a thing". Although this is far from a typical description of an epileptic seizure, there are a number of features in it which are suggestive to a clinician, namely episodic, stereotyped events with loss of awareness and for which there is subsequent amnesia.

At times, Evans herself seems to concur with the possibility that epilepsy facilitated creativity in her own work: she speaks of writing "many poems in the hospital ward" not to mention "hundreds of letters". "In my writing … words and phrases … began to race over the pages without stopping", although she notes a "fatal voluminousness" in her output (hypergraphia may be one feature of complex partial seizures, often associated with temporal lobe pathology[36]). She speaks of a "quickness of mind", and of an "intuitive imagination" as an attribute of "horror-stricken sufferers".

In contrast, the adverse effects of epilepsy on cognition are now well recognised. These may be multifactorial, related to epileptic seizures per se, to the underlying brain pathology responsible for the seizures, and to anti-epileptic drug treatment, as well as to concurrent depression, anxiety, and sleep disturbance occasioned by the illness itself.[37–39] Indeed, the effects of medication were all too apparent to Margiad Evans:

> … since taking drugs I cannot keep awake for those free quiet hours which were my most creative. True my power of concentration is lost also.
>
> … the drugs I have to take to prevent the discharges of the epilepsy make me apathetic, have faded and dulled and dimmed the powers of imagination and concentration.

Although "grateful for the treatment", she also acknowledges that she "cannot work against drugs … although I should perhaps have died mentally last summer without … these drugs, it is better to die than to continue so wearily, dulled, blunted, stricken".

If the "cloud of epilepsy" affected her poetry favourably, itself a questionable contention, its effect on her prose was undoubtedly adverse. Empirically, she published no books after *A Ray of Darkness*, and despite the "many poems" written she states that "the only poem I wrote in the hospital I really liked I lost", possibly the one entitled *Cassandra desolated*. A projected work on Emily Brontë, an author for whom Margiad Evans had a long-standing interest, was abandoned.

Furthermore, William Lennox's encomium of *A Ray of Darkness* (it "carries the bonus of being beautifully and deftly expressed") could not be applied, even by the most generous critic, to *The Nightingale Silenced*, a less coherent work, difficult to read and interpret, and with many repetitions, some almost verbatim (possibly representing two drafts of the same work). This may explain why *The Nightingale Silenced* remains unpublished more than 50 years after the author's death.

Conclusion

A Ray of Darkness and *The Nightingale Silenced* manifest the author as witness of her own subjectivity, writing an "adventure of body and mind" which was "the story of my epilepsy", a mental journey ("The Margiad", perhaps?[40]) which produced a novel literary account. This history, or perhaps more correctly "herstory", of epilepsy ends tragically, the inescapable conclusion being that the progressive nature of the brain pathology underlying her seizures robbed Margiad Evans of her creative powers as well as, eventually, her life. Epilepsy was perhaps just one more facet, along with gender, sexuality, and a border identity,[41] of "the isolation and the inevitable 'otherness' of the artist"[42] which characterised the oeuvre of Margiad Evans. Nevertheless, her works on epilepsy remain as a bridge between the discourses of the humanities and the sciences.

Acknowledgements

Thanks are due to Jim Pratt, Peggy Williams' nephew, for permission to quote from his typescript of *The Nightingale Silenced*, and to Kirsti Bohata of the Centre for Research into the English Literature and Language of Wales, Swansea. Adapted from: Larner AJ. "A ray of darkness": Margiad Evans's account of her epilepsy (1952). *Clin Med* 2009;9:193–194; Larner AJ. Margiad Evans (1909–1958): a history of epilepsy in a creative writer. *Epilepsy Behav* 2009;16:596–598; and Larner AJ. A "herstory" of epilepsy in a creative writer: the case of Margiad Evans. In Bohata K, Gramich K (eds.). *Rediscovering Margiad Evans: marginality, gender and illness*. Cardiff: University of Wales Press, 2013:129–141.

References

1. Dearnley M. *Margiad Evans*. Cardiff: University of Wales Press, 1982.
2. Lloyd-Morgan C. *Margiad Evans*. Bridgend: Seren Press, 1998.
3. Prys-Williams B. *Twentieth-century autobiography. Writing Wales in English*. Cardiff: University of Wales Press, 2004:32–57.
4. Evans M. *A ray of darkness*. London: John Calder, [1952] 1978.

5. Cooper R, Bird J. *The Burden: fifty years of clinical and experimental neuroscience at the Burden Neurological Institute.* Bristol: White Tree Books, 1989:67.
6. Panayiotopoulos CP. *The epilepsies. Seizures, syndromes and management.* Chipping Norton: Bladon Medical Publishing, 2005.
7. Fisher RS, van Emde BW, Blume W et al. Epileptic seizures and epilepsy: definitions proposed by the International League Against Epilepsy (ILAE) and the International Bureau for Epilepsy (IBE). *Epilepsia* 2005;46:470–472.
8. Larner AJ, Smith SJM, Duncan JS, Howard RS. Late-onset Rasmussen's syndrome with first seizure during pregnancy. *Eur Neurol* 1995;35:172.
9. Larner AJ. "Neurological literature": headache (part 4). *Adv Clin Neurosci Rehabil* 2008;7(6):17.
10. Larner AJ. Illusory visual spread or visuospatial perseveration. *Adv Clin Neurosci Rehabil* 2009;9(5):14.
11. Larner AJ. Has Shakespeare's Iago deceived again? http://bmj.com/cgi/eletters/333/7582/1335, 2 January 2007.
12. Lawson R. The epilepsy of Othello. *J Mental Sci* 1880;26:1–11.
13. Heaton KW. Faints, fits and fatalities from emotion in Shakespeare's characters: survey of the canon. *BMJ* 2006;333:1335–1338.
14. Stirling J. *Representing epilepsy. Myth and matter.* Liverpool: Liverpool University Press, 2010:4.
15. Larner AJ. Syncope. In: Cox TM et al. (eds.). *Oxford Textbook of Medicine* (5th edition). Oxford: Oxford University Press, 2010:4838–4841.
16. Larner AJ. "Neurological literature": epilepsy. *Adv Clin Neurosci Rehabil* 2007;7(3):16.
17. Larner AJ. Demise of botany in the medical curriculum. *J Med Biogr* 2008;16:1–2.
18. Iniesta I. On the good use of epilepsy by Fyodor Dostoevsky. *Clin Med* 2008;8:338–339.
19. Larner AJ. Dostoevsky and epilepsy. *Adv Clin Neurosci Rehabil* 2006;6(1):26.
20. Baxendale S. Epilepsy at the movies: possession to presidential assassination. *Lancet Neurol* 2003;2:764–770.
21. Ford SF, Larner AJ. Neurology at the movies. *Adv Clin Neurosci Rehabil* 2009;9(4):48–49.
22. *John Bull Magazine*, 18 October 1952:8.
23. Lennox WG, Lennox MA. *Epilepsy and related disorders.* London: JA Churchill, 1960:182,191,192,269,297,711.
24. Pratt J. Margiad Evans: centenary of an artist with epilepsy. Paper delivered to the 28th International Epilepsy Congress, Budapest, 28 June-2 July 2009.
25. Iniesta I. Epilepsy and literature. *Medical Historian* 2008–2009;20:31–53 [at 36–38].
26. *The Nightingale Silenced*, National Library of Wales, MSS23367B. All quotations are taken from the typescript prepared by JE Pratt, dated 17/04/2009.
27. Rosa VP, Filho GMA, Rahal MA, Caboclo LOSF, Sakamoto AC, Yacubian EMT. Ictal fear: semiologic characteristics and differential diagnosis with interictal

anxiety disorders. *Journal of Epilepsy and Clinical Neurophysiology* 2006;12:89–94.

28. Wieshmann UC, Niehaus L, Meierkord H. Ictal speech arrest and parasagittal lesions. *Eur Neurol* 1997;38:123–127.
29. Clare Morgan showed a slide depicting some written notes by ME on what appeared to be EEG paper on which calibration traces are seen, presumably thrown out as scrap paper. Clare Morgan, 'Margiad Evans: a writer in her time', Margiad Evans Centenary Conference, National Library of Wales, Aberystwyth, 15 May 2009.
30. Griffiths TD. Capturing creativity. *Brain* 2008;131:6–7.
31. Bogousslavsky J, Boller F (eds.). *Neurological disorders in famous artists* (Frontiers of Neurology and Neuroscience Volume 19). Basel: Karger, 2005.
32. Bogousslavsky J, Hennerici M (eds.). *Neurological disorders in famous artists Part 2* (Frontiers of Neurology and Neuroscience Volume 22). Basel: Karger, 2007.
33. Bogousslavsky J, Hennerici M, Bazner H, Bassetti C (eds.). *Neurological disorders in famous artists Part 3* (Frontiers of Neurology and Neuroscience Volume 27). Basel: Karger, 2010.
34. Thomas RH, Mullins JM, Waddington T, Nugent K, Smith PEM. Epilepsy: creative sparks. *Pract Neurol* 2010;10:219–226.
35. Zamyatin Y. *We*. London: Penguin, [1924] 1993:18.
36. Larner AJ. *A dictionary of neurological signs* (3rd edition). New York: Springer, 2011:184.
37. Blake R, Wroe S, Breen E, McCarthy R. Accelerated forgetting in patients with epilepsy: evidence for impairment in memory consolidation. *Brain* 2000;123:472–483.
38. Loring DW, Marino S, Meador KJ. Neuropsychological and behavioural effects of antiepilepsy drugs. *Neuropsychol Rev* 2007;17:413–425.
39. Larner AJ. Neuropsychological neurology: the neurocognitive impairments of neurological disorders. Cambridge: Cambridge University Press, 2008:115–124.
40. Atwood M. *The Penelopiad*. Toronto: Knopf, 2005.
41. Gramich K. *Twentieth-century women's writing in Wales. Land, gender, belonging*. Cardiff: University of Wales Press, 2008.
42. Morgan C. Exile and the Kingdom: Margiad Evans and the mythic landscape of Wales. *Welsh Writing in English. A Yearbook of Critical Essays* 2000;6:89–118 [at 90].

Roald Dahl (1916–1990): tales of the unexpected (neurological contributions)

Roald Dahl (1916–1990) is best known as an author of children's books, although his oeuvre also extends to other works, including screenplays, ghost tales and novels. It may therefore seem surprising at first sight that he might have made any contributions to neurology. However, in the second volume of his autobiography, *Going solo* (1986), he declares "All my life I have taken an intense and inquisitive interest in every form of medicine", perhaps in part because of the head injury he suffered as a pilot in World War 2. Recovering in Alexandria, he was blind for some time, and reports "Both my senses of smell and of hearing had become very acute since my blindness, and I had developed an instinctive habit of translating sounds and scents into a coloured mental picture".[1] This account suggests the phenomenon of hyperpilaphesie, but not of true ("strong") synaesthesia.

Dahl's book *George's marvellous medicine* (1981) contains the epigraph (in the hardback edition, but not in subsequent paperback editions) "This book is for doctors everywhere". This bald statement is not further elaborated upon, but certainly the book may be read as a salutary lesson about the grave consequences of unregulated experimentation in clinical pharmacology. The author advises readers not to try the recipes reported in the book.

These descriptions may hardly be termed "contributions", but two personal tragedies certainly did lead to developments of clinical import. Whilst living in New York in 1960, Dahl's son Theo, aged 3–4 months, was involved in a road traffic accident which caused some brain damage and secondary hydrocephalus, the latter requiring shunting. Problems with blocked shunts occurred. The family returned to England and Theo came under the care of Kenneth Till, a neurosurgeon at Great Ormond Street Hospital (1956–80). Prompted by Dahl, and in collaboration with Stanley Wade, an hydraulic engineer, a new type of shunt valve was designed. Reported in the *Lancet* by Kenneth Till, under the rubric of "New Inventions", the special characteristics were reported to be "low resistance, ease of sterilisation, no reflux, robust construction, and negligible risk of blockage". The author acknowledged that the valve was "designed by Mr Stanley C. Wade … with the assistance of Mr Roald Dahl and myself".[2] The Wade-Dahl-Till (or WDT) valve became widely used (http://medgadget.com/archives/2005/07/water_on_the_br.html).

Kenneth Till subsequently wrote a preface for a new edition of Valerie Eaton Griffith's book entitled *A stroke in the family. A manual of home therapy* (www.strokescheme.ie/articles/reviews/family.htm), wherein lies another Dahl connection. In 1965, Dahl's first wife, the American actress Patricia Neal, suffered a stroke due to a ruptured intracranial aneurysm, one of the consequences of which was marked aphasia, a potential career-ending misfortune for an actress (her illness and recovery are recorded in a book by Barry Farrell[3]). Dahl appealed to Valerie Eaton Griffith, who lived in the same village, for help. With Dahl, she devised a rota of volunteer carers to engage the patient in conversation and hence to stimulate language recovery. This approach, different from formal speech therapy, was documented in Griffith's book (initially published in 1970, with an introduction by Roald Dahl[4]). It earned the approbation, as "treatment of a surreptitious character", of no less a neurological figure than Macdonald Critchley,[5] and still has advocates today.[6]

In his first volume of autobiography, *Boy: tales of childhood* (1984), Dahl portrays a schoolmaster, "Captain Hardcastle", who may have suffered from Tourette syndrome since he seems to manifest both vocal and motor tics.[7] This teacher, encountered by Dahl in 1925–6 when he was nine years old, was almost certainly the inspiration for "Captain Lancaster", also a teacher, who appears in the book *Danny the champion of the world* (1975): "I could hear him snorting and snuffling through his nose like a dog outside a rabbit hole." In the film version, Captain Lancaster (as portrayed by Ronald Pickup) has a larger role than in the book but neither snorting nor snuffling are in evidence.

Why should Dahl have recalled this particular teacher, and incorporated him into a book almost 50 years after the event? I would like to suggest that one possibility is that Dahl himself had some characteristics suggestive of an obsessive-compulsive spectrum condition, albeit without tics. For example, when writing in his famous hut at bottom of the garden at Gypsy House, he had to have a particular type of paper, lined yellow American Legal, and both a particular brand (Dixon Ticonderoga HB) and an even number of pencils ("because odd numbers were unlucky"), supplied by his publishers in the USA. When, in 1980, his publishers became unable to supply this particular type of pencil, but something "very similar" instead, Dahl wrote to say that the substitute pencils "don't have erasers on top. They are too hard. And they are the wrong colour".[8,9]

Dahl's desire for routine and order is further exemplified in an account given by his daughter, Tessa:

> He had a routine. Every single day of his life was the same. He got up at the same time, he took the children to school, he made his thermos of coffee, he went up to the hut, he worked to a certain time, he listened to *The World at One* [a radio news programme], he had his Bloody Mary, he had his second Bloody Mary, he had his lunch, he had his nap, he watched the horse racing, he put on his bets, he got up, he took his coffee back to the

> hut. He was up there till about quarter to six. He'd start sniffing the scotch at six, then he'd either drive up to London or he'd have supper at home, then he'd take the dogs out they'd go out and pee and he'd go to bed. Imagine disrupting that... he'd been doing that for over twenty years.[10]

In a short story, *The Wish*, Dahl described a child who was terrified of stepping on the cracks in the pavement or the wrong colour in the carpet. Dahl's official biographer states that, like this child, the author had a premonition of disaster. He also speaks of "an obsessive need" that Dahl had to clarify the storyline of *Charlie and the Chocolate Factory* (1964).[11]

Although these scattered references cannot establish a diagnosis in the way that formal consultation may do, nonetheless they are suggestive of behaviours seen in the obsessive compulsive spectrum. Most might be described as impulsions, to distinguish them from obsessions and compulsions, namely repetitive behaviours which are performed not to avoid harm or reduce anxiety (like compulsions) but to achieve a sense of rightness, completion, or satisfaction. These behaviours do not seem to have impaired Dahl's productivity as a writer, indeed they may have facilitated it.[12] One wonders whether other writers might manifest similar behaviours. Just as Patricia Neal's aphasia may have influenced Dahl's creative processes, for example in the neologisms of *The BFG* (1982),[13] so also his desire for sameness and orderliness might have facilitated his creativity.

The Roald Dahl Foundation (www.roalddahlfoundation.org) continues to provide charitable grants for neurological conditions affecting young people including epilepsy; acquired brain injury due to benign brain tumour, encephalitis, head injury, hydrocephalus, meningitis, and stroke; and neurodegenerative conditions causing progressive intellectual or neurological deterioration.

Acknowledgements

Thanks to Elizabeth Larner for drawing my attention to the Wade-Dahl-Till valve. Adapted from: Larner AJ. Tales of the unexpected: Roald Dahl's neurological contributions. *dv Clin Neurosci Rehabil* 2008;8(1):22. Reprinted, abridged, as: Tales of unexpected [*sic*]: Roald Dahl's neurological contributions. *The Encephalitis Society Newsletter* 2008;Autumn (number 44):12.

References

1. Dahl R. *Going solo.* London: Puffin 2001:106,107.
2. Till K. A valve for the treatment of hydrocephalus. *Lancet* 1964;1:202.
3. Farrell B. *Pat and Roald.* New York: Random House, 1969.

4. Griffith VE. *A stroke in the family. A manual of home therapy.* New York: Delacourte Press, 1970.
5. Critchley M. The chronic aphasiac, a sociological problem. In: *The divine banquet of the brain and other essays.* New York: Raven Press, 1979:83–87 [at 86–87].
6. Hale S. *The man who lost his language. A case of aphasia* (Revised edition). London: Jessica Kingsley, 2007:50,57.
7. Larner AJ. Three historical accounts of Gilles de la Tourette syndrome. *Adv Clin Neurosci Rehabil* 2003;3(5):26–27.
8. Donkin A. *Dead famous: Roald Dahl and his chocolate factory.* London: Scholastic, 2002:167–168.
9. Sturrock, D. *Storyteller. The life of Roald Dahl.* London: Harper Press, 2010:269,286,378,504.
10. Sturrock, 2010: 462–463.
11. Sturrock, 2010:367,396.
12. Larner AJ. *Roald Dahl's marvelous medicine* by Tom Solomon. *Medical Historian (Journal of the Liverpool Medical History Society)* 2018;**28**:67–70.
13. Donkin, 2002:156–157.

Doctors

Edward Jenner (1749–1823): on the intellect

Surely no medical practitioner can be unaware of the name and work of Dr Edward Jenner (1749–1823). A Gloucestershire country doctor, he pioneered smallpox vaccination, work for which he is rightly adjudged one of the immortals of medical history, and the anniversary of which is still noted.[1] Even the Royal College of Physicians of London, which assiduously excluded him during life, seems prepared to acknowledge him "one of the greatest doctors in history".[2] Besides smallpox, some may know of Jenner's work on the nesting habits of the cuckoo (*Cuculus canorus*), the work for which he was appointed a Fellow of the Royal Society. Few, if any, may be aware that he also had ideas on the classification of the intellectual faculties.

Jenner's thoughts were published in an article, bearing the long-winded title of:

Classes of the Human Powers of Intellect – Hints for a Classification of the Powers of the Human Mind as they appear in various Descriptions of Men – Examples of Excellence rare – General Division into seven Classes – Difficulty of analysing all the Varieties of Intellect in Individuals

This article [hereafter *Classes of the Intellect*] was first published in the London weekly periodical *The Artist* (no. XIX, Saturday 18th July 1807), published by Prince Hoare, foreign secretary of the Royal Academy. Thirteen years later it was reprinted as a pamphlet by the Cheltenham publisher Griffiths, a friend of Jenner's who was facing financial difficulties in the summer of 1820. The reprint was without any revisions, notwithstanding Jenner's statement in the original that "I may hereafter treat more copiously" of the subject. Jenner's first biographer, Baron,[3] does not mention the work at all, and more recent biographers, Saunders[4] and Fisher,[5] mention it only in passing. In his bibliography of Jenner's publications, Le Fanu lists it under "Medical Digressions".[6] I am not aware of any previous publications devoted to it

The Artist was, as its name implies, a non-scientific periodical, although it did have a scientific editor, Tiberius Cavallo (1749–1809), who was interested in the therapeutic aspects of electricity. *The Artist* consisted of essays by artists, writers and politicians; Jenner was the only physician to contribute.

Jenner's paper ran to seven pages, about two thousand words. The classification of intellect, "or, to speak more correctly, of the various degrees of intellectual capacity, which distinguish the human animal", which Jenner "hinted" at was into seven classes, *viz.*:

1. The Idiot: "the mere vegetative being"
2. The Dolt: "the weak, silly, poor creature"
3. Mediocrity: "the large mass of mankind"
4. Mental Perfection: "From this point Intellect again diverges"
5. Eccentricity: "I have in this class a very numerous acquaintance"
6. Insanity: "the most affecting of all conditions"
7. The Maniac: "the wreck of the mental faculties"

Although no doubt based on Jenner's personal observations, *Classes of the Intellect* lacks (and does not pretend to) scientific rigour, or any kind of empirical verification, so unlike the experimental method, learned by Jenner from his mentor John Hunter (1728–1793), which marks his work on smallpox vaccination (and, for that matter, the nesting habits of the cuckoo). It has been suggested that the article was written as a diversion or distraction, perhaps light-hearted, from the struggle to establish smallpox vaccination which occupied so much of Jenner's time and energy, and on which subject he was under attack from various critics.[4,5] No contemporaneous reaction to the article is, to my knowledge, recorded.

From the vantage of hindsight, it is probable that many of us may recognise from personal experience some verisimilitude in this scheme, and indeed may find some attractions in it. Yet nonetheless it is difficult to disagree with Le Fanu's analysis of *Classes of the Intellect* as a "slight essay in psychology … showing a scientific bent to classification, it is little more than a *jeu d'esprit*".[6] Fisher calls it "a fair summary of the common eighteenth-century [*sic*] wisdom on mental attributes, elevated slightly by being ordered into classes".[5]

The nineteenth century saw the origin of many of our currently accepted neuroscientific concepts,[7] and so it is reasonable to ask how Jenner's ideas compared with those of the time. The early nineteenth century saw a gradual increase in research interest devoted to the nervous system such that many physiologists saw it as pre-eminent. Moreover, hierarchical views of nature, espoused particularly by adherents of *Naturphilosophie*, popular in the early nineteenth century, envisaged not only a hierarchy of animal forms reaching its apogee in the human body, but also within the human body itself, with the nervous system its apex. The first four of Jenner's categories seem to form a hierarchy but, as Saunders points out,[4] the next three seem to depart from this pattern. This perhaps reflects the difficulties of attempting to conflate physiological variation with pathological aberration.

As Fisher implies,[5] Jenner's ideas were perhaps more akin to those of earlier epochs, when the urge to classify was strong, as exemplified in the work of Linnaeus in the eighteenth century and of John Ray in the seventeenth century. Analogies may be seen between Jenner's classification and the idea of a "Great Chain of Being", as seen for example in the work of Edward Tyson published on the threshold of the eighteenth century.[8] Noting the morphological similarities and differences between an "orang-outang" (in fact, a chimpanzee) and man, Tyson conceived a gradation of forms, in which man was placed above brute animals, of which the chimpanzee was his nearest relative, but below the angels. Jenner's grading may also be seen to span from the sublime to the fatuous.

Acknowledgment

Adapted from: Larner AJ. Jenner, on the intellect. *Adv Clin Neurosci Rehabil* 2003;3(2):29.

References

1. Larner AJ. Smallpox. *N Engl J Med* 1996;335:901.
2. Hamblin T. How ironic that college says Jenner is the greatest doctor. *Hospital Doctor* 2003;27 February:19.
3. Baron J. *Life of Edward Jenner, Physician Extraordinary to His Majesty George IV, etc* (2 volumes). London: Henry Colburn, Vol. I, 1827; Vol. II, 1838.
4. Saunders P. *Edward Jenner: the Cheltenham years, 1795–1823. Being a chronicle of the vaccination campaign.* Hanover and London: University Press of New England, 1982:201–202, 408.
5. Fisher RB. *Edward Jenner 1749–1823.* London: Andre Deutsch, 1991:184.
6. Le Fanu W. *A bio-bibliography of Edward Jenner 1749–1823.* London: Harvey & Blythe, 1951:84–85, in which the publication date of the Cheltenham edition is queried as 1807; in Le Fanu's second edition (Winchester: St Paul's Bibliographies, 1985:95–96) this is corrected to 1820, following Saunders (*op. cit.* ref. 3:408).
7. Clarke E, Jacyna LS. *Nineteenth-century origins of neuroscientific concepts.* Berkeley: University of California Press, 1987.
8. Larner AJ. Edward Tyson and "The Anatomy of a Pygmie", 1699. *J Med Biogr* 2000;8:78–82.

Caleb Hillier Parry (1755–1822): neurological observations

Caleb Hillier Parry (1755–1822) was a schoolfellow of Edward Jenner during the latter's education in Cirencester, Gloucestershire, between 1758 and 1761. The friendship established during these years was to be lifelong. Parry was the original dedicatee of Jenner's seminal 1798 pamphlet describing smallpox vaccination, and Parry returned the compliment in his book on rabies and tetanus published in 1814.

After qualifying in Edinburgh, Parry set up in practice in Bath in 1779, which was to be his home for the rest of his life. He was the first president of the short-lived "Gloucestershire Medical Society" (1788–1793), meeting at the Fleece Inn in Rodborough near Stroud, of which Jenner was also a member. Like Jenner, Parry was an observant clinician, and an experimentalist, and they also shared interests in other aspects of natural history, including geology.[1,2]

With the benefit of hindsight, Parry's most significant clinical contribution was probably his 1799 book on angina, the first devoted to the subject, in which he drew on Jenner's (unpublished) work showing that the symptom was associated with "malorganisation" of the coronary arteries.[3] Parry also encountered cases of exophthalmic goitre, the first in 1786, some fifty years before the account of Graves (1835) which achieved eponymous fame for the latter. However, Sir William Osler acknowledged Parry's priority, and the nomenclature "Parry's disease" has found favour in some quarters. These works have attracted attention in journals devoted to cardiology and endocrinology, respectively.[4,5]

Parry believed his most important contribution was his theory of "determination of the blood", in essence that flow of blood, usually excessive, contributed to organ dysfunction. He thought this was particularly applicable to diseases of the nervous system. Although this theory is now of historical interest only, Parry did make various contributions of value to neurological practice. Long sections of two of his major works were devoted to the nervous system.[6,7] I am not aware of previous articles on Parry in journals devoted specifically to neurology (Jenner too had neurological interests[8]).

1. Carotid artery compression for seizures

Parry's studies of carotid artery compression date from the late 1780s. In addition to the observation (1799) that carotid compression slowed the heart beat, a manoeuvre still used in clinical practice for the emergency treatment of some tachyarrhythmias, he also reported the use of carotid compression to treat episodes of loss of consciousness. Motivated by his theory that nervous system disease resulted from excessive blood flow to the brain ("determination"), he reported improvement in a young woman with bizarre episodes of convulsive movements and impairment of consciousness (in retrospect it is possible that these were induced by hyperventilation) following carotid compression, although the effects were only transient.[9]

Other cases with features more suggestive of partial-onset epileptic seizures were also reported to be controlled by carotid compression.[9,10] This is of possible interest in light of current investigations of implantable vagal stimulators for the control of refractory seizures, although Parry specifically denied that his technique of carotid compression produced pressure on the vagus.[11]

Parry also had other suggestions for how to deal with "fits". Consulted by a carpenter about his 15 or 16 year-old daughter who was having fits, Parry reports that:

> ... he and his wife had made it a rule never to contradict her, but uniformly indulged her in every wish ... I urged this man to change his method of proceeding and, instead of this absurd indulgence, to give her a good shaking, or else throw a bason [*sic*] of cold water in her face, immediately on the approach of the next fit.

In the event, the carpenter could not bring himself to follow these recommendations, but apparently spoke sharply to his daughter instead, and the fits ceased.[12]

2. Headache

Parry gives a clear description of his own migraine aura without headache (or migraine equivalent):

> After violent fatigue, more especially when accompanied with fasting eight or ten hours, ... I have frequently experienced a sudden failure of sight. The general sight did not appear affected; but when I looked at any particular object, it seemed as if something brown, and more or less opake [*sic*], was interposed between my eyes and it, so that I saw it indistinctly or sometimes not at all. Most generally it seemed to be exactly in the middle of the object, while what my sight comprehended all round it, was as distinct and clear as usual; in consequence of which, if I wished to see any thing, I was obliged to look on one side ... After it had continued a few

minutes, the upper or lower edge ... appeared bounded by an edging of light of a zig-zag shape, and coruscating nearly at right angles to its length ... they would remain for twenty minutes sometimes to half an hour ... They were in me never followed by headach [*sic*] ..."[13]

Parry also presents cases which are suggestive of migraine exacerbation during holiday periods,[14] and of migrainous stroke.[15]

The young woman with bizarre convulsive episodes (see above) also had "fits of delirium ... preceded by a sense of fulness and throbbing pain in the head, accompanied with a great degree of heat and flushing about the head (what the common people in this country call opening and shutting) and neck", and also "an unusual sensibility with regard to light and sound". Carotid compression, as well as helping the seizures, also "nearly or totally removes the hemicrania of the side on which the compression is made; the headach [*sic, passim*] which is called nervous; that also which is intituled bilious, ... " restoring the patient to "perfect use of her senses and powers of reasoning. At the same time the headach, and the undue sensibility with regard to light and sound, which had always taken place in the intervals of the paroxysms, were altogether wanting, and the patient declared that in every respect she was free from complaint". Moreover, whereas the beneficial effect on the seizures was brief, "I have, however, seen some instances in which the nervous and bilious headachs have been for a considerable time, and even permanently, relieved".[16] Modern accounts of the efficacy of carotid or superficial temporal artery compression in migraine have appeared.[17]

It was suggested by Kelly in 1948 that Parry's 1792 paper[9] contained a description of the condition known as "histaminic cephalgia",[18] which itself would now be included under the rubric of cluster headache[19] or perhaps trigeminal autonomic cephalgia.[20] However, the case contains no mention of unilaterality, pacing behaviour, nocturnal attacks, miosis, ptosis, conjunctival injection, lacrimation or nasal congestion, so it seems that the case for Parry describing cluster headache is not established. However, another patient, Mrs R., had "nervous headach [*sic*] over the forehead, eyes, and occiput ... accompanied with fulness [*sic*] and stuffing of the nose like a cold, coming and going off in a short time".[21]

3. Facial hemiatrophy

... Miss F., aged twenty-eight, ... thirteen or fourteen years ago, when at school, was rather suddenly seized with some degree of hemiplegia of the left side ... from the period of the attack the left side of the face began to grow more thin than the right, and the eye to become less prominent, and therefore to appearance smaller ... from the same period, her hair on the

> upper part of the left side of her head, which was before of a dark brown colour, began to grow white ... when she protrudes her tongue it turns to the left.[22]

This is from Parry's account of hemifacial atrophy, still sometimes known as Parry-Romberg syndrome (the German's account appeared some years later, 1846). The condition is still seen occasionally by neurologists, sometimes associated with ipsilateral brain atrophy, vascular malformations, and partial-onset seizures, as well as various ophthalmological and dermatological features. There are probably various causes.[23]

4. Miscellaneous

Other neurological conditions which may be encountered in Parry's writings include:

- Visual hallucinations on alcohol withdrawal;
- Dropped hands from lead poisoning, in painters and plumbers (but never cider drinkers!);
- Tic douloureux;
- Wry neck, "suspended by attention to other objects".

He also writes (in 1815) of "shaking palsy", in which the "head and limbs shake, more especially on any muscular exertion", a description perhaps more suggestive of essential tremor than Parkinson's disease.

It is reassuring to find that, like some of his neurological successors, Parry sometimes struggled with clinical-anatomical correlation: a description of right facial weakness with involvement of taste, suggestive of a Bell's palsy, is ascribed to "affection of the second and third branches of the Trigeminus". As there was no difficulty moving the eyeball "it follows that the first (ophthalmic) branch was unaffected"![24]

Parry's medical practice was effectively ended in 1816, at the age of 61 years, by a stroke which resulted in aphasia and right hemiparesis (presumably a left middle cerebral artery territory event). Jenner reported:

> He looked at me earnestly for some time, then grasped my hand and by piteous moans and sighs expressed how strongly he felt his situation,

perhaps in part from his clinical familiarity with right hemiplegia.[25] Communication remained difficult for the rest of his life but his two unmarried daughters who helped to care for him were able to interpret, and hence he was able to dictate reminiscences which they wrote down. It is also recorded that he was able to correct with his left hand a manuscript written by his son, Edward (noted for his exploration of the Arctic), an achievement perhaps reminiscent of the scientist Ernst Mach who learned how to type with his left hand after a left hemisphere stroke.[26]

Acknowledgment

Adapted from: Larner AJ. Neurological contributions of Caleb Hillier Parry. *Adv Clin Neurosci Rehabil* 2004;4(3):38–39.

References

1. Glaser S. *The spirit of enquiry. Caleb Hillier Parry MD, FRS.* Stroud: Alan Sutton, 1995.
2. Larner AJ. Caleb Hillier Parry (1755–1822); clinician, scientist, friend of Edward Jenner (1749–1823). *J Med Biogr* 2005;13:189–194.
3. Hart FD. William Heberden, Edward Jenner, John Hunter and angina pectoris. *J Med Biogr* 1995;3:56–58.
4. Fye WB. Caleb Hillier Parry. *Clin Cardiol* 1992;15:619–621.
5. Volpé R. Caleb Hillier Parry 1755–1822. *The Endocrinologist* 1994;4:157–159.
6. Parry CH. *Elements of pathology and therapeutics, being the outlines of a work, intended to ascertain the nature, causes, and most efficacious modes of prevention and cure, of the greater number of the diseases incidental to the human frame; illustrated by numerous cases and dissections.* Bath: Cruttwell, 1815:226–367 (paragraphs DXIX-DCCCLII). [Hereafter *Elements.*]
7. Parry CH. *Collections from the unpublished medical writings of the late Caleb Hillier Parry M.D. F.R.S.* (3 volumes). London: Underwoods, 1825: volume I:260–590. [Hereafter *Collections.*]
8. Larner AJ. Jenner, on the intellect. *Adv Clin Neurosci Rehabil* 2003;3(2):29.
9. Parry CH. On the effects of compression of the arteries in various diseases, and particularly in those of the head; with hints towards a new mode of treating nervous disorders. *Memoirs of the Medical Society of London* 1792;3:77–113. [Hereafter *Memoirs.*]
10. Parry CH. On a case of nervous affection cured by pressure of the carotids; with some physiological remarks. *Philosophical Transactions of the Royal Society* 1811;101:89–95; see also *Elements*, 1815: 315 (paragraph DCCXXXVII).
11. *Collections*, 1825; volume I:322.
12. Ibid., volume I:368.
13. Ibid., volume I:557–559.
14. Ibid., volume I:279.
15. Ibid., volume I:480–481; see also *Elements*, 1815:373 (paragraph DCCCLVIII).
16. *Memoirs*, 1792:85,82,89,86,97 respectively; see also *Elements*, 1815:305 (paragraph DCCXVI).

17. Drummond PD, Lance JW. Extracranial vascular changes and the source of pain in migraine headaches. *Ann Neurol* 1983;13:32–37.
18. Kelly EC. *Encyclopedia of medical sources.* Baltimore: Williams & Wilkins, 1948:317.
19. Sjaastad O. *Cluster headache syndrome.* London: WB Saunders, 1992:1–34 [especially 1–18].
20. Matharu MS, Goadsby PJ. Trigeminal autonomic cephalgias. *J Neurol Neurosurg Psychiatry* 2002;72(supplII):ii19–ii26.
21. *Collections*, 1825; volume I:331.
22. Ibid., volume I:478–480. *Elements*, 1815:404 (paragraph DCCCLXXI) mentions this same case but only the eye and hair changes.
23. Larner AJ, Bennison DP. Some observations on the aetiology of hemifacial atrophy ("Parry-Romberg syndrome"). *J Neurol Neurosurg Psychiatry* 1993;56:1035–1036.
24. *Collections*, 1825; volume I:545–546; see also *Elements*, 1815:254–255 (paragraph DXCII).
25. *Collections*, 1825; volume I:492–510.
26. McManus C. *Right hand, left hand. The origins of asymmetry in brains, bodies, atoms and cultures.* London: Phoenix, 2003:185–187.

Dr John Forbes (1787–1861) and the Brontës

2016 marked the 200th anniversary of the birth of Charlotte Brontë (1816–1855), an anniversary that prompted a re-reading of Elizabeth Gaskell's 1857 biography, the first to commemorate the author of *Jane Eyre*. Within Gaskell's pages, three references were noted to Dr John Forbes,[1] a physician who has been of enduring historical interest to Dr Robin Agnew. However, a re-reading of Agnew's short biography of Forbes (2nd edition) revealed no mention of the Brontës.[2] This omission had been previously noted,[3] was partially addressed in the updated entry for Forbes in the *Oxford Dictionary of National Biography*,[4] and moreso in the 3rd edition of Agnew's biography (2018).

Gaskell's biography

Firstly, the context. According to Gaskell's biography,[1] John Forbes made his first appearance in Charlotte Brontë's life in 1849, when her youngest sister and only surviving sibling, Anne (born 1820), fell ill. Gaskell reports that:

> "A system of treatment was prescribed, which was afterwards ratified by the opinion of Dr Forbes." (p.299).

A little later, quoting from one of Charlotte's letters addressed to her friend, Ellen Nussey,

> "A few days ago I wrote to have Dr Forbes' opinion ... He warned us against entertaining sanguine hopes of recovery. The cod-liver oil he considers a peculiarly efficacious medicine. He, too, disproved of change of residence for the present." (p.305).

Eventually, however, Anne's desire to leave her home at Haworth parsonage and go to Scarborough in the hope that sea air might restore her health was granted, but she died there on Monday 28 May 1849.

Gaskell's final allusion to Forbes related to an event in May of 1851. Charlotte was visiting London, a guest of her publisher George Smith (1824–1901), head of the firm of Smith, Elder & Co., during which time she attended a lecture given by the author William Makepeace Thackeray (1811–1863), the second of his series of lectures on *The English Humorists of the Eighteenth*

Century. After the lecture, various individuals introduced themselves to Charlotte:

> "Then came Dr Forbes, whom I was sincerely glad to see." (p.380).

These snippets are tantalisingly brief. Subsequent Brontë scholarship has fortunately shed more light on the matter. But before examining this, we may ask why it was that Charlotte should seek the opinion of Dr Forbes.

Dr John Forbes

Dr John Forbes life and work have been previously described.[2,4–7] To summarise briefly, by the late 1840s, Forbes was living in London, having moved there in 1840. Prior to this he had worked as a naval surgeon, and then graduated MD in Edinburgh before moving to practise in Penzance and Chichester. During his 18 years in Chichester he had established a reputation in diseases of the chest, based in part on his book *Original Cases with Dissections and Observations illustrating the use of the Stethoscope and Percussion in the Diagnosis of Diseases of the Chest* published in 1824. He had previously translated Laennec's seminal work on stethoscopy from French. In London, Forbes had developed a career in medical journalism, was editor of the *Medical Review*, physician to the Queen's household and, most importantly, one of the first authorities in England on consumptive cases. He had officially retired in 1848, but evidently was still available for consultations.

Further Brontë scholarship

In her magisterial account of the Brontës, Juliet Barker has, like Gaskell, three references to John Forbes.[8] This account is informed by access to Charlotte Brontë's letters, as collected and edited in three volumes by Margaret Smith,[9] which gives the fullest picture of Forbes' interaction with the Brontës. Accordingly, this is the source of the references upon which this account is based.

Although all biographers agree that Forbes was involved with Anne Brontë's medical management, Charlotte obviously knew of him before this, because the first reference to him in her correspondence (II:150) is dated 9 December 1848 when her sister Emily was very ill:

> "I know it would be useless to consult Drs Elliotson or Forbes; my Sister would not see the most skilful physician in England if he were brought to her just now – nor would she follow his prescription."

Indeed it was not until shortly before her death on 19 December 1848 that Emily consented to see a doctor, by which time her case was hopeless.

When Anne fell ill in early 1849, she was examined at Haworth parsonage by a Dr Thomas Pridgin Teale (1800–1867), a physician from Leeds with experience in cases of consumption, who recommended treatment with clysters and cod-liver oil. Charlotte wrote to George Smith (II:170–1) on 22 January 1849 " ... on the subject of your friend, Dr Forbes ..." (apparently Forbes was a schoolfellow of Smith's father; III:109n8), asking if she could:

> " ... obtain, through you, Dr Forbe's [*sic*] opinion on the regimen prescribed [by Teale] ... It would be a satisfaction to know whether Dr Forbes approves these remedies – or whether there are others he would recommend in preference."

A recent biography of Anne Brontë claims that Smith offered "to pay at his own expense for ... Dr John Forbes ... to visit Anne and provide a suitable treatment",[10] taking as its reference an earlier Anne Bronte biography,[11] but there is nothing in Charlotte's correspondence to corroborate this statement.

Evidently Dr Forbes was prompt in his response, for in her letter to Ellen Nussey of ca. 29 January 1849 (II:172–3) Charlotte states:

> "A few days ago I wrote to have Dr Forbes' opinion – he is one of the first authorities in England on consumptive cases ... the remedies were precisely those he would have recommended himself – he warned us against entertaining sanguine hopes of recovery. The cod-liver oil he considers a peculiarly efficacious medicine."

Writing to WS Williams, George Smith's reader at the Smith, Elder & Co. publishing house located in London's Cornhill, on 1 February 1849 (II:174) Charlotte reports that "remedies prescribed by Mr Teale and approved ... by Dr Forbes are working a good result", and to Laetitia Wheelwright on 15 March 1849 (II:190) she reports on "a system of treatment ... ratified by the opinion of Dr Forbes." Sadly, though, just over two months later Anne was dead.

Although both Gaskell[1] and Barker[8] next mention Forbes in relation to the Thackeray lecture of May 1851, it is possible that Charlotte may in fact have met John Forbes before this. During her visit to London in December 1849 she stayed at the house of George Smith, who arranged a dinner in her honour on 4 December to which Thackeray was invited. It is possible, according to Margaret Smith, that Forbes was also a guest at this dinner (II:300n8, also II:383n2 and II:594n2). This may explain why, in a letter to WS Williams, dated 12 April 1850, Charlotte states (II:382):

> "It was very kind in Dr Forbes to give me his book",

probably referring to *A Physician's Holiday, or a Month in Switzerland in the Summer of 1848* which was published in 1849 (by John Murray).

It was not the last such gift. Writing to George Smith on 31 March 1851 (II:593), Charlotte tells him that:

> "Dr Forbes will tell you and tell you truly that successful labour to a good end is one of the best gifts of Heaven to Man"

and the following month (19 April 1851) asks Smith (II:607):

> "Will you have the goodness to forward the enclosed note to Dr Forbes – ... it is an acknowledgement of the gift of his little book – the Lecture which I like very much".

The book referred to in both these excerpts is *Of Happiness in its relations to work and knowledge. An introductory lecture delivered before the members of the Chichester Literary Society, October 25th, 1850, and published at their request*, which was published by Smith, Elder & Co. in 1850 (this was also the theme for Forbes's MD thesis at Edinburgh in 1817) and reviewed in the *Provincial Medical and Surgical Journal* (the forerunner of the *British Medical Journal*) in 1851.[12]

Letters of 31 May and 2 June 1851 allude to Charlotte's attendance at Thackeray's lecture: to her father, Patrick Brontë, she reports "Dr Forbes came up afterwards" (II:625), "whom I was sincerely glad to see" she told Ellen Nussey (II:628). It looks as though Gaskell chose to run together quotes from these two letters (vide supra).

It is not until 1853, the year that Forbes was knighted, that he once again appears in Charlotte Brontë's correspondence. Writing to Ellen Nussey from London on 19 January 1853, where she was again staying with George Smith, Charlotte reports (III:108):

> "... to-day if all be well – I go with Dr Forbes to see Bethlehem Hospital."

It is not entirely clear if this visit did take place; the relevant hospital visitors book is apparently lost.[3] Gaskell states (p. 422) that Charlotte visited Bethlehem (alias Bedlam), but does not mention Forbes in this context.[1] Both Juliet Barker (p. 843) and Margaret Smith (II:151n2) hold that the visit did occur.

Standard histories of the hospital do not mention Charlotte Brontë,[13,14] but one book on the subject of Bedlam devotes some pages, describing "Mad Women", to the account in *Jane Eyre* (1847) of Bertha Mason,[15] the (now) proverbial mad woman in the attic, apparently oblivious of the fact that Charlotte's had visited the hospital. Certain it is, however, that Charlotte subsequently gave Forbes an inscribed copy of her novel *Villette* (1853) "in acknowledgement of kindness" (III:109n8), now in the Berg Collection of the New York Public Library.

A subsidiary question, perhaps worthy of a brief digression, is why Charlotte wanted to visit Bethlehem Hospital. By 1853 the hospital had long ceased to be the place of public resort for entertainment, as graphically illustrated in Hogarth's *The Rake's Progress.* A suggestion, entirely speculative, which might be considered relates back to Elizabeth Gaskell. Her brother-in-law, Samuel Gaskell (1807–1886), was the nominal head of the four Lunacy Commissioners who inspected Bethlehem Hospital in June 1851 and subsequently issued a highly critical report (*Report and Evidence of the Lunacy Commission to the Home Secretary on Bethlehem Hospital*, contained in the *7th Annual Report of the Lunacy Commissioners*) in February 1852 which initiated a gradual process of reform at the hospital.[16] Might it be possible that Samuel Gaskell and his work may have arisen in conversation between Elizabeth Gaskell and Charlotte Brontë? It would certainly have been topical when Charlotte visited Elizabeth in Manchester at the end of June 1851.

One further book by John Forbes was seen by Charlotte. On 28 May 1853 she acknowledges to WS Williams the receipt of a box of books (III:170), which included (III:170n1) Forbes's *Memorandums Made in Ireland in the Autumn of 1852*, published by Smith, Elder & Co. in 1853. Writing to George Smith on 14 July 1853 Charlotte acknowledges (III:184) the "great pleasure I derived from reading Dr Forbes *Memorandum* (sent in the last Cornhill-parcel)". Smith, Elder & Co. also published Forbes's subsequent travel book, *Sight-seeing in Germany and the Tyrol in the Autumn of 1855.*

Conclusion

It is evident that, although the contacts between Charlotte Brontë and Dr John Forbes as documented in the correspondence between 1849 and 1853 were limited, they shared a mutual respect of each other's powers of observation.

Acknowledgment

Adapted from: Agnew RAL, Larner AJ. Dr John Forbes and the Brontës. *Medical Historian (Journal of the Liverpool Medical History Society)* 2017;27:37–42.

References

1. Gaskell E. *The life of Charlotte Brontë.* Oxford: World's Classics, 2009 [1857]:299,305,380.
2. Agnew RAL. *The life of Sir John Forbes (1787–1861). Royal physician, medical journalist and translator of Laënnec – a Victorian polymath* (2nd edition). Bernard Durnford, 2009.
3. http://museumofthemind.org.uk/blog/post/just-visiting-charlotte-Bront%C3%AB-2–of-2, (accessed 12/08/16).
4. http://www.oxforddnb.com.libezproxy.open.ac.uk/view/article/9841, (accessed 12/08/16).
5. Agnew R. A memoir of Sir John Forbes (1787–1861). *J Med Biogr* 2014;22:190–194.
6. Agnew RAL. Sir John Forbes (1787–1861). *Medical Historian* 1995–1996;8:38–45.
7. Agnew R. The prelude to stethoscopy – some pioneer stethoscopists of the nineteenth century. *Medical Historian* 2002–2003;14:25–33.
8. Barker J. *The Brontës* (2nd edition). London: Abacus, 2010:690,797,843.
9. Smith M. (ed.). *The Letters of Charlotte Brontë* (3 volumes). Oxford: Clarendon Press, 1995–2004.
10. Holland N. *In search of Anne Brontë.* Stroud: The History Press, 2016:241–242.
11. Gérin W. *Anne Brontë.* London: Allen Lane, 1959:304–305.
12. Anonymous. Of Happiness in its relations to Work and Knowledge. An Introductory Lecture delivered before the Members of the Chichester Literary Society, October 25th, 1850, and published at their request. *Prov Med Surg J (1840)* 1851;15:40–41.
13. Andrews J, Briggs A, Porter R, Tucker P, Waddington K. (eds.). *The history of Bethlem.* London: Routledge, 1997.
14. Chambers P. *Bedlam. London's hospital for the mad.* Hersham: Ian Allen Publishing, 2009.
15. Arnold C. *Bedlam. London and its mad.* London: Pocket Books, 2008:229–231.
16. Larner AJ. Dr Samuel Gaskell (1807–1886): a brief biography, and thoughts on his possible influence on Elizabeth Gaskell's writings. *Gaskell Society Newsletter* 2016;62:11–18.

Dr Samuel Gaskell (1807–1886): a medical and literary legacy?

Introduction

It is well known that two figures renowned in the history of science emerged from Lancaster in the nineteenth century: William Whewell (1794–1866) and Richard Owen (1804–1892).[1,2] Contributions to medical science from Lancaster in the nineteenth-century may be less well known. This brief article makes the case for Dr Samuel Gaskell, in terms of both a medical and, possibly, literary legacy.

Brief biography

Samuel Gaskell's biography has been documented on occasion.[3–6] He was born in Warrington on 10th January 1807. His desire to study medicine was initially thwarted on account of poor eye sight, apparently caused by an attack of measles. For some years he was apprenticed to a publisher and bookseller in Liverpool, but this was eventually remitted allowing Samuel to pursue his medical education in Manchester and Edinburgh. In 1834 he was appointed as house apothecary at the Manchester Royal Infirmary and Lunatic Asylum and it was presumably during this time that his interest in the treatment of the insane developed.

In 1840 he was appointed medical superintendent of the Lancaster County Asylum, following election by the county magistrates. Lancaster Asylum had opened in 1816, part of a wave of new asylum building throughout England following the 1808 County Asylums Act. During his years in Lancaster, Gaskell instituted changes in the administrative regime, as documented in his annual asylum reports, and he became an active member of the Association of Medical Officers of Asylums and Hospitals for the Insane, founded in 1841. He gained the Fellowship of the Royal College of Surgeons by election in 1844.

In early 1849 Gaskell was appointed as one of the Commissioners in Lunacy, an influential position which required him to move to London. The Lunacy Commission was founded by the Lunacy Acts of 1845 to provide a permanent inspectorate able to visit any asylum or madhouse, public or private, in England and Wales with the power to order changes to patient care if provision was deemed inadequate. The thoroughness of Gaskell's inspections was noted, and did not always endear him to proprietors and superintendents of madhouses. He has been described as “possibly the most influential commissioner in the commission’s history”.[7] A road accident in 1865 forced his early retirement from his post of Commissioner in 1866 due to “mental infirmity”.

Medical legacy

Samuel Gaskell is credited with ending the system of physical restraint of patients in Lancaster Asylum. This approach was common at the time, not only in Lancaster but also in many of the asylums of the day, although there were notable exceptions, particularly the pioneering approach of the Tuke family at the Retreat near York.[8]

Along with the Visiting Physician, Dr Edward De Vitré (1806–1878), simultaneously elected to Lancaster Asylum, Gaskell was a proponent of the system of “moral treatment” which had been developed in England by Dr John Conolly (1794–1866) at Middlesex County Lunatic Asylum at Hanwell. This was part of a revolution in the care of mental illness during this period, which sought not only to abolish restraint but also to encourage recovery through the provision of adequate care, diet, and employment, in a therapeutic (i.e. clean) environment with access to exercise and recreation.

A detailed study of the Lancaster Asylum records covering the period of Gaskell’s superintendency was undertaken by John Walton,[9] from which he concluded that “[t]he overall impression is of a genuine attempt by the medical officers [Gaskell and De Vitré] to introduce a system of “moral treatment” in the fullest sense, and to change the whole spirit in which the asylum was conducted. There is sufficient evidence to suggest that, up to a point, they succeeded”. In addition to the removal of locks, chains and restraining devices, iron bars and gates were dispensed with, and a building programme sought to increase space, remove walls, and improve light and ventilation (for example by lowering and enlarging windows).

Gaskell is also said to have allocated orphan children to the care of female patients “to develop in the women the great principle of maternal love”, an innovation which was noted on a visit by the Earl of Shaftesbury, the chairman of the Lunacy Commission from its establishment in 1845 until his death in 1885. Shaftesbury’s approbation for Gaskell’s work undoubtedly prompted his appointment as one of the Commissioners in Lunacy in 1849.

Lancaster Asylum was later renamed Lancaster County Mental Hospital and then Lancaster Moor Hospital, finally closing in 2000. Gaskell’s role in the development of mental health services in Lancaster is still remembered to this day.[10]

Literary legacy?

Samuel Gaskell was the younger brother of the Reverend William Gaskell (1805–1884), Unitarian minister at Cross Street Chapel in Manchester, and the husband of the novelist Elizabeth Gaskell (1810–1865). Samuel was the best man at the Gaskell's wedding in 1832. He makes occasional appearances in Mrs Gaskell's extant correspondence, as an occasional advisor on the health of the Gaskell's first child, Marianne, and as a holiday companion for William on his walking trips. (William Whewell was also an occasional correspondent of Mrs Gaskell.)

It seems that Elizabeth grew close to her brother-in-law, feeling that she could be more open with him than with her husband. Naturally then, one might wonder whether knowledge of Samuel's profession had any influence on Elizabeth's creative life. A number of characters with mental infirmity may be discovered in her works,[6] but the most suggestive possibility of a link with Samuel occurs in the short story *Half a life-time ago* (1855),[11] in which Lancaster Asylum is specifically named.

The heroine of the story, Susan Dixon, promises her dying mother that she will be as a mother to her brother Willie, a boy named after his father. (These names and relationships were full of personal significance for Elizabeth Gaskell, as her own son Willie had died as an infant in 1845, an event which apparently prompted her husband to suggest she start writing to assuage her grief.) In the story, a feverish illness robs Willie of the "little wit … he ever possessed", his verbal skills regress to consist largely of vocalisations, and "he had to have the same care taken of him that a little child of four years old requires". Michael Hurst, Susan's intended husband, takes Willie, unbeknown to Susan, to see a Dr Preston in Kendal, "the first doctor in the county", who is reported by Michael to think that Willie "will get badder from year to year" and advises sending him off to Lancaster Asylum. Susan, aware of "stories of the brutal treatment offered to the insane; stories that were, in fact, but too well founded", and of "horrible stories … about madhouses", will not agree, pledging herself to look after her brother, and so losing her chance of marriage to Michael Hurst.

This passing reference to Lancaster Asylum in *Half a life-time ago* may, of course, be entirely incidental to Elizabeth's family relationship to its erstwhile superintendent. As the county asylum, the building would probably have been a familiar name, even to residents of Manchester. Moreover, the Gaskell family regularly spent holidays in Silverdale near Lancaster (the Gaskell Memorial Hall in the centre of the village is named after her); Elizabeth's correspondence suggests visits in 1850, 1852, and 1855, as well as 1858 and 1861. However, other textual evidence may be relevant here: *Half a life-time ago* is set "fifty or fifty-one years ago" which would place it in the first decade of the nineteenth century, well before Samuel's medical career and the movement to reform the running of madhouses and the care of the insane. There is anachronism here, in that Lancaster Asylum was only opened in 1816, although there is no doubt that in the period 1816–1840 conditions there were grim,[9] and hence all too possibly a subject of "stories of the brutal treatment offered to the insane".

Conclusion

In addition to his contributions to the care of patients with mental illness, at both a local and a national level, it is possible that Samuel Gaskell may have influenced some of the writings of his more eminent sister-in-law, the author Elizabeth Gaskell.

Acknowledgements

Thanks to Dr Quenton Wessels of Lancaster Medical School, Faculty of Health and Medicine, Lancaster University, for helpful comments on this manuscript. Adapted from: Larner AJ. Dr Samuel Gaskell at Lancaster Asylum: a medical and literary legacy? *Morecambe Bay Medical Journal* 2016;7(7):177–178.

References

1. Wilson DB. William Whewell, Galileo, and reconceptualising the history of science and religion. *Notes Rec R Soc Lond* 2011;65:343–358.
2. Wessels Q, Taylor AM. Anecdotes to the life and times of Sir Richard Owen (1804–1892) in Lancaster. *J Med Biogr* 2017;25:226–233.
3. Freeman HL. Samuel Gaskell. In: Elwood WJ, Tuxford AF (eds.). *Some Manchester doctors. A biographical collection to mark the 150th anniversary of the Manchester Medical Society 1834–1984.* Manchester: Manchester University Press, 1984:89–92.
4. Scull A, Mackenzie C, Hervey N. *Masters of Bedlam. The transformation of the mad-doctoring trade.* Princeton: Princeton University Press, 1996:161–186.
5. Shaw H, Wessels Q, Taylor AM, Chin-Quee E. The asylums and pioneers of psychiatric care. In: Wessels Q (ed.). *The medical pioneers of nineteenth century Lancaster.* Berlin: epubli GmbH, 2016:99–121.
6. Larner AJ. Dr Samuel Gaskell (1807–1886): a brief biography, and thoughts on his possible influence on Elizabeth Gaskell's writings. *Gaskell Society Newsletter* 2016;62:11–18.
7. Anonymous. Biographies of Medical Lunacy Commissioners 1828–1912. http://studymore.org.uk/6biom.htm#M11 (last accessed 08/03/2016).
8. Kibria AA, Metcalfe NH. A biography of William Tuke (1732–1822): founder of the modern mental asylum. *J Med Biogr* 2016;24:384–388.

9. Walton J. The treatment of pauper lunatics in Victorian England: the case of Lancaster Asylum, 1816–1870. In: Scull A (ed.). *Madhouses, mad-doctors, and madmen. The social history of psychiatry in the Victorian era.* Philadelphia: University of Pennsylvania Press, 1981:166–197.
10. Fearnley E. Care and confinement: A reflective overview of mental health service development in Lancaster and the UK. *Cumbria Partnership Journal of Research Practice and Learning,* 2014;4/1:56–58; http://www.cumbriapartnership.nhs.uk/assets/uploads/cpft-journal/CPFT_Journal_4_-_1_-Fearnley_p56.pdf (last accessed 08/03/2016).
11. Gaskell E. *Cousin Phillis and other stories* (ed. H. Glen). Oxford: Oxford World's Classics, 2010:89–129.

Charles Dickens (1812–1870) *qua* neurologist

It is well recognised that acute observers of nature may record medical conditions, unwittingly or not, sometimes prior to their description (and hence legitimation) by members of the medical professions. A number of examples of relevance to neurology are evident in the work of painters.[1,2] Likewise, in the writings of non-medical authors, subsequent medical readers have felt able to discern accounts corresponding to conditions recognised clinically. Perhaps nowhere is this more evident than in the works of Charles Dickens (1812–1870), famed for his close observation of the human condition. Not only does Dickens provide insights into contemporary workings of the medical profession,[3–6] but there is also a tradition of distinguished clinical neurologists attempting to explain some of the vivid character descriptions in his works in terms of neurological diagnoses, including Lord Brain,[7] Macdonald Critchley,[8] and David Perkin.[9] Justification for some further possible tentative Dickensian diagnoses, if any be needed, may be found in Critchley's statement that "Both as a stylist, and as a recorder of the *comédie humaine*, Charles Dickens is still insufficiently acclaimed".[8]

The classic "Dickensian diagnosis" is that of Joe the fat boy, in the *Posthumous Papers of the Pickwick Club* (1837), whose obesity, ruddy complexion, hypersomnolence, and dropsy prompted use of the term "Pickwickian syndrome" to describe similar cases, only more recently superseded by "obstructive sleep apnoea-hypopnoea syndrome". Dickens's powers of observation, in respect of this case, have been claimed to exceed those of his physician contemporaries.[10] However, Cosnett, reviewing sleep disorders in Dickens's works,[11] suggests that Joe in fact has a diencephalic tumour or suffers the consequences of a head injury, but he identifies Mr Willet in *Barnaby Rudge* (1841) as a possible case of obstructive sleep apnoea syndrome.

To be sure, some of Dickens' insights have been acknowledged, for example an account in *David Copperfield* (1850) which may describe the phenomenon of *déjà vu*:[12,13]

> We have all some experience of a feeling which comes over us occasionally, of what we are saying and doing having been said or done before, in a remote time – of our having been surrounded dim ages ago, by the same faces, objects, and circumstances – of our knowing perfectly what will be said next, as if we suddenly remembered it.

Other characters and descriptions of possible neurological significance may be identified in Dickens's oeuvre. Although there are dangers associated with making such inferences (anachronism, hegemonism), nonetheless they may give some insights into the history of neurology since the accuracy of the descriptions (as judged retrospectively) prompts the belief that they are based on observation of actual patients. (We have no difficulties accepting this premise when viewing the work of painters.) Here previous relevant publications are reviewed and some further cases of possible neurological interest suggested.

Lord Brain, famed for his textbooks of neurological diagnosis and diseases, identified several "Dickensian diagnoses".[7] For example, Sir Leicester Dedlock (*Bleak House*, 1853), William Dorrit (*Little Dorrit*, 1857), and Mrs Skewton (*Dombey and Son*, 1848) are all adjudged to suffer cerebrovascular accidents. We would perhaps not be quite so ready to ascribe Mrs Skewton's head tremor, evident before her stroke, to "cerebral arteriosclerosis", other than as a diagnosis of exclusion ("senile tremor"). The tremor of Mr Dolls (*Our Mutual Friend*, 1865) may simply reflect alcohol withdrawal but might conceivably be essential tremor. The villagers who witness Betty Higden's blackout (*Our Mutual Friend*, book 3, chapter 8) are uncertain whether she has suffered a faint or a fit, a familiar enough diagnostic dilemma even today. The old lady's rapid recovery and flight from the scene suggest it was a syncopal event. An epileptic seizure is the likely cause of death of Anthony Chuzzlewit (*Martin Chuzzlewit*, 1844).[7]

Both Grandfather Smallweed (*Bleak House*), who needs to be carried everywhere, and Mrs Clennam (*Little Dorrit*), who is confined to a chair in her room, have been cited as examples of paraplegia by Lord Brain.[7] As regards the latter, there is an interesting description following her dramatic recovery of the ability to walk at the end of the novel (chapter 31):

> There Mrs Clennam dropped upon the stones; and she never from that hour moved so much as a finger again, or had the power to speak one word. For upwards of three years she reclined in her wheeled chair, looking attentively at those about her, and appearing to understand what they said; but, the rigid silence she had so long held was evermore enforced upon her, and, except that she could move her eyes and faintly express a negative and affirmative with her head, she lived and died a stone.

This description may call to the neurologist's mind the locked-in syndrome (de-efferentation) following a ventral brainstem stroke, which typically leaves patients alert and able to perceive sensory stimuli, but unable to move other than some preservation of eyelid and sometimes ocular movements; the head movements apparent in Mrs Clennam would be unusual. Bauby, a famous sufferer of locked-in syndrome (and now the subject of a motion picture), cited a possible literary case of this condition in Alexandre Dumas's novel *The Count of Monte Cristo* (1894),[14] but not this possible, and prior, case report by Dickens.

The Smallweeds (*Bleak House*) are a peculiar clan. Mrs Smallweed, wife of Grandfather, is "weak in her intellect" and accordingly has been identified as suffering from dementia.[7] Macdonald Critchley cites two fragments of her speech as examples of senile verbigeration (inappropriate recurrent utterances, speech iteration).[15] And what can one make of young Mr Bartholomew Smallweed, aka Small, or Chick Weed?

> Whether Young Smallweed ... was ever a boy, is much doubted .. of small stature and weazen features ... he is a weird changeling, to whom years are nothing ... a kind of fossil Imp (Chapter 20)
>
> There has been only one child in the Smallweed family for several generations. Little old men and women there have been, but no child ... until grandmother ... became weak in her intellect, and fell (for the first time) into a childish state (Chapter 21).

This early appearance of features typically associated with ageing in the apparent absence of cognitive impairment has suggested to my erstwhile colleague, Dr Varun Singh, a diagnosis of progeria (Hutchinson-Gilford progeria syndrome, HGPS).[16] Short stature, skin changes, facial features that resemble aged persons, but with normal cognitive development are typical of this syndrome. Classical HGPS follows an autosomal dominant pattern of inheritance, although almost all cases represent spontaneous mutations.[17]

Krook (*Bleak House*), brother of Mrs Smallweed, is famed for his untimely demise by means of spontaneous combustion, a storyline which involved Dickens in some controversy, not all his readers wishing to suspend disbelief. But a possible pre-mortem diagnosis may be suggested by this description of Krook:

> He was short, cadaverous, and withered, with his head sunk sideways between his shoulders, and the breath issuing in visible smoke from his mouth, as he were on fire within. His throat, chin and eyebrows were so frosted with white hairs, and so gnarled with veins and puckered skin, that he looked from his breast upwards, like some old root in a fall of snow.

Dilatation or engorgement of neck and face veins is one of the characteristic physical findings in superior vena cava obstruction.

Cousin Feenix (*Dombey and Son*) is described as "meaning to go in a straight line, but turning off sideways by reason of his wilful legs", diagnosed by Brain as an ataxic gait.[7] Perkin has mentioned a number of other Dickensian characters with apparent gait disturbances, but without proferring diagnoses.[9] Perhaps Sairey Gamp's difficulties (*Martin Chuzzlewit*) result from her partiality to gin.

Lord Brain also mentions Dickens's descriptions of the sequelae of head injury, as in Mrs Joe Gargery (*Great Expectations*, 1861) and Eugene Wrayburn (*Our Mutual Friend*). Cases of "mental defectives" are also in evidence, such as Maggy (*Little Dorrit*), and the title character of *Barnaby Rudge*.[7] Exactly what diagnosis one might apply to these individuals with learning disability is uncertain, but it has been argued that Barnaby Rudge has autism.[18]

Mrs Gradgrind (*Hard Times*, 1854) famously fails to locate her pain any more precisely than "somewhere in the room", which has been taken as an example of the difficulty of locating pain of visceral origin, so familiar in clinical practice. For this description Dickens earns the chastisement of Oliver Sacks, who informs us that "one cannot have a pain except in oneself".[19]

The field of movement disorders might be expected to provide a rich source of materials for a novelist as observant as Dickens, and indeed a number of publications have been devoted to this topic.[20–23] In *David Copperfield* (1850), Uriah Heep's writhings have suggested a generalised dystonia, Mr Creakle the schoolmaster may have a spasmodic dysphonia,[21] and the sleepy waiter at the Golden Cross Inn (chapter 19) restless legs syndrome.[7,21] Cosnett has suggested that two characters in *Little Dorrit* are worthy of note in this context: the description of Jeremiah Flintwinch is highly suggestive of spasmodic torticollis, and Mr Pancks manifests features concordant with those of Gilles de la Tourette syndrome.[20] To this list one might perhaps add Frederick Dorrit, uncle of the title character of *Little Dorrit*, who is described (chapter 8) as "stooped a good deal", turning round in a "slow, stiff, stooping manner", and speaking with a "weak and quavering voice", features which might be construed as parkinsonism. A clearer description of parkinsonism, with an accompanying eye movement disorder, highly suggestive of progressive supranuclear palsy, has been identified in *The Lazy Tour of Two Idle Apprentices* (1857), written jointly by Dickens and his friend Wilkie Collins.[22] This latter account predates by more than 100 years the eponymous description of Steele et al. (1960). Likewise Mr Pancks predates Gilles de la Tourette's (1885) description.[20]

A few passages give insight into nineteenth century attempts at neurorehabilitation, rudimentary though these were. Most famous perhaps is the little crutch used by Tiny Tim Cratchitt in *A Christmas Carol* (1843); his limbs are also supported by an "iron frame". Jenny Wren, the dolls' dressmaker in *Our Mutual Friend*, also uses a crutch. Prostheses are also in evidence: the wooden leg of Silas Wegg (*Our Mutual Friend*) is illustrated by Marcus Stone as little more than a stump (book 3, chapters 7 and 14) which proves a significant hindrance when climbing the dust heaps in search of Mr Boffin's buried treasure. Captain Cuttle, in *Dombey and Son*, has "a hook instead of a hand attached to his right wrist" which conveniently doubles as a toasting-fork (chapter 49), and is illustrated being thus used by "Phiz" (Hablot K Browne). Curiously, two other illustrations of Captain Cuttle clearly show the hook on the left hand! A remarkable account of a wheeled chair, used by Mr Omer to facilitate his failing mobility, is to be found in *David Copperfield* (chapter 51): this easy chair on wheels "runs as light as a feather, and tracks as true as a mail-coach". Mrs Clennam (*Little Dorrit*) reclined in a wheeled chair after her final relapse into silence and immobility.

Richard Carstone (*Bleak House*) rejects several career opportunities, including medicine, before becoming embroiled in the legal case of Jarndyce and Jarndyce, all the proceeds of which are consumed by lawyers' fees before judgement is finally given, during which time Carstone's health fails leading to his untimely death. Perhaps unwittingly, Dickens, familiar as he was with the workings of the law from his time at Doctors' Commons as a young man, may be reporting here a case of "Chancery cachexia", described as such by the nineteenth century Irish physician Jonathan Osborne (Chancery was formerly one of the courts of justice, presided over by the Lord High Chancellor).[24] In his paper on the subject,[25] Osborne described a clergyman whose fatal wasting was "occasioned by the delays and vexations in legal proceedings" in much the same way that Richard Carstone fades away having pursued his suit against the advice of John Jarndyce, and preyed upon by the venal lawyer Mr Vholes who makes much money at Carstone's expense.

Miss Havisham (*Great Expectations*, 1861) merits an eponymous syndrome in the writings of Macdonald Critchley,[8] as the prototype of comparable cases of young women, usually of aristocratic or well-to-do parentage, who suffer a major shock or rebuff and who then become reclusive, opt out of life, and try to make time stand still. Queen Victoria's behaviour after the death of Prince Albert is cited as a possible example.

It has been suggested that Dr Manette in *A Tale of Two Cities* (1859) is an example of dissociative amnesia.[26]

George Orwell (1903–1950) contends that Dickens sees human beings with the most intense vividness yet, as a caricaturist, with a narrowness of vision; the mark of his writing is seen as the unnecessary detail. These may be the very qualities which permit us to see some of his characters "like pictures", "fixed like painted miniatures",[27] and hence in certain cases as exemplars of neurological diseases.

Acknowledgment

Adapted from: Larner AJ. Charles Dickens *qua* neurologist. *Adv Clin Neurosci Rehabil* 2002;2(1):22; and Singh V, Larner AJ. Some more Dickensian diagnoses. *Adv Clin Neurosci Rehabil* 2009;9(2):19–20.

References

1. Smith PEM. Neurology in the National Gallery. *J R Soc Med* 1999;92:649–652.
2. Smith PEM. Fainting painting. *Pract Neurol* 2005;5:106–109.
3. Waldron Smithers D. *Dickens's doctors.* Oxford: Pergamon Press, 1979.
4. Dauber LG. Dickens and doctors: physicians in fiction of Charles Dickens. *NY State J Med* 1981;81:1522–1526.
5. Andrews M. Dickens and the medical profession *NZ Med J* 1985;98:810–813.
6. Cosnett JE. Dickens and doctors: vignettes of Victorian medicine. *BMJ* 1992;305:1540–1542.
7. Brain R. Dickensian diagnoses. *BMJ* 1955;ii:1553–1556 (also published in Brain R. *Some reflections on genius and other essays.* London: Pitman Medical, 1960:123–136).
8. Critchley M. *The divine banquet of the brain and other essays.* New York: Raven Press, 1979:136–140.
9. Perkin GD. Disorders of gait. *J Neurol Neurosurg Psychiatry* 1996;61:199.
10. Douglas NJ. Sleep apnoea/hypopnoea syndrome. In: Seaton A, Seaton D, Leitch AG (eds.). *Crofton and Douglas's respiratory diseases.* Oxford: Blackwell Scientific, 2000 (5th edition):1250–1263.
11. Cosnett J. Charles Dickens and sleep disorders. *Dickensian* 1997;93(3):200–204.
12. Lennox WG, Lennox MA. *Epilepsy and related disorders.* London: J&A Churchill, 1960 (2 volumes):275,704.
13. Warren-Gash C, Zeman A. Déjà vu. *Pract Neurol* 2003;3:106–109.
14. Bauby J-D. *The diving-bell and the butterfly.* London: Fourth Estate, 1997:55–56.
15. Critchley M. *The citadel of the senses and other essays.* New York: Raven Press, 1986:127 (also published in *Arch Neurol* 1984;41:1135–1139 [at 1138]).
16. Singh V. Reflections: neurology and the humanities. Description of a family with progeria by Charles Dickens. *Neurology* 2010;75:571.
17. Hennekam RCM. Hutchinson-Gilford progeria syndrome: review of the phenotype. *Am J Med Genet* 2006;140A:2603–2624.
18. Grove T. Barnaby Rudge: a case study in autism. *Dickensian* 1987;83:139–148.
19. Sacks O. Foreword. In: Ramachandran VS, Blakeslee S. *Phantoms in the brain. Human nature and the architecture of the mind.* London: Fourth Estate, 1998:vii-ix.
20. Cosnett JE. Dickens, dystonia and dyskinesia. *J Neurol Neurosurg Psychiatry* 1991;54:184.

21. Garcia-Ruiz PJ, Gulliksen LL. Movement disorders in David Copperfield [in Spanish]. *Neurologia* 1999;14:359–360.
22. Larner AJ. Did Charles Dickens describe progressive supranuclear palsy in 1857? *Mov Disord* 2002;17:832–833.
23. Schoffer KL, O'Sullivan JD. Charles Dickens: the man, medicine, and movement disorders. *J Clin Neurosci* 2006;13:898–901.
24. Breathnach CS. Jonathan Osborne (1794–1864), MD, FRCPI, a crypto-neurologist. *J Med Biogr* 2009;17:144–148.
25. Osborne J. Chancery cachexia. An account of an individual whose disease and death were occasioned by the delays and vexations belonging to legal proceedings under our present system of jurisprudence. *London Medical Gazette* 1839–40;25:398–399 [extracted in *Edinburgh Medical and Surgical Journal* 1840;53:247–249].
26. Dieguez S, Annoni J-M. Stranger than fiction: literary and clinical amnesia. In: Bogousslavsky J, Dieguez S (eds.). *Literary medicine: brain disease and doctors in novels, theater, and film* (Frontiers of Neurology and Neuroscience Volume 31). Basel: Karger, 2013:137–168 [at 158].
27. Orwell G. Charles Dickens. In: *The Penguin essays of George Orwell.* Harmondsworth: Penguin, 1991:41–84.

Reading David Livingstone (1813–1873)

It is perhaps difficult at this remove of time to appreciate fully the profound appeal that Dr David Livingstone (1813–1873) had for many mid-Victorians, but some contemporary accounts may give us a flavour. For example, on the evening of 14th December 1874 the diarist Francis Kilvert (1840–1879), curate in the parish of Langley Burrell, Wiltshire, took "21 of our schoolchildren into Chippenham to the Temperance Hall to see a Panorama of the African travels of Dr Livingstone", of which "One of the most favourite [*sic*] pictures with the children was the Funeral of Dr Livingstone in Westminster Abbey." Kilvert commented "What pleasure these few pence have given to twenty-one young hearts". He had also given a lecture on the subject of Livingstone's funeral a few weeks earlier.[1]

The enormous success of Livingstone's printed works when they first appeared[2–4] may also give some indication, a response that seems not to have been confined exclusively to Great Britain. Growing up in the rural American Midwest, in De Smet, Dakota, the author Laura Ingalls Wilder (1867–1957) recalls in her account of the hard winter of 1880–1, when her family was confined to the house in the cold and dark of blizzards that could last several days, that her father would read to them about "Livingstone's Africa" from a big green book: "Please read about the lions, Pa" she pleaded.[5] The French author Alphonse Daudet (1840–1897), suffering locomotor ataxia as a consequence of neurosyphilis in the 1880s and 1890s, recorded in his occasional personal journal entitled *La Doulou* ("pain") that he was "spending time with good old Livingstone in darkest Africa. The monotony of his endless and virtually pointless journey, the constant obsession with barometric pressure and meals that rarely arrive, and the silent, calm unfolding of vast landscapes – all this makes for truly wonderful reading. My imagination doesn't require anything more of the book than to provide a framework within which it can wander."[6]

It is difficult to imagine many people reading Livingstone for pleasure in this day and age, but nonetheless a few readers are ready to battle their way through the ¾ million words in three his major works. Dr John Beard has examined both primary and secondary sources in an attempt to read the motives which sustained Livingstone's life work.[7] Clearly this is potentially hazardous territory to explore, the texts providing only clues from which inferences may be drawn. However, since readers can hardly fail to note the considerable privation and hardship which Livingstone endured during his travels, including frequent personal illness and the death of his wife, it is not an unreasonable question to pursue. Livingstone's explicit and oft-repeated assertion that all he did (including undergoing surgery[8]) was in order to serve Christ and for the promulgation of the Gospel must be tempered by the observation, made by both some contemporaries and by posterity, that he was unsuited to and largely unsuccessful in missionary work.

Beard argues that Livingstone's principal interest, dating from boyhood, lay in scientific observation, for example of fauna, flora, geology, and meteorology, as reflected (and as noted in the quote from Daudet[6]) in his voluminous writing, and also in his tolerance of tribal customs which drew the opprobrium of other missionaries. That Livingstone himself had some insight into the possible disparity between his stated and actual motivations is also clear, in which respect he perhaps does not differ from many of us.

Livingstone's published books, letters and journals may also be read as providing a more or less detailed contemporary account, although in no way systematic, of issues related to medicine. For instance, it is possible, taking Livingstone as representative of medical training, understanding, knowledge and practice between the 1840s and 1870s, to make some inferences about these topics with respect to African fever,[9] ophthalmology,[10] otolaryngology,[8] and neurology.[11] This reflects the vast resource which Livingstone's writings constitute, as is true of other medical travellers,[12] and their openness to further readings.

Acknowledgment

Adapted from: Larner AJ. Reading Livingstone. *J Med Biogr* 2009;17:63.

References

1. Plomer W (ed.). *Kilvert's diary Volume three: 14 May 1874–13 March 1879. Selections from the diary of the Rev. Francis Kilvert.* London: Jonathan Cape, 1940:107, 121–122.
2. Livingstone D. *Missionary travels and researches in South Africa; including a sketch of sixteen years' residence in the interior of Africa, etc.* London: John Murray, 1857.
3. Livingstone D, Livingstone C. *Narrative of an expedition to the Zambesi and its tributaries: and the discovery of the lakes Shirwa and Nyassa 1858–1864.* London: John Murray, 1865.
4. Waller H (ed.). *The last journals of David Livingstone in Central Africa, from 1865 to his death. Continued by a narrative of his last moments and sufferings obtained from his faithful servants Chuma and Susi.* London, 1874 (2 volumes).
5. Ingalls Wilder L. *The Long Winter.* Harmondsworth: Puffin 1968 [1940]:178–179.

6. Barnes J (ed./trans.). *Alphonse Daudet. In the land of pain*. London: Jonathan Cape, 2002:8.
7. Beard JAS. What motivated Dr David Livingstone (1813–1873) in his work in Africa? *J Med Biogr* 2009;17:95–99.
8. Larner AJ. David Livingstone's uvulectomy. *J Med Biogr* 2006;14:104–108.
9. Larner AJ. Charles Meller and John Kirk: medical practitioners and practice on Livingstone's Zambesi expedition, 1858–64. *J Med Biogr* 2002;10:129–134.
10. Larner AJ. Ophthalmological observations made during the mid-19th century European encounter with Africa. *Arch Ophthalmol* 2004;122:267–272.
11. Larner AJ. Dr David Livingstone (1813–1873): some neurological observations. *Scott Med J* 2007;53(2):35–37.
12. Larner AJ, Fisher HJ. Dr Gustav Nachtigal (1834–1885): a contribution to the history of medicine in mid-nineteenth-century Africa. *J Med Biogr* 2000;8:43–48.

David Livingstone (1813–1873): some neurological observations

Dr David Livingstone was a medical missionary in southern Africa for over ten years before commencing the explorations which were to bring him to widespread public attention. The three major journeys he undertook were the Transcontinental Expedition of 1853–1856, crossing Africa from west (Angola) to east (Mozambique); the Zambezi Expedition of 1858–1864; and the final journey of 1866–1873, ostensibly searching for the sources of the river Nile, an ambition brought to a close by his death at Chitambo's village in May 1873. Throughout his time in Africa, Livingstone kept journals[1–5] and corresponded extensively;[3,6,7] much of this material is now published. He also wrote up the first two of his expeditions for contemporaneous publication.[8,9]

All these works provide a rich resource for the study of Africa in the mid-nineteenth century, including the history of medicine,[10] since Livingstone was a qualified doctor.[11] Although as early as 1843, he reported that he was keen to give up all medical practice so that he could devote his energies entirely to evangelization,[12] nonetheless there is much medical information in his writings. We also have accounts from two other doctors who accompanied Livingstone on the Zambesi Expedition, John Kirk and Charles Meller, both also Scots.[13]

As for other European travellers in Africa, fever was the major health problem faced by Livingstone: it is mentioned in passing in all of his works. The first attack seized him in May 1853 and 2 years later he reported having suffered 27 attacks in all.[14] He recognised that there were different forms of fever. For the most part this was probably malaria, which was apparently often associated with "stoppage", hence Livingstone's favoured remedy of quinine in combination with a purgative, a view which he communicated to the medical press.[15] Fever with diarrhoea may possibly have been dysentery.

Neuropsychiatric features associated with fever were observed by Livingstone, both in himself and others. Fever was "preceded by great lassitude . . . for a few days", so much so that this became a diagnostic point:

> . . . a peculiar kind of irritability produced by the climate, possibly by malaria, as it often, though not always, preceded an attack of fever. It has been noticed and experienced so frequently that we set it down as a symptom of fever when a man thinks himself insulted or slighted, and takes on airs.[16]

Headache was one of the cardinal features of fever. In some forms "there was only pain in the head, which a dose of quinine removed"; in other attacks, for example affecting his servants, "all complain of pain, violent generally, in the head and neck". This was sometimes relieved by spontaneous rectal bleeding, but not by venesection, which perhaps prompted Livingstone's belief that "a mild purgative with quinine seems the most effectual medicine." Cases of fever, headache, spinal pain and haematuria have been suggested to be bilharzia.[17]

Fever induced not only physical but also cognitive impairment:

> The fever makes me perfectly useless as far as mental work is concerned. I cannot perform a simple calculation or lay in a few new words . . . I have been reduced so low by it I forget the days of the week, the names of those about me . . .

This could progress to more serious impairments of consciousness: "I have had fever . . . once with inflammation of part of the head (meningitis), which kept me down for 25 days and left me nearly blind and almost deaf." One wonders if this was delirium. Behavioural change was noted in others, for example Baines, who had "muttering deliriums, involuntary wetting of the bed clothes, on the verge of coma." Clark had mania and epileptic fits; after a few days Livingstone notes: "Clarke [*sic*] better; after croton oil and colocynth and calomel pill, quinine acted as a sedative and his senses returned."[18]

Other neurological complications of fever were also recorded, including what sound like visual hallucinations, again perhaps reflecting delirium:

> . . . ugly phantoms . . . are often seen in continued fever . . . and prevent sleep.
>
> . . . if I look at any piece of wood, the bark seems covered over with figures and faces of men, and they remain, though I look away and turn to the same spot again.

Also vertigo:

> . . . fits of vertigo, probably from exhaustion, troubled me for some time; everything seemed to rush to the left, and I had to lay hold on something to prevent a fall.
>
> Exhaustion produced vertigo, causing me, if I looked suddenly up, almost to lose consciousness.[19]

One wonders if this latter was in fact related to the treatment of fever, rather than fever *per se*, since therapy might also be complicated by neurological symptoms. Quinine, recognised to abort the headache associated with fever, was given in doses sufficient to cause "cinchonism", namely ringing in the ears and deafness. Indeed, it was recommended that quinine be given 2–3 hourly until deafness was produced, the greater the deafness the speedier the restoration of the patient. The absence of such symptoms following large doses of cheaper unbleached quinine indicated to Kirk its impure nature.

Despite these problems, Livingstone was upbeat about the health prospects of Africa for any European immigrants, including other neurological illnesses:

> The fever is certainly the great bugbear of this field. But it must ever be borne in mind that it is the only one. There are few other diseases ... 3 cases of mania, ... one of senile dementia, in 15 years, do not require notice.
>
> I have seen but one well marked case of hydrocephalus, three of epilepsy ... none of hydrophobia or delirium tremens.
>
> Consumption is unknown, and so is scrofula and madness.[20]

Having had some training at the Moorfields Eye Hospital before travelling to Africa,[11] Livingstone may have had some familiarity with ophthalmological problems. For example, he noted that when diet contained "so very much starch the eye became affected, as in the case of animals fed on pure gluten or amylaceous matter only."[21] This nutritional eye disease may be xerophthalmia from vitamin A deficiency, the experiments referred to being those undertaken in dogs by Magendie in 1816. However, Livingstone was at a loss to explain an outbreak of "moon-blindness" amongst his faithful African followers from the Makololo tribe, which afflicted many of them when, after waiting 4 years (1856–1860) for Livingstone's return to escort them back to their own country, and having established new business interests and married new wives, they were about to be repatriated:

> Four or five of our men were affected with moon-blindness at Tette; though they had not slept out of doors there, they became so blind that their comrades had to guide their hands to the general dish of food; the affection is unknown in their own country. When our posterity shall have discovered what it is which, distinct from foul smells, causes fever, and what, apart from the moon, causes men to be moon-struck, they will pity our dulness [*sic*] of perception.

It is possible that this was functional or "hysterical" blindness.

Another mysterious disorder encountered by Livingstone was earth- or clay-eating (geophagia or geophagy):

> 29th November [1870]. – *Safura* is the name of the disease of clay or earth eating, at Zanzibar; it often affects slaves, and the clay is said to have a

> pleasant odour to the eaters, but it is not confined to slaves, nor do slaves eat in order to kill themselves; it is a diseased appetite, and rich men who have plenty to eat are often subject to it. The feet swell, flesh is lost, and the face looks haggard; the patient can scarcely walk for shortness of breath and weakness, and he continues eating until he dies.

Livingstone noted that "clay built in walls is preferred, and Manyuema women when pregnant often eat it", and may also have observed the associated weakness when he reported "A Banyamwezi carrier, who bore an enormous load of copper, is now by safura scarcely able to walk".[22] Livingstone thought it might be a functional or hysterical disorder.[23]

Reports of geophagia have been found dating back to Hippocrates,[24] and the loss of flesh associated with geophagia which was noted by Livingstone was re-reported almost a century later as "Cachexia Africana".[25]

Another inexplicable illness amongst the natives on the Zambesi expedition was noted when members of the party ascended the summit at Ndonda, estimated to be at 3440 feet above sea level:

> The air which was so exhilarating to Europeans had an opposite effect on five men who had been born and reared in the malaria of the Delta of the Zambesi. No sooner did they reach the edge of the plateau of Ndonda, than they lay down prostrate, and complained of pains all over them.

Both scarification and western medicines were without therapeutic effect:

> ... in two days one of them actually died in consequence of, as far as we could judge, a change from a malarious to a purer and more rarified atmosphere.[26]

One wonders about the possibility of acute mountain sickness in unacclimatized individuals but the stated elevation, estimated from the boiling point of water, is far too low for this (Dr Charles Clarke, personal communication, 23/08/2006).

In enumerating these examples, it is not suggested that Livingstone was a neurologist (or "proto-neurologist" or "crypto-neurologist"); his training predated the foundation of the first hospital dedicated to neurological disorders in Queen Square, London, in 1860. He probably knew little of neurological illnesses, as has been suggested for ophthalmology and otorhinolaryngology.[27,28] Moreover, his observations were frequently no more than incidental to his travelogue. Nonetheless, being some of the earliest medical records of disease in Africa, they provide some insights into neurological problems and their treatment in mid-nineteenth century southern Africa. Certainly his travels had a huge impact on his contemporaries,[29,30] and also resulted in the description of new species, as acknowledged in the Linnean binomial taxonomy, such as Livingstone's fruit bat *Pteropus livingstonii* from the Comoros Islands, and Meller's duck *Anas melleri* from Madagascar.[31]

Acknowledgments

Adapted from: Larner AJ. Dr David Livingstone (1813–1873): some neurological observations. *Scott Med J* 2008;53(2):35–37; and Larner AJ. Neurological signs: geophagia (geophagy) and pica (pagophagia). *Adv Clin Neurosci Rehabil* 2009;9(4):20.

References

1. Schapera I (ed.). *Livingstone's private journals 1851–1853.* London: Chatto & Windus, 1960.
2. Schapera I (ed.). *Livingstone's African journal 1853–1856.* London: Chatto & Windus, 1963 (2 volumes).
3. Wallis JPR (ed.). *The Zambesi Expedition of David Livingstone 1858–1863.* London: Chatto & Windus, 1956 (2 volumes).
4. Shepperson G (ed.). *Livingstone and the Rovuma.* Edinburgh: Edinburgh University Press, 1965.
5. Waller H (ed.). *The last journals of David Livingstone in Central Africa, from 1865 to his death. Continued by a narrative of his last moments and sufferings obtained from his faithful servants Chuma and Susi.* London, 1874 (2 volumes).
6. Schapera I (ed.). *David Livingstone: family letters 1841–1856.* London: Chatto & Windus, 1959 (2 volumes).
7. Schapera I (ed.). *Livingstone's missionary correspondence 1841–1856.* London: Chatto & Windus, 1961.
8. Livingstone D. *Missionary travels and researches in South Africa; including a sketch of sixteen years' residence in the interior of Africa, etc.* London: John Murray, 1857.
9. Livingstone D, Livingstone C. *Narrative of an expedition to the Zambesi and its tributaries: and the discovery of the lakes Shirwa and Nyassa 1858–1864.* London: John Murray, 1865.
10. Gelfand M. *Livingstone the doctor: his life and travels. A study in medical history.* Oxford: Basil Blackwell, 1957.
11. Morris DE. The medical career of Dr David Livingstone. *Scott Med J* 1984;29:183–186.
12. Seaver G. *David Livingstone: his life and letters.* London: Lutterworth, 1957:62.
13. Larner AJ. Charles Meller and John Kirk: medical practitioners and practice on Livingstone's Zambesi expedition, 1858–64. *J Med Biogr* 2002;10:129–134.
14. Schapera (*op. cit.* ref. 6):261; Livingstone (*op. cit.* ref. 8):169–170.

15. Livingstone D. On fever in the Zambesi. *Lancet* 1861;ii:184–186.
16. Schapera (*op. cit.* ref. 2):40; Wallis (*op. cit.* ref. 3):359.
17. Schapera (*op. cit.* ref. 7):157; Schapera (*op. cit.* ref. 1):103–104,149; Gelfand (*op. cit.* ref. 10):94.
18. Schapera (*op. cit.* ref. 2):135, also Gelfand (*op. cit.* ref. 10):80; Schapera (*op. cit.* ref. 6):261; Wallis (*op. cit.* ref. 3):311,228.
19. Schapera (*op. cit.* ref. 2):14; Waller (*op. cit.* ref, 5):II.2; Schapera (*op. cit.* ref. 7):251,255.
20. Schapera (*op. cit.* ref. 7):291,292; Schapera (*op. cit.* ref. 6):261; also Gelfand (*op. cit.* ref. 10):32–33.
21. Schapera (*op. cit.* ref. 7): 292; Livingstone (*op. cit.* ref. 8): 389, 431; also Gelfand (*op. cit.* ref. 10): 96, 97.
22. Waller (*op. cit.* ref, 5):II.83–II.84.
23. Livingstone & Livingstone (*op. cit.* ref. 9):176; Gelfand (*op. cit.* ref. 10):257.
24. Woywodt A, Kiss A. Geophagia: the history of earth-eating. *J R Soc Med* 2002;95:143–146.
25. Mengel CE, Carter WA, Horton ES. Geophagia with iron deficiency and hypokalemia. Cachexia Africana. *Arch Intern Med* 1964;114:470–474.
26. Livingstone & Livingstone (*op. cit.* ref. 9):518–520.
27. Larner AJ. Ophthalmological observations made during the mid-19th century European encounter with Africa. *Arch Ophthalmol* 2004;122:267–272.
28. Larner AJ. David Livingstone's uvulectomy. *J Med Biogr* 2006;14:104–108.
29. Larner A. Kilvert and Livingstone. *Journal of the Kilvert Society* 2008;Issue 27:17.
30. Larner AJ. Reading Livingstone. *J Med Biogr* 2009;17:63.
31. Larner AJ. Medical memorials in the Linnean binomial taxonomy. *J Med Biogr* 2010;18:123.

Lewis Carroll (Charles Lutwidge Dodgson, 1832–1898): an Oxford neurologist?

The University of Oxford may boast of many renowned neurologists, neuroscientists and philosophers of the mind during its long history. Christ Church, the author's college, may particularly claim, amongst its many great alumni,[1] Thomas Willis (1621–1675), who coined the word "neurology",[2] and Richard Lower (1631–1691) who performed the dissections for Willis's 1664 *Cerebri Anatome*,[3] as well as Robert Hooke (1635–1703) whose pioneering work in microscopy, as illustrated in his *Micrographia* (1665), paved the way for many neuroscientific advances. To this list might be added Robert Burton (1577–1640), author of *The Anatomy of Melancholy* (1621), and John Locke (1632–1704), author of *An Essay Concerning Human Understanding* (1689).

At first glance, the mathematician Reverend Charles Lutwidge Dodgson (1832–1898), specialising in symbolic logic, may seem an unlikely candidate for admission to this Christ Church neuroscience pantheon. However, a careful examination of those of his works published under the pseudonym of Lewis Carroll, particularly *Alice's Adventures in Wonderland* (1865) and *Through the looking-glass and what Alice found there* (1872), reveals a number of possible neurological cases.

Case 1: Girl with a distorted body image

Carroll reports the case of a girl, Alice, who experienced distortions of body image, or corporeal awareness (*Wonderland*, chapters 1,2,4), in which she felt she was shutting up and then opening out like a telescope (as illustrated by Sir John Tenniel), such that her head was pressed against the ceiling and she had to stoop to stop her neck from being broken.

These phenomena, microsomatognosia and macrosomatognosia respectively, have subsequently been labelled the "Alice in Wonderland" syndrome.[4] Since they have been reported to occur in the context of migraine,[5] and as Dodgson was known to suffer from migraine, some neurologists have believed it possible that Carroll was writing from his own experience.[6,7] Objections to this claim have been lodged, based on the rarity of somaesthetic auras as a feature of migraine, and also on chronological grounds, there being no account in Dodgson's diaries of the onset of migraine until after he had written the Alice books.[8] However, an earlier drawing with evidence of a right paracentral negative scotoma, a fairly common visual aura of migraine, may undermine this latter objection.[9,10]

It should be remembered that other conditions may also give rise to micro- or macrosomatognosia, including epilepsy, encephalitis, cerebral mass lesions, schizophrenia, and drug intoxication. As famously pointed out by Jefferson Airplane in the song "White Rabbit", from the 1967 album *Surrealistic Pillow*, the latter might be relevant to Alice, since her experiences occur after drinking from a phial (labelled "DRINK ME") and after eating cake ("EAT ME").

Case 2: Egghead unable to recognise faces

An egg, in which Alice perceives the face of Humpty Dumpty (*Looking-glass*, chapter 6), reports difficulty with facial recognition. After their conversation, as Alice is about to depart, Humpty Dumpty says he would not be able to recognise Alice if they did meet again: "Your face is the same as everybody has". However, he makes it clear that he can perceive individual eyes, nose and mouth.

Humpty Dumpty may suffer from prosopagnosia, a rare form of visual agnosia, which may be developmental or acquired, characterised by impaired recognition of familiar faces or equivalent stimuli.[11] Recognition of individual facial features, including direction of eye gaze and facial expression may be preserved in prosopagnosia.

Case 3: Neurobehavioural syndrome in a hatter

At a mad tea party (*Wonderland*, chapter 7), Alice encounters a hatter who behaves very oddly: making personal remarks, posing a riddle to which he does not know the answer, and mistaking the lyrics of a well-known nursery rhyme. He reappears as the King's Messenger Hatta (*Looking-glass*, chapters 5,7), who is punished before his trial, indeed even before committing any crime.

Use of mercury in the felt hat industry, as a stiffener of rabbit fur, meant that hatters were liable to mercury poisoning, the neurological consequences of which included sensorimotor peripheral neuropathy, tremor (often circumoral), stomatitis, skin rash, and a neuropsychiatric syndrome characterised by timidity, seclusion, easy blushing, irritability, quarrelsomeness and mood lability (erethism), prompting the simile "as mad as a hatter". As has been noted, Carroll's Mad Hatter displays none of these features of mercury poisoning,[12] and hence use of the term "Mad Hatter's disease" as a synonym for mercury poisoning, as encountered in some publications,[13] may be questioned.

Tenniel's illustration of the Mad Hatter/Hatta is said to resemble one Theophilus Carter, a furniture dealer based near Oxford, who was known to

Dodgson, and known in the locality as the Mad Hatter because he always wore a top hat and was prone to eccentric ideas.

Discussion

It might be argued that these cases simply reflect flights of Carroll's powerful imagination, and that any *post hoc* resemblance to neurological disorders occurs quite by chance, and moreover that any such claim for neurological relevance is deeply anachronistic. Although this is possible, it cannot be doubted that, wittingly or not, Dodgson had some personal interest in neurological phenomena. For example, he had a developmental stammer. Although ordained a deacon, his unwillingness to preach and to progress to holy orders has been attributed to this speech defect. Carroll parodied this in the character of the Dodo ("Do-do-Dodgson"; *Wonderland*, chapters 2,3).

Carroll was a noted mirror writer,[14] penning occasional "looking glass" letters principally to amuse children who corresponded with him. The poem Jabberwocky first appears (*Looking-glass*, chapter 1) mirror reversed, in a Looking-glass book; only by holding it up to the mirror is Alice able to read it. Mirror writing may be associated with stammering, and is much commoner in left handers: Dodgson apparently wrote with his right hand but may originally have been left handed. Moreover, Gardner states that Dodgson was "handsome and asymmetric – two facts that may have contributed to his interest in mirror reflections. One shoulder was higher than the other, his smile was slightly askew, and the level of his blue eyes not quite the same".[15]

Acknowledgment

Adapted from: Larner AJ. Lewis Carroll: an Oxford neurologist? *Oxford Medical School Gazette* 2007;57(2):44–45.

References

1. Butler C (ed.). *Christ Church, Oxford. A portrait of the house.* London: Third Millenium, 2006.
2. Hughes JT. *Thomas Willis 1621–1675. His life and work.* London: Royal Society of Medicine Press, 1991.
3. Larner AJ. A portrait of Richard Lower. *Endeavour* 1987;11:205–208.
4. Todd J. The syndrome of Alice in Wonderland. *Can Med Assoc J* 1955;73:701–704.
5. Lippman CW. Certain hallucinations peculiar to migraine. *J Nerv Ment Dis* 1952;116:346–351.
6. Critchley M. *The citadel of the senses and other essays.* New York: Raven Press, 1986:203.

7. Kew J, Wright A, Halligan PW. Somesthetic aura: the experience of "Alice in Wonderland". *Lancet* 1998;351:1934.
8. Blau JN. Somesthetic aura: the experience of "Alice in Wonderland". *Lancet* 1998;352:582.
9. Podoll K, Robinson D. Lewis Carroll's migraine experiences. *Lancet* 1999;353:1366.
10. Restak RM. Alice in migraineland. *Headache* 2006;46:306–311.
11. Larner AJ. Lewis Carroll's Humpty Dumpty: an early report of prosopagnosia? *J Neurol Neurosurg Psychiatry* 2004;75:1063.
12. Waldron HA. Did the Mad Hatter have mercury poisoning? *BMJ* 1983;287:1961.
13. O'Carroll RE, Masterton G, Dougall N, Ebmeier KP, Goodwin GM. The neuropsychiatric sequelae of mercury poisoning: the Mad Hatter's disease revisited. *Br J Psychiatry* 1995;167:95–98.
14. Schott GD. Mirror writing: Allen's self observations, Lewis Carroll's "looking glass" letters, and Leonardo da Vinci's maps. *Lancet* 1999;354:2158–2161.
15. Gardner M (ed.). *The annotated Alice. The definitive edition.* London: Penguin, 2001:xvi-xvii.

Gustav Nachtigal (1834–1885): contributions to the history of medicine in mid-nineteenth century Africa

Between 1869 and 1874, Dr. Gustav Nachtigal travelled extensively in the interior of northern and central Africa, visiting areas within the modern-day borders of Libya, Niger, Nigeria, Cameroon, Chad, Sudan and Egypt. Throughout this journey, Nachtigal recorded his many experiences and interests, encompassing geography, meteorology, history, ethnography, medicine, linguistics, and more – even feminine hairstyles. His collected data later appeared as a 3–volume travel narrative, *Sahara und Sudan*, translated complete into English over 100 years later.[1]

Nachtigal's continuous medical work within Africa had multiple importance: as a tribute of gratitude to his hosts for a hospitable reception, totally dependent as he was on their goodwill for his safety; as a key to access people even in places where he was distrusted as a Christian or a possible spy; and as a deterrent safeguard, inasmuch as mysterious healing powers, such as he apparently possessed, might imply a corresponding capacity to harm. Nachtigal's medical observations provide insights not only into the medical problems of Europeans travelling in Africa, but also indigenous African medical practices in the pre-colonial era. Little has been written on this aspect of Nachtigal's work.[2]

Biography

Nachtigal was born in Eichstedt, near Stendahl, on 23rd February 1834, the son of a Lutheran pastor who died from tuberculosis when Gustav was only five; a brother, Theodor, also succumbed to this disease. Nachtigal received his medical training in Berlin, Halle, Würzburg (here he was a pupil of Virchow),[3] and Griefswald, qualifying in 1858. Three years later he fell ill with pulmonary haemorrhages, presumably tuberculosis. Fearing the fate of his father and brother, he followed the advice of Professor Niemeyer, one of his teachers at Griefswald, and in 1862 travelled to Algiers (i:230n). About this time, Algeria, under French control and, with regular steamships from Marseilles, was becoming popular with Europeans for holidays and healing.[4] Nachtigal later moved to Tunis, becoming physician to the Bey, as well as an army doctor and interpreter for a Tunisian mission to Europe. He witnessed the calamitous changes in Tunisia between 1863 and 1869, through cholera (part of the fourth world pandemic), typhus, drought, civil strife, and foreign interference (i:4–6).[5]

When Nachtigal was on the point of returning finally to Germany in 1869, his health now fully restored, the opportunity unexpectedly arose to convey gifts from the Prussian King Wilhelm to the Sheikh of Borno (a state beside Lake Chad, in modern day Nigeria) acknowledging the Sheikh's welcome to previous German travellers. Nachtigal left Tripoli in February 1869, shortly before his 35th birthday, on a journey which would last more than 5 years and cover over 10,000 kilometres.[6] He travelled first to Murzuq (southern Libya), where he was delayed awaiting a southbound caravan. Against friends' advice, he undertook an arduous journey to the mountainous region of Tibesti or Tu (northern Chad), the first European to visit this region and return.[7] He received a hostile reception from the people, nearly losing his life, yet still was consulted for medical advice. After returning to Murzuq, he could proceed to his primary objective, Kuka (or Kukawa), capital of Borno, to deliver the royal gifts. From his Kuka base, Nachtigal made further journeys, north-east to Borku (Chad), south to Bagirmi (Cameroon and Chad), before travelling eastwards to the kingdoms of Wadai (Chad) and Darfur (Sudan), eventually reaching Cairo in November 1874.

There were long sedentary periods in various locations, chiefly Murzuq, two visits, altogether nearly nine months, and Kuka, nearly 15 months over three visits. In addition to a detailed, almost day-by-day, account, including many medical details, each of these regions, Fezzan and Borno, has a "climate and diseases" chapter (i:124–143; iii:186–207). Nachtigal saw many patients, he reports 50 per day in Borno (ii:274), and about 1000 patients in Kuka during the rainy season, June to September 1870 (iii:195–196; here Nachtigal mentions substantially limiting his medical work later, to husband both time and medicaments; see also iii:186), and this despite the Bornoans' unwillingness to consult a Christian physician (ii:274). Nachtigal's excellent medical training, and his familiarity with disease in Africa even before his journey, suggests that his medical observations in *Sahara and Sudan* may be largely trusted, although his nineteenth-century diagnostic categories may not entirely coincide with those of today.

Other long halts were less productive medically, whether through extreme isolation in the desert (Borku, over three months), or Nachtigal's own fraught circumstances and illness (with the Bagirmi king, nearly four months), or because the published material appeared posthumously (Abeshr, capital of Wadai, eight months over three visits, and El-Fasher, capital of Darfur, nearly four months).[8]

Illness Experienced

The diverse African environments were not always conducive to European travellers' health, as witnessed by the high mortality rate on early African expeditions.[9] Nachtigal certainly suffered his share of ailments. Coming to North Africa a dying man, he was restored to health, able to withstand the repeated assaults of disease on his travels. These experiences may have profoundly shaped his attitudes to the sick people he encountered: he wrote of experience, information, satisfaction, joy (i:97).

Shortly after arriving in Murzuq in 1869, he noted its unhealthy proximity to marshy ground (i:84). He soon contracted malaria, which dogged him intermittently throughout his African travels (i:131). He used quinine, more curatively than prophylactically (i:132; iii:197–198), carefully withholding a stock for himself (ii:271; iii:196). Once, travelling north of Lake Chad, periodically unconscious through (presumably malarial) fever, Nachtigal faced the desperate prospect of an all-night forced march through potentially hostile territory. When he fell dizzy from his horse, his companions somehow fastened him atop two chests carried by a camel. Seeing "that in spite of this I fell to the ground, and several times pulled the whole load down with me, they were at last, after seven hours of agony, moved by pity to take rest for the night" (ii:326). In the desert, sunburn blistered his feet and shins on more than one occasion (i:197; ii:510).

Inflammation of the eyes ascribed to the effects of sand-laden winds was a common affliction for Nachtigal and his fellow travellers (i:47,65211, 213,215,216,327; ii:42,361,363; iv:106) causing pain, suppuration, and intolerance to light and necessitating bandaging. Rubbing painful eyes might also lead to transmission of diseases of the eyelids and conjunctiva. Antimony powder, or kohol, was used by Nachtigal (and local healers) for the treatment of ophthalmia (i:193,436).

Nachtigal's most serious affliction occurred during the Tibesti journey; the guide lost his way and the party ran out of water. Nachtigal graphically describes progressive dehydration: hoarseness, strangury, feelings of impending death. At the last moment a well was discovered and they were saved (i:223–231). Another close encounter with potentially fatal illness occurred when an intestinal disorder was contracted whilst Nachtigal was held almost a prisoner at the war-camp of the fugitive Bagirmi king (iii:364). Gastrointestinal upsets from unfamiliar food or brackish well water were a recurrent problem.

Illness Observed

Fevers were common, usually from malaria, although typhus, smallpox, and syphilis also occurred. Nachtigal noted variable susceptibility to the effects of fever; for example, during a fever epidemic in Borno in 1870, "northerners" were more affected than locals (ii:270–272; iii:196–198). Inflammation of skin (including leprous ulceration) and eyes was exceptionally common, as were joint problems, respiratory problems, and gastroenterological upsets (diarrhoea and dysentery). However, Nachtigal noted the rarity of cancer of the stomach and liver, and of gastric ulcers (i:135; iii:199). Syphilis was apparently uncommon in Tibesti, but trauma was a frequent cause of morbidity and mortality, despite local surgical skills (i:393). Diseases of the nervous system were the least commonly observed ailments.

Nachtigal frequently encountered leprous conditions, particularly the form called in Arabic baras(s), manifesting as discoloration and atrophy of the skin. He noted their lower frequency in Murzuq, "rarity, or relative absence" in Tibesti, and in Borku they were "almost entirely absent" as compared to the coastal regions. The greatest prevalence of such conditions, however, was observed in Borno, south of the desert. Nachtigal attributed these differences to terrain and, most of all, climate, the hot dry conditions of the desert interior having a protective effect (i:136,391; ii:425; iii:205–206).[10] Further east, in Darfur, Nachtigal mentions two rulers holding power for years despite "the ravages of leprosy"; in one case apparently supernatural punishment – "the vengeance of fate" – for the king's misdeeds (iv:283,305). Only one indigenous remedy for leprosy is mentioned, "carbonised, powdered pig's teeth", in Wadai. Nachtigal's own preferred treatment, apparently successful in two cases, was internal arsenic (iii:206).

A belief in the hereditary nature of tuberculosis was evident in Borno and the desert. This must have had particular resonances for Nachtigal, with his own family history, and perhaps also from his medical training since an hereditary predisposition to tuberculosis had long been suspected; the 18th century nosologist William Cullen (1710–1790) had stated that "phthisis … arising from a hereditary taint is almost certainly fatal".[11] Nachtigal reports "only one case in which the hereditary predisposition was clearly demonstrable … a young woman with galloping consumption, whose mother and seven siblings had perished of phthisis" (iii:199).

Smallpox was encountered in both Fezzan ("not infrequently brought in … from the south by slave caravans") and Borno ("virtually endemic") (i:133 & n.; iii:203). Vaccination was known to the north coast Arabs; from them it had reached Fezzan where it was "sometimes practised", preferably on earlobes or temples. In Borno, it was not even moderately extensively used.

Blindness, frequently as a consequence of inflammatory eye disease, was often encountered, in Fezzan (i:138), Kuka (ii:160), Bornu (iii:201), and Wadai (iv:58). Ritual blinding was a feature of political life in some of the states visited by Nachtigal such as Bagirmi (iii:327,412) and Wadai (iv:174,179).

Indigenous Health Beliefs and Practices

A dichotomy between natural and supernatural ideas of disease causation has been suggested by some medical ethnologists and historians, supernatural ideas being particularly prominent in non-literate societies.[12] The two categories are certainly evident in Nachtigal's observations, but the division is artificial, the two categories forming a continuum for the indigenous populations of mid-nineteenth century Africa.

Hot/cold contrasts, as well as being an integral feature of ancient Greek humoralism, are found in many non-literate societies free of Greek influence, as a system to explain disease causation and treatment without recourse to supernatural agencies. Nachtigal encountered such a system in Fezzan: heat, represented by "the blood", often carried the responsibility for illness, and necessitated treatment of a type different from that for ailments resulting from a "chill". Foods were judged "healthy" or "unhealthy", "hot" or "cold". Accordingly, "if the patient accepts these explanations of his condition, which to him are very clear, he also adopts a treatment which for him is rational, seeks to paralyse the influence of hot food by 'cold', takes 'hot' things against a chill" (i:142). Hence, heat in the form of hot baths or the cautery iron was an appropriate treatment for rheumatism (i:135–136).

The natural treatments most commonly mentioned by Nachtigal are butter and the cautery iron, although he alludes also to plant and mineral remedies. The therapeutic uses of butter, especially melted butter, taken internally or externally, were extensive. Specific uses mentioned by Nachtigal include malaria, syphilis, rheumatism, jaundice, and to promote haemostasis. Rancid butter is mentioned as being particularly salubrious for eye diseases. In Wadai, Nachtigal observed the treatment of the senior eunuch, suffering from a spear thrust penetrating the lung: a small bottle-gourd, holding about an ounce of heated butter, was emptied into the wound, not losing a drop. At the first session, witnessed by Nachtigal, this was done seventeen times; the treatment was repeated every other day. After a death-struggle of nearly four weeks, the eunuch died at last (iv:121,126).

Hardly less popular than butter was the cautery iron: Nachtigal mentions its use in fever, phthisis, lung inflammation, dysentery – where the iron was applied to the buttocks – rheumatism, brain inflammation, and pain in any location. The cautery was used with "barbaric energy" in Tibesti where, butter being scarce, it was often the only available treatment, leaving many Teda people with "innumerable, often colossal, scars" (i;393,308). It is possible that these favoured remedies may reflect the existence of a hot/cold opponent system of disease causation – "cold" as a cause of illness, particularly chronic illness, necessitating "hot" therapy, such as the cautery iron – as seen in pre-industrial societies in Asia and Latin America, and still in modern day Morocco.[13]

Traumatic injuries being so frequent, surgical skills were highly developed in many of the localities Nachtigal visited. For example, surgery was "the most highly developed part of the ... art of healing" in Tibesti, where skin and muscle wounds could be sutured using acacia thorns. More serious bleeding necessitated the cautery iron or boiling butter. In skull fractures, the cerebral membranes were examined if possible: if undamaged, the out-of-line bone parts were cut away; if breached, the prognosis was hopeless and treatment therefore withheld. The Teda could also reduce common dislocations and make light and effective splints to immobilize broken bones (i:393). In Darfur, Nachtigal commented on a local surgeon's setting of a broken bone, "I could not have done better myself" (iv:369–370), an experience contrasting with Livingstone's observation in sub-Saharan Africa shortly before that the "surgical skill of [the] natives [is] at [a] low ebb".[14] Another operation described by Nachtigal several times is childhood uvulectomy, often combined with removal of the first budding eye teeth, performed for hygienic and prophylactic reasons (i:135,393; ii:376,419,449; iii:201). The practice continues in some areas even today.[15] Nachtigal extracted many teeth, ruined by a diet of dates (ii:62,71).

Nachtigal mentions various plant and mineral remedies: henna as an astringent for ulcers and inflammation, incorporated in a poultice for carbuncles, and as an abortifacient; colocynth as a cathartic and in the treatment of syphilis; senna for scabies; tamarind water for smallpox; antimony for ophthalmia. Occasionally there is "a certain prejudice" against particular plants, which are used "with a certain reluctance", for example senna and colocynth, as laxatives, in Fezzan (i:142–143).

Alongside these "natural" remedies, there flourished also "supernatural" treatments, indicating a pluralistic (to Western eyes) system of health beliefs and remedies. Almost all Nachtigal's journey was through states which were, at least nominally, Muslim, affording him many opportunities to learn of indigenous Muslim beliefs about disease causation.[16] In Fezzan, for example, "... it is partly the spirits, jinn [singular jinnii, whence our genie], who are blamed, but the evil eye ... causes still more mischief" (i:142). All diseases of the brain and nervous system were ascribed either to the devil, ibliis, or perhaps more frequently to the jinn (i:140). In Darfur, Sultan Giggeri had an epileptic seizure (in 1682, diagnosis at a time distance) on the first day of his reign, and was immediately replaced: no one "possessed by the devil" might rule (iv:280). Among Pagan tribes south of Bagirmi, "direct diabolic influences are assumed with epileptics, who for this reason are said . . . to be killed" (iii:391). Measures in Fezzan were less drastic: "In the event of epileptic or other seizures, red colours are avoided, the patient is covered with black cloth, and given indigo to smell, and care is taken that no adults come near him" (i:141).

The Borno people believed that all Christians had a supernatural mastery over the powers of nature, which may explain both their willingness to consult Nachtigal over medical matters and their reluctance to accept medicines from him (ii:273–275). The power to heal could also be used to do harm: when Lamino, a senior Borno official, and friend and patient of Nachtigal, died, Nachtigal feared lest he be blamed for the death (ii:300 & n.,168n.). In Tibesti, his arrival was expected to precipitate "some frightful public calamity, perhaps a disastrous natural catastrophe, a devastating pestilence or a general cattle epidemic" (i:312). Nachtigal was blamed for drought in Wadai (iv:78; ii:270 & n.; see also iii:20). The heal/harm interplay applied also to treatments: both the cautery and boiling butter were used for the barbaric practice of ritual blinding as well as for therapeutic purposes.[17]

To counter malevolent supernatural forces, the recourse was to religion, especially to the healing power of the Qur'an. Sacred texts in small leather bags or pouches were worn about the neck, arms or turban, as amulets or talismans. During the 1870 fever epidemic in Borno (probably malaria), more of these amulets were worn, and public prophylactic recitations of the Qur'an were held (ii:271–272 & n.; see also ii:297). Aside from prophylaxis, amulets might also be a fashion statement; in Fezzan men wore them "certainly as much to decorate their persons as to give them protection against sorcery, sickness and wounds" (i:210; see also iv:65 referring to women in Wadai). Qur'an texts could be written on sick people's skin, or "administered" internally in water used to elute verses from a wooden slate (i:393–394). Such activities required literacy: the fuqahaa – literally those skilled in jurisprudence, but also commonly applied to more limited intellectual achievement, for instance any man succeeding in reading the Qur'an once – made a living providing therapeutic Qur'an formulae. Nachtigal himself was once asked for one (iii:274; see also iii:230). Perhaps because of the cost entailed in employing a faqiih, it seems from Nachtigal's accounts that supernatural remedies such as these were only called upon when simpler natural remedies, knowledge of which could be handed down from generation to generation, had failed. Sacrifices in times of sickness or to avoid sickness were mentioned in Darfur, but Nachtigal believed these to be a throwback to pagan times. The continuing use of Qur'an verses in amulets, written on the skin, and in slate water[18] and of a hot/cold opponent system[13] is indicative of their continuing utility in African societies as explanatory and therapeutic systems.

Conclusion

Nachtigal's contribution to the exploration and understanding of Africa was recognized in his own lifetime with the award of the Gold Medal of the Royal Geographical Society of London in 1882. Soon after his untimely death, at sea off the West African coast in 1885, Nachtigal was described by Kumm, another traveller, as "without doubt one of the most, fruitful African explorer[s]",[19] or even himself the most fruitful. In recent decades, however, Nachtigal has been in eclipse. His birthplace, in what was East Germany, has been neglected.[20] His reputation in Communist eyes was undermined by the last year of his life when he helped represent Germany in the colonial scramble for Africa.[21] His masterpiece *Sahara und Sudan* was finally fully translated into English only in 1987, almost exactly a century after the final, posthumous volume of the original German. A reappraisal of his contribution to the understanding of Africa in general, and of its medical culture in particular, is certainly overdue.

Sahara and Sudan provides a wealth of detail on many subjects, including medicine. The illustrations given above, only a fraction of the total, may indicate the potential utility of travel narratives in elucidating medical history. Clearly they are far from ideal sources, neither comprehensive nor systematic, tending to be incidental, opportunistic, hampered by the inadequacy of informants and by the limitations of the authors' own interests – for instance, Nachtigal reports very little about organized religion (though he discussed it often with his African acquaintances), which clearly overlapped significantly with the wider healing enterprise. However, in the absence of significant indigenous records, travellers' accounts may provide some insights.[22] Doctors' accounts may be peculiarly useful: not only were they interested in medical problems, and carefully trained as scientific observers, but they could also, through their medical skills, achieve privileged access to indigenous peoples; witness Nachtigal's access to people, attending for medical advice even in Tibesti where his life was in jeopardy. A doctor who knew the local languages, paid heed to local customs, adopted practical local dress, and lived for months, even years, as a European on his own, in the closest proximity to local people, was particularly well placed to learn of the lives of indigenous peoples, and hence to enlighten our studies even today.

Acknowledgments

Adapted from: Larner AJ, Fisher HJ. Dr. Gustav Nachtigal (1834–1885): a contribution to the history of medicine in mid-nineteenth century Africa. *J Med Biogr* 2000;8:43–48; and Larner AJ. Ophthalmological observations made during the mid-19th-century European encounter with Africa. *Arch Ophthalmol* 2004;122:267–272.

References

1. Nachtigal G. *Sahara und Sudan.* Three volumes, 1879–1889. English translation by Fisher AGB, Fisher HJ. *Sahara and Sudan.* Four volumes, 1971–1987, London, Christopher Hurst. All references to Nachtigal's writing are to this translation.
2. Fisher AGB, Fisher HJ. A Christian amongst Muslims: Nachtigal in Muslim black Africa. In: Ganslmayr H (ed.). *Gedenkschrift Gustav Nachtigal 1874–1974.* Bremen, 1977:14–32 [especially 28–30]; Fisher HJ. A doctor in nineteenth century Africa. *Oxford Medical School Gazette* 1985;36(3):13–15.
3. Ackerknecht EH. *Rudolf Virchow: doctor, statesman, anthropologist.* Madison: University of Wisconsin Press, 1953:232. See also Nachtigal, iii:xvii & n.
4. See, for example, Knox AA. *The new playground, or wanderings in Algeria.* London, 1881. Knox was there 1879–1880 (476). He mentions "the almost interminable books about Algeria" (482); also the "remarkable discovery" by "the French scientific men", that the Algerine climate is "prejudicial, if not fatal to Germans . . . A delicate German will pine and die there" (111). Happily, Nachtigal was apparently indelicate. See also Curtin PD. *Death by migration: Europe's encounter with the tropical world in the nineteenth century.* Cambridge: Cambridge University Press, 1989:76–77,87 (Table 4.2b),140–143, showing significantly higher tuberculosis death rates among European troops in France than in North Africa.
5. Gallagher NE. *Medicine and power in Tunisia 1780–1900.* Cambridge: Cambridge University Press, 1983:passim. Gallagher (124) says that Nachtigal departed for the Sudan "because of the famine and cholera of 1867"; the actual reason for the Sudan departure, as we shall see in a moment was more positive; and one biography (Wiese J. *Gustav Nachtigal.* Berlin, 1914:29–30) reports Nachtigal returning to Tunis from a short European visit precisely because of new outbreaks of illness in Tunis.
6. For a brief journey summary, see Fisher AGB, Fisher HJ. Nachtigal's companions. *Paideuma* 1987;33:231–262.
7. Tibesti remains inaccessible for the Western traveller even today; see *The Independent* 1997;29 November.
8. For further biographical details on Nachtigal, see Wiese, 1914:passim.
9. Livingstone D. On fever in the Zambesi. *Lancet* 1861;ii:184–186; Coupland R. *Kirk on the Zambesi: a chapter of African history.* Oxford, Clarendon Press,

1928; Cook GC. Doctor David Livingstone FRS (1813–1873): "the fever" and other medical problems of mid-nineteenth century Africa. *J Med Biogr* 1994;2:33–43.

10. Iliffe J. *The African poor: a history.* Cambridge: Cambridge University Press, 1987:215, reports that "in the 19th century leprosy sufferers were excluded from Kukawa, the capital of Bornu". Nachtigal does not mention such exclusion, though he lived in Kukawa for more than a year, and emphasises the frequency of leprosy in Borno, where, he adds, lepers are not "excluded from human society, but . . . are avoided as much as possible" (iii:206).
11. Quoted in Bynum WF. *Science and the practice of medicine in the nineteenth century.* Cambridge: Cambridge University Press, 1994:23; the belief in a hereditary predisposition to tuberculosis was still widely emphasised even after Koch's discovery of the tubercle bacillus in 1882; see Bynum, 1994:131.
12. For examples, see Ullmann M. *Islamic medicine.* Edinburgh, Edinburgh University Press, 1978:1–10; Gallagher, 1983:7–9; Abdalla IH. Diffusion of Islamic medicine into Hausaland. In: Feierman S, Janzen JM (eds.). *The social basis of health and healing in Africa.* Berkeley, University of California Press, 1992:177,180–185; Greenwood B. Cold or spirits? Ambiguity and syncretism in Moroccan therapeutics. *Ibid.*, 286–295.
13. Greenwood, 1992:285–314.
14. Cook, 1994:38.
15. For modern accounts of uvulectomy, see Maclean U. *Magical medicine: a Nigerian case study.* London, 1971:65ff; and Einterz EM, Einterz RM, Bates ME. Traditional uvulectomy in northern Cameroon. *Lancet* 1994;343:1644.
16. See also Fisher HJ. Hassebu: Islamic healing in black Africa. In: Brett M (ed.). *Northern Africa: Islam and modernization.* London, Frank Cass, 1973:23–47.
17. Butter is specified in Bagirmi (iii:411–412), a hot iron in Wadai (iv:174–175), where this task is entrusted to the chief of the blacksmiths, who, in a startling instance of the healing/harming conundrum, "must be well-read in the Qur'an", and is "the physician for the whole royal family", in which capacity he is permitted to enter the royal harem (iv:179). Mistrusted brothers, and sometimes other relatives too, potential rivals to a newly installed ruler, were regularly blinded, in one eye or both, in several of the states Nachtigal visited. Prospective victims, of course, often sought safety in flight.
18. For modern accounts, see Greene G. *Journey without maps.* London, 1936 (reprinted Harmondsworth, Penguin, 1978:109); Lamarque L. *Recherches historiques sur la médecine dans la régence d'Alger.* Algiers, 1951:120–122; Buck AA, Anderson RI, Sasaki TT, Kawata K. *Health and disease in Chad: epidemiology, culture and environment in five villages.* Baltimore, Johns Hopkins Press, 1970:55.
19. Kumm HKW. *From Hausaland to Egypt.* London, 1910:2.
20. Fisher HJ. A pilgrimage in honour of a forgotten German. *Frankfurter Allgemeine*, 1996;19 September [in German].
21. Büttner T, Loth H. *Geschichte Afrikas.* East Berlin, 1976;i:284,310; ii:19.

22. LI Conrad makes a similar suggestion regarding Bedouin Arab medicine in the accounts of 19th and 20th century travellers in Arabia in his chapter on Arab-Islamic medicine. In: Bynum WF, Porter R (eds.). *Companion Encyclopedia of the History of Medicine.* London: Routledge, 1993:676–727 [especially 686,720–721 & n43).

Clifford Allbutt (1836–1925): an early account of neuromyelitis optica

The many achievements of Sir Thomas Clifford Allbutt (1836–1925) as a clinician, teacher, administrator, medical historian, pioneer of the pocket-sized thermometer, and long-serving Regius Professor of Physic in the University of Cambridge[1] are still acknowledged more than 80 years after his death, but his neurological contributions may be less familiar.

To be sure, Bearn states in his monograph on Allbutt that he had an "early interest in neurology"[1] fostered by the neuropathologist Jacob Lockhart Clarke (1817–1880) at St George's Hospital in London where Allbutt trained, and augmented by studies in Paris in the 1860s under G.B.A. Duchenne de Boulogne and, briefly, Charcot. He is also generally credited, along with William Gowers, with pioneering the use of the ophthalmoscope, first described by Hermann von Helmholtz in 1851,[2] in the United Kingdom. Indeed he wrote a monograph on the subject of ophthalmoscopy which included accounts of its use in diseases of the nervous system.[3] This familiarity with ophthalmoscopy facilitated what may possibly be the single neurological first accruing to Allbutt: the description of the syndrome now adumbrated by the term neuromyelitis optica.

In a paper entitled "On the ophthalmoscopic signs of spinal disease", published in the *Lancet* of 15th January 1870, Allbutt reported:

> Of acute myelitis I have examined five cases, and in 1 only did eye disorder supervene. This remarkable case was of very long duration, and was followed by partial recovery; in it sympathetic disorder of the eye came on many weeks (twelve or thirteen weeks at least) after the subsidence of the acuter symptoms.[4]

These brief details, later characterised as indicative of optic nerve oedema in the course of acute myelitis,[5] were thus given merely in passing, the rest of the paper being concerned with accounts of the ophthalmoscopic changes seen in cases of spinal injury and chronic degenerations of the cord, including "locomotor ataxy" (presumably syphilitic), along with speculations about the relationship of concurrent spinal and ophthalmic disorder.

At the time of this publication, Allbutt was physician to the Leeds Infirmary, in Yorkshire in the north of England, an appointment which he had held since 1864. As he originated from nearby Dewsbury, this local connection may have prompted his return to the north from London following his training. He remained in Leeds until 1889, then becoming a Commissioner in Lunacy, an appointment facilitated by his friendship with James Crichton Browne (1840–1938), then superintendent of the West Riding Pauper Lunatic Asylum in Wakefield, Yorkshire. Following the death of Sir George Paget in 1892, Allbutt was offered the Regius Chair in Physic in Cambridge which he eventually accepted. A prolonged battle ensued before he was elected as physician to Addenbrooke's Hospital in Cambridge in 1900.[1] Perhaps the most outstanding of his many achievements during these years was editing the eight-volume textbook *System of Medicine* published between 1896 and 1899, three volumes of which were devoted to diseases of the nervous system. He also had a keen interest in the history of medicine, writing particularly on Greek and Roman medicine.[1]

It was in 1894, nearly a quarter of a century after Allbutt's *Lancet* paper, that Eugène Devic (1858–1930), working in Lyon, France, reported a further similar case, with pathological examination of the cord and optic nerves demonstrating demyelination and necrosis with some cellular infiltration. Along with Fernand Gault, his doctoral student, he also reviewed sixteen other cases previously reported in the literature.[5,6] However, Allbutt's paper was not among these citations. Devic termed this disorder "neuro-myélite optique", but a consequence of this work was that eponymous fame devolved upon him, with the term Devic's disease ("maladie de Devic") being proposed in 1907 by Acchiote.[5]

This formulation did not subsequently meet with universal approval. In particular, Macdonald Critchley (1900–1997) had reservations, such that he included the condition in an essay on "mythical maladies of the nervous system":

> The theme of neuromythology could be extended considerably to include some other syndromes that have been described but where growing doubts lead to an attitude of scepticism short, however, of frank disavowal. In such a batch belong Devic's disease ...[7]

Critchley was wise to leave the door partly open, since the passage of time has confirmed the pathophysiological distinctness of Devic's disease. This disorder is now universally known as neuromyelitis optica (NMO), an inflammatory demyelinating disorder of the central nervous system associated with antibodies to aquaporin-4 and amenable to immunosuppressant treatment with agents such as azathioprine, mycophenolate and rituximab to prevent relapses.[8]

In his monograph, Bearn discusses Allbutt's contributions to ophthalmoscopy[1] but remarkably fails to mention the 1870 *Lancet* paper with the first presumed report of neuromyelitis optica, this despite the fact that many articles on Devic's disease acknowledge Allbutt's precedence. Though brief, Allbutt's account, quoted above, indicates a condition characterised by successive involvement of the spinal cord, with only partial recovery, and optic nerve, and the possible linkage of the two is implied by the description of the latter as a "sympathetic disorder". Certainly the features described would be consistent with current clinical criteria for neuromyelitis optica. Perhaps "Allbutt's NMO" is as good a term as "Devic's NMO" and has the advantage of being historically correct. That said, there are a number of earlier reports in the medical literature of cases which have attracted retrospective diagnoses of NMO.[9–11] Of particular note is that one of these reports was from Jacob Lockhart Clarke,[9] Allbutt's early mentor. It would be intriguing to know if Allbutt was aware of this publication (as would seem likely) or may even have seen the patient described, either event perhaps sensitizing him to the observation of a further case.

Acknowledgment

Adapted from: Jacob A, Larner AJ. Clifford Allbutt (1836–1925). *J Neurol* 2013;260:346–347.

References

1. Bearn AG. *Sir Clifford Allbutt. Scholar and physician.* London: Royal College of Physicians, 2007.
2. Larner AJ. Hermann Ludwig Ferdinand von Helmholtz (1821–1894). *Eye (Lond)* 1994;8:717.
3. Allbutt TC. *On the use of the ophthalmoscope in diseases of the nervous system and of the kidneys and also in certain general disorders.* London: Macmillan and Co., 1871.
4. Allbutt TC. On the ophthalmoscopic signs of spinal disease. *Lancet* 1870;1:76–78.
5. Miyazawa I, Fujihara K, Itoyama Y. Eugene Devic (1858–1930). *J Neurol* 2002;249:351–352.
6. Devic E. Myélite subaiguë compliquée de névrite optique. *Bull Med* 1894;8:1033–1034.
7. Critchley M. *The citadel of the senses and other essays.* New York: Raven Press, 1986:87.
8. Jacob A, McKeon A, Nakashima I et al. Current concepts of neuromyelitis optica (NMO) and NMO spectrum disorders. *J Neurol Neurosurg Psychiatry* 2013; 84: 922–930.
9. Jarius S, Wildemann B. An early case of neuromyelitis optica: on a forgotten report by Jacob Lockhart Clarke, FRS. *Mult Scler* 2011;17:1384–1386.

10. Jarius S, Wildemann B. "Noteomielite" accompanied by acute amaurosis (1844). An early case of neuromyelitis optica. *J Neurol Sci* 2012;313:182–184.
11. Jarius S, Wildemann B. An early British case of neuromyelitis optica (1850). *BMJ* 2012;345:e6430.

Richard Caton (1842–1926): the beginnings of electroencephalography

Richard Caton was brought up in Yorkshire and trained in medicine in Edinburgh. He came to Liverpool in the late 1860s, and by the 1870s, as a Lecturer in Physiology, had embarked on experimental work recording the electrical currents of the cerebral cortex in dogs and apes using unipolar electrodes and the string galvanometer.[1–5]

On 21st January 1875 Caton delivered a paper to the Liverpool Medical Society entitled "On the Electrical Relations of Muscle and Nerve" which drew on the work of the celebrated German physiologist Emil Du Bois-Reymond (1818–1896) to demonstrate the properties of a frog nerve-muscle preparation.[6] This presentation may have been made at the Liverpool Medical Institution (LMI), where, in addition to his other activities related to Liverpool medicine, he was certainly an active member.[7] Caton's report seems a little incongruous in the proceedings, following as it does an exhibit by Dr Michael Harris of two fetuses completely joined at the thorax and abdomen, an exhibit by Mr AMS Hamilton of a stomach and oesophagus, the latter obstructed by a fibrous stricture, and a case narrated by Dr Glynn of an aneurism [*sic*] of the second part of the aorta pressing on the left bronchus.

Later in the same year (4th August 1875), Caton presented data at the 43rd British Medical Association meeting, held in Edinburgh, on "The Electric Currents of the Brain", an entirely more original piece of work. It is probable he would have preferred to present his work at the Royal Society, as a more appropriate forum for such "cutting edge" scientific research, but this did not happen. The choice of Edinburgh may perhaps have been because his funding was a grant from the British Medical Association. His presentation made little impact on his clinical audience: it is all too easy to imagine the bewilderment of clinicians listening to his presentation, and perhaps wondering what electrodes in animal brains had to do with medical practice. Moreover, animal experimentation had caused controversy at the BMA meeting of the previous year when the French neurologist Valentin Magnan showed the effects of absinthe on two dogs, provoking a prosecution.[8]

Caton's experimental work was subsequently published in the *British Medical Journal* in 1875,[9] (the *Journal of Physiology*, an altogether more suitable outlet, was not founded until 1878) in a paper later characterised by Danilevsky as "distinguished by its unwarranted brevity", and in 1877.[10] These papers mark the beginnings of the study of electroencephalography (EEG), which after many trials and various insights[11] was to reach clinical fruition in 1924 with the first recording of the human EEG by Hans Berger (1873–1941) in Jena, who acknowledged the importance of Caton's work.[12]

It is perhaps worth quoting from Caton's 1875 paper to give a flavour of his work, and his discoveries:

> In every brain hitherto examined, the galvanometer has indicated the existence of electric currents. The external surface of the grey matter is usually positive in relation to the surface of a section through it. Feeble currents of varying direction pass through the multiplier when the electrodes are placed on two points of the external surface, or one electrode on the grey matter, and one on the surface of the skull.

The possible functional significance of these currents was also alluded to. In the 1877 paper, the effects of sleep and death on the currents was also examined. The experimental technique was difficult, with more than half of the animals examined proving to be failures because of factors such as brain swelling and haemorrhage.

Caton was appointed Professor of Physiology in Liverpool in 1884, and in 1887 presented his work at the 9th International Congress of Medicine in Washington, D.C.[13] However, in 1891 he resigned the chair, not before persuading the local magnate George Holt to endow a full-time chair in physiology, and thereafter undertook no further work on the brain. (Holt also endowed a chair in pathology, in 1894. His bronze relief may be seen on the stairs between the 1st and 2nd floors of the Victoria Art Gallery and Museum in Liverpool.)

Caton's clinical interests in later years were more in the realm of cardiology, writing on rheumatic fever and its treatment, as well as in medical history: his Harveian Oration of 1904 combined the two.[14,15] He also became more involved with medical and local politics, serving as President of the LMI in 1896–7 and as Lord Mayor of Liverpool in 1907–8. A splendid portrait of him in mayoral garb hangs at the LMI. Posthumously a ward was named for him at the Walton Centre for Neurology and Neurosurgery, the regional neuroscience centre in Liverpool. Perhaps surprisingly his various contributions did not merit his inclusion in the *Dictionary of National Biography* (2004).

Acknowledgment

Adapted from: Larner AJ. Some Liverpool contributions to neurology and medicine. *Medical Historian* 2008–2009;20:79–84.

References

1. Lord Cohen of Birkenhead. Richard Caton (1842–1926) Pioneer Electrophysiologist. *Proc R Soc Med* 1959;52:645–650.
2. Schoenberg BS. Richard Caton and the electrical activity of the brain. *Mayo Clin Proc* 1974;49:474–481.
3. Haas LF. Hans Berger (1873–1941), Richard Caton (1842–1926), and electroencephalography. *J Neurol Neurosurg Psychiatry* 2003;74:9.
4. Ormerod W. Richard Caton (1842–1926): pioneer electrophysiologist and cardiologist. *J Med Biogr* 2006;14:30–35.
5. Sykes AH. Dr Richard Caton (1842–1926): Medicine, education and civic affairs in Liverpool. *Medical Historian* 2010–2011;22:11–27.
6. Caton R. On the Electrical Relations of Muscle and Nerve. *Liverpool and Manchester Medical and Surgical Reports* 1876;4:274–275.
7. Shepherd JA. *A History of the Liverpool Medical Institution.* Liverpool: Liverpool Medical Institution, 1979: 146,151,153,170,171,172,185,189.
8. Snow SJ. *Blessed days of anaesthesia. How anaesthetics changed the world.* Oxford: Oxford University Press, 2008:157.
9. Caton R. The Electric Currents of the Brain. *Br Med J* 1875;ii:278.
10. Caton R. Interim report on investigation of the electric currents of the brain. *Br Med J* 1877;Supplement:62.
11. Brazier MAB. *A history of the electrical activity of the brain. The first half-century.* London: Pitman, 1961.
12. Chancellor A. Electroencephalography: maturing gracefully. *Pract Neurol* 2009;9:130–132.
13. Caton R. Researches on electrical phenomena of cerebral grey matter. *Ninth International Congress Medicine* 1887;3:246–249.
14. Caton R. 1. The medicine and the medicine God of the Egyptians: contemporary views of the circulation. 2. Prevention in valvular disease. *Lancet* 1904;i:1769–1772.
15. Lord Cohen of Birkenhead. The Liverpool Medical School and its physicians (1642–1934). *Med Hist* 1972;16:310–320 [at 317–318].

Robert Lawson (ca.1846–1896): alcoholic amnesia before Korsakoff

Various descriptions of what would now be called Korsakoff Syndrome may be found in the medical literature predating the eponymous reports of Sergei Korasakoff (1854–1900) which date from 1887 onwards. Of these, it has been stated that the "most promising account"[1] may be that of Dr Robert Lawson, published in 1878 in the journal *Brain* in its inaugural year of publication.[2] As Lawson is likely to be an unfamiliar name to most neurologists, and does not appear in the *Oxford Dictionary of National Biography*, this brief account of his life and work is offered.

At the time of his paper in *Brain*, Lawson was working as Medical Superintendent of the Wonford House Lunatic Hospital in Exeter in the County of Devon in the south west of England. Opened in 1869, Wonford House succeeded the St Thomas Hospital for Lunatics of 1801, by then too small, both institutions dating their origin to a bequest of £200 made in 1795 to build a lunatic ward at the Devon and Exeter Hospital. Further funds were later made available through William Buller (1735–1796), Bishop of Exeter (1792–1796), in order to build a separate lunatic asylum. According to Lawson's obituary, his appointment in Exeter was only for a "short time".[3] The *Medical Directory* for 1879 (accessed Liverpool Medical Institution, 23/07/2010) records Lawson as Deputy Commissioner in Lunacy for Scotland, the post in which he died in 1896 after 18 years of service, and does not mention Exeter at all.

Despite this provincial appointment, Lawson's academic credentials were sound. Born at Kirriemuir in Scotland, the son of a draper according to the 1851 Census records (viewed online 16/09/2011), he was an Edinburgh graduate (1871) and, according to the *Medical Directory* for 1879, "Asst. to Prof. of Pract. of Med. and Med. Psychol. Univ. Edin. 1871–72", namely Thomas Laycock (1812–1876), a major figure in the development of ideas about cerebral reflexes.[4] Professor Laycock selected Lawson as his "class assistant for 1871–2 and imbued him with the shrewd and original thinking for which the chair of medicine was then celebrated".[3] After "practising for a short time in London", Lawson was appointed in 1874 as Assistant Medical Officer to the West Riding Pauper Lunatic Asylum in Wakefield, in Yorkshire in the north of England, an institution then under the direction of James Crichton Browne (1840–1938).[5] Here, Lawson investigated the use of hyoscyamine, reporting good results in recurrent, acute and subacute mania, monomania of suspicion and the excitement of senile dementia, and even reporting cures of patients with chronic mania and often with chronic alcoholism, finding that hyoscyamine worked where bromide of potassium and tincture of cannabis had failed.[6]

Interestingly, before his move to the West Riding Pauper Lunatic Asylum, Crichton Browne had worked as an assistant physician in asylums in Exeter under John Charles Bucknill (1817–1897), one of the founding editors of *Brain*. These connections may possibly help to explain why Lawson sent his paper, "On the symptomatology of alcoholic brain disorders",[2] to this nascent journal of neurology. The patients reported on were from London and York, consistent with Lawson's "short time" in Exeter. Towards the end of this paper, Lawson states:

> There is another well-pronounced class of cases which owe their origin to excess in alcoholic drinks, and which possess some interesting features. In this class the patients … generally bring with them a history of excessive drinking suddenly abandoned. The feature of such cases which is sufficiently striking to give character to them is the almost absolute loss of memory for recent events. The patients … show little dementia as far as simple processes of reasoning are concerned, but are absolutely destitute of memory for passing events. When the medical officer makes his visit (perhaps the third in the course of the day), and asks, "Have you seen me before?" the patient asserts that he or she has not; and the constant and ineffectual repetition of this question at short intervals, shows that the capability of retaining new impressions has completely disappeared. (ref 2, pp191–192).

This is a clear description of the amnesic syndrome. Lawson acknowledged there may be other causes of such a "complete failure of memory", citing a case in which the "exciting cause was the shock produced on the patient by the death of her husband". He also distinguished these cases from those with dementia, since the "patients are not dirty in their habits, sometimes employ themselves, are interested in immediate impressions, but retain no recollection of recent experiences".[2]

Once Lawson was established in Scotland in 1878, his publications largely ceased, no doubt because of the onerous role he had undertaken: "… his work led him to the most remote parts of Scotland, where he had to visit and report upon the boarded-out cases of lunacy", producing annual reports which gave "graphic accounts of his journeyings".[3] Lawson's obituary states that he "early showed a marked literary capacity" and also described him as "illumined by intimate acquaintance with the master minds of literature".[3] These facts may explain his 1880 publication on the epilepsy of Othello,[7] wherein he seems happy to accept Iago's account that the Moor "has fallen into an epilepsy" (*Othello*, IV;i:50), Shakespeare's only use of the word "epilepsy". In this interpretation, Lawson is followed by several modern (non-neurological) commentators,[8,9] although the description of the circumstances of Othello's collapse and his rapid recovery to resume his argument with Iago may be thought to point more towards a diagnosis of syncope than epileptic seizure.[10] Of note, Bucknill also apparently thought Iago's statement "a mere falsehood" (ref 7, p3).

Robert Lawson thus merits remembrance for his lucid description of an amnesic syndrome related to excessive alcohol consumption, although thorough accounts of its pathology and pathogenesis related to thiamine deficiency lay many years in the future.

Acknowledgment

Adapted from: Larner AJ, Garner-Thorpe C. Robert Lawson (?1846–1896). *J Neurol* 2012;259:792–793.

References

1. Draaisma D. *Disturbances of the mind.* Cambridge: Cambridge University Press, 2009:163–164.
2. Lawson R. On the symptomatology of alcoholic brain disorders. *Brain* 1878;1:182–194.
3. Anonymous. Dr Robert Lawson. *J Mental Sci* 1896;42:474.
4. Leff A. Thomas Laycock and the cerebral reflex: a function arising from and pointing to the unity of nature. *Hist Psychiatry* 1991;2:385–407.
5. Jellinek EH. Sir James Crichton-Browne (1840–1938): pioneer neurologist and scientific drop-out. *J R Soc Med* 2005;98:428–430.
6. Lawson R. On the physiological actions of hyoscyamine. *West Riding Pauper Lunatic Asylum Medical Reports* 1875;5:40–84.
7. Lawson R. The epilepsy of Othello. *J Mental Sci* 1880;26:1–11.
8. Heaton KW. Faints, fits and fatalities from emotion in Shakespeare's characters: survey of the canon. *BMJ* 2006;333:1335–1338.
9. Stirling J. *Representing epilepsy. Myth and matter.* Liverpool: Liverpool University Press, 2010:4.
10. Larner AJ. Has Shakespeare's Iago deceived again? http://bmj.com/cgi/eletters/333/7582/1335, 2 January 2007.

Charles Clouston (1847–1883) and Francis Kilvert

A number of doctors are mentioned in the diary of Francis Kilvert (1840–1879) covering the period 1870–1879. Some of these are included in Tony O'Brien's magnum opus *Who's who in Kilvert's Diary*,[1] both those personally known to Kilvert (Dr Peter Giles, p.86) and those known only by reputation (Sir Henry Thompson, p.30; Sir William Jenner, p.72–73). The omission of Dr David Livingstone (1813–1873), whose link with Kilvert's diary has been noted,[2] is a little surprising. As befitting his pastoral role as a clergyman, Kilvert's diary entries sometimes noted illness in his parishioners.[3]

However, another, more serious, omission from O'Brien's work, is that of Dr Clouston. O'Brien mentions Kilvert's longstanding "neuralgia", possibly a form of periodic headache and facial pain disorder known as cluster headache,[4,5] in the context of his visits to his dentist, Charles Gaine, but has nothing to say on Dr Clouston. In July 1872 Kilvert suffered one of his episodic bouts of pain, and wrote a note asking Clouston to come. After a sleepless night (7th-8th July 1872), Kilvert changed the wording of his note, "begging the doctor to come as soon as possible" but as he gave this missive to the postboy the pain resolved (in Kilvert's words, the "abscess broke", although there are no grounds for believing that this was the correct diagnosis), and the note was not sent (Diary, volume II:234). Things must have been very bad to prompt the writing of this note, since Kilvert seems to have eschewed medical intervention for his neuralgia. He was ready to resort to self-help measures (including alcohol consumption) for this problem, but seems to have been unwilling to bother the doctor, a possibility which may be exemplified by the fact that he did not seek help from Dr Clouston even when he saw him in the town of Hay-on-Wye on the same day, 6th December 1871, that he was having symptoms (II:94).

Another professional activity in which we see Clouston is mentioned in Kilvert's diary entry for 14th April 1870. John Watkins of the Cwm was, according to Kilvert, "a good deal more crazed lately wandering about the country and scarcely master of himself". Watkins was attended by Clouston, who "thought him a case for the [Abergavenny] Asylum from the wildness of his talk" but Watkins managed to slip the net, appearing normal when seen by Trumper the magistrate.[6]

Clouston was perhaps a friend or at least an acquaintance of Kilvert's since he is one of the dinner guests on 14th November 1871. On 7th February 1872 a lady mistook Kilvert for Dr Clouston, who "begged her not to regard the matter as I was used to being mistaken for Dr Clouston" (II:134), so presumably the latter was bearded.

What more is known of Dr Clouston? Besides Kilvert's diary, the sources are rather limited, and include appearances in the *Medical Directory* (the annual list of medical practitioners licensed to practice medicine by the General Medical Council, the statutory body charged since 1858 with oversight of the nation's doctors) and an obituary in the *British Medical Journal*,[7] as well as publications by Clouston himself,[8,9] and various internet entries related to genealogy. In the *Medical Directory* of 1871 (accessed Liverpool Medical Institution, 13/07/2010) one finds reference on page 328 to "CLOUSTON, CHAS. STEWART, Hay, Breconsh.", undoubtedly Kilvert's man, the entry noting that he was a graduate of the University of Edinburgh and also held the post of Medical Officer to the Radnorshire District Hay Union ("the workhouse").

Charles Stewart Clouston was born at Sandwick in Orkney, on 28th May 1847. He was the fifth child and third son of the Reverend Charles Clouston, LLD (1800–1884), a Minister in the Church of Scotland at the parish of Sandwick, and Margaret Clouston. Clouston's obituary states that his father was "now the venerable father of the Church of Scotland, and the oldest member of the College of Surgeons of Edinburgh".[7] The Medical Register confirms that Clouston senior gained the Licentiate Diploma of the Royal College of Surgeons of Edinburgh (RCSEd) in 1819, when aged 19, qualifying him to practice "the arts of anatomy, physiology and surgery". At the time of his son's death, Clouston senior was 83 years old, and therefore quite possibly the eldest living member of the RCSEd. Clouston junior studied medicine at the University of Edinburgh, qualifying MB, CM in 1868, but never became a Licentiate of the RCSEd like his father.

Clouston's obituary states that following graduation he "first went to Hay".[7] This was presumably to build up a practice, but in addition his income would have been supplemented by appointment to the post of "Medical Officer to the Radnorshire District Hay Union", the local workhouse. The Hay Poor Law Union dated to 1836, shortly after the introduction of the New Poor Law of 1834, and represented 25 constituent parishes, eleven in the county of Brecon (including two in Hay), five in the county of Hereford (including Bredwardine), and nine in the county of Radnor (including Clyro). In Hay, Clouston "built up a practice, as large as he could possibly overtake, and was universally esteemed as a man and as a physician".[7] His marriage to Emma Traill (1848–1916), in July 1875 at St Andrews, Fife, presumably indicates that he was earning a sufficient income to support a wife and family. Clouston's paternal grandmother was born Traill, so there may have been a family connection to his wife. Emma was the daughter of William Traill MD.

From Hay, Clouston "removed to Gunnersbury, London", but the date is not specified in the obituary other than as "a few years ago",[7] hence the date of his departure from Hay is unclear. The Medical Register of 1880 gives his address as 2 Marlborough Road, Gunnersbury, Chiswick, so he must have moved before 1880. He does not appear amongst the Hay workhouse staff listed in the 1881 Census, but as the Medical Officer was a non-resident post this does not particularly help.

Clouston "did not rest contented with relying on former rules of practice, but made accurate observations for himself on many subjects", perhaps an indication that he had "inherited his father's scientific tastes".[7] Evidence of this may be found in the two papers he published in *The Practitioner* (*A Journal of Therapeutics and Public Health*) in 1882, both entitled "On the salicylate treatment of rheumatism",[8,9] and subtitled as his graduation (MD) thesis to the Medical Faculty of the University of Edinburgh in 1881. The papers detail 27 cases of "subacute articular rheumatism" treated with salicylate. Clouston noted that the severity of pain was much lessened after about five or six hourly doses of 10–12 grains of salicylate, with resolution of pain in 2–4 days, with reduction in elevated body temperature (pyrexia) and heart rate (tachycardia). A noted side effect of salicylate treatment was tinnitus (ringing in the ears), "like the sound of a train or like machinery at work". Clouston recommended hourly salicylate treatment "till pain is relieved, or singing in the ears comes on".

A number of unknowns are to be noted with these publications. No correspondence address is given, nor any information on the source of salicylate, both of which would be anticipated in a similar publication today. Although it is difficult to extrapolate disease categories over time, it is possible that "subacute articular rheumatism" might represent cases of septic (infective) arthritis, a condition associated with joint pain, pyrexia, and tachycardia. The antipyretic action of salicylates might be anticipated to be of symptomatic benefit in such cases, although not addressing the underlying infective cause. Acute flare-ups of rheumatoid arthritis are another diagnostic possibility.

All Clouston's cases were stated to have been "encountered in private practice". Prior to the advent of the National Health Service in 1948, all medical practice was private (i.e. undertaken for a fee payable by the patient) unless performed under charitable auspices, for example in a local voluntary hospital, access to which was limited to subscribers or those given a ticket by a subscriber. Whether any of the patients described in Clouston's papers date from his time in Hay, perhaps collected over a number of years, is not stated, but since the publications postdate his move to Gunnersbury this may not be the case. Of note, these publications predate by some years the synthesis of acetylsalicylic acid, better known as aspirin, by Eichengrün and colleagues in

1897 at the dye manufacturer Friedrich Bayer & Co, which initiated the global use of aspirin.

Clouston's time in Gunnersbury was limited, since he fell "a victim to professional duty, for he caught a bad attack of scarlet fever some years ago from a patient, to which his later illness can be traced". He "suffered from pneumonia in November last [1882], and this was succeeded by a series of obscure hepatic [liver], renal [kidney], and purpuric [bruising] symptoms". He "went up to the Orkneys in June [1883], to see if his native air would not restore his health", and one wonders whether he may have consulted medical opinion from his father and/or father-in-law. However, regrettably, "he steadily got worse, and died in the manse where he was born, calm, cheerful and resigned to the will of Providence" on 16 September 1883, aged 36, "cut off in the very prime of his life".[7] [Some internet entries on Clouston date his death as 16 December 1883, but this cannot be correct since his *British Medical Journal* obituary appears in the issue for 29 September 1883.] The obituary notes that Clouston left "five young children".[7] Charles Traill Clouston, his only son, died at Ficksburg, South Africa on 9 April 1902 at the age of 23, at which time his mother was living at 4 Kinburn Place, St Andrews.

Clouston was described as a "man of sound judgment and of high professional honour, as well as marked general ability and culture".[7] One has the impression from the limited entries in Kilvert's diary that he was an acquaintance, rather than a close friend, of Kilvert.

Acknowledgments

Adapted from: Larner AJ. Kilvert and the medical profession. *Journal of the Kilvert Society* 2010;Issue 31:53; and Larner AJ. Hay's "universally acclaimed" junior doctor. *Journal of the Kilvert Society* 2012;Issue 35:187–188.

References

1. O'Brien T. *Who's who in Kilvert's Diary*. Llandrindod Wells: Kilvert Society, 2010.
2. Larner A. Kilvert and Livingstone. *Journal of the Kilvert Society* 2008;Issue 27:17.
3. Larner AJ. Kilvert and cholera. *Journal of the Kilvert Society* 2009;Issue 28:22–23.
4. Larner A. Headache, face-ache and neuralgia. The neurological case of the Reverend Francis Kilvert. *Journal of the Kilvert Society* 2008;Issue 26:18–19.
5. Larner AJ. Francis Kilvert (1840–1879): an early self-report of cluster headache? *Cephalalgia* 2008;28:763–766.
6. Walk A, Hare E. Psychiatry in the 1870s: Kilvert's mad folk. *Psychiatric Bull* 1979;3(9):150–153.

7. Obituary. Charles Stewart Clouston, M.D. Edin. *Br Med J* 1883;ii:654.
8. Clouston CS. On the salicylate treatment of rheumatism. *The Practitioner* 1882;28(157):321–336.
9. Clouston CS. On the salicylate treatment of rheumatism. *The Practitioner* 1882;28(158):401–419.

Charles Féré (1852–1907): neurological contributions

Many of the neurologists who were protégés of Jean-Martin Charcot (1825–1893) at the Salpêtrière hospital in Paris in the late nineteenth century remain familiar names to neurologists today, for example Joseph Babinski (1857–1932),[1] Pierre Marie (1853–1940),[2] and Georges Gilles de la Tourette (1857–1904).[3] Many of these individuals may be seen in André Brouillet's celebrated painting entitled "Un leçon clinique à la Salpêtrière" of 1887, which now hangs in a corridor near the Musée d'Histoire de la Médecine in Descartes University, 12 rue de l'Ecole de Médecine, in Paris. Perhaps few neurologists,[4] though, will have heard of Charles Féré, also a Charcot protégé at the Salpêtrière, who is also to be seen in Brouillet's painting, second left from Charcot: his slightly wistful, enquiring appearance perhaps gives some clues as to his character.

Charles Samson Féré was born in Auffay in Normandy, midway between Dieppe and Rouen, on 13th June 1852, the only child of a wealthy family of farmers. Féré first studied medicine in Rouen in 1870 before moving to Paris in 1872 where Paul Broca (1824–1880) was apparently one of his teachers.[5] He initially aspired to surgery but coming under the influence of the great Charcot at La Salpêtrière he decided to pursue an interest in neuropathology. His thesis of 1882 was devoted to the *Functional disorders of vision by cerebral lesions (amblyopia and crossed hemianopsia)*. He was appointed Assistant Physician at the Salpêtrière in 1884 and then Chief Physician at the Bicêtre in 1887 where he remained until his death on 22nd April 1907 at the age of 54 years. His laboratory was described as "a shrine visited by a constant flow of scientific pilgrims from all parts of France and from foreign countries".[6]

As his obituaries record,[6,7] his interests were broad and his output prolific, ranging through the disciplines of biology, psychology, psychiatry and anthropology as well as neurology. His publications include books entitled *Animal magnetism* (with Alfred Binet, 1887, with observations on hypnosis and hallucinations, of which the latter has attracted some recent attention[8]), *Degeneration and criminality* (1888), *The pathology of emotions: physiological and clinical studies* (1892), *The neuropathic family* (1894), and *The sexual instinct: evolution and dissolution* (1899). As one of his obituarists wrote, these works were "familiar to those interested in psychiatry".[7] Another stated that "He studied the problems of heredity, evolution and degeneration",[6] all major concerns not only of nineteenth century biology but also of society in general.

Concordant with these disparate interests, Féré was a member of many learned societies, including those devoted to biology, psychology, anthropology and medicine.

In addition to these publications, Féré also made contributions in several branches of neurology which may be considered worthy of our remembrance. For example, in 1881 he published a review of Charcot's teachings on migrainous infarction,[9] noting that the symptoms of aura, though usually transient, could be prolonged and even permanent, which was ascribed to constriction and thrombosis of cerebral vessels secondary to migrainous vasospasm.[10] The eponym "Charcot-Féré syndrome" has been suggested for this unusual phenomenon,[11] now largely considered a diagnosis of exclusion.

Féré's 1890 textbook on epilepsy was entitled *Les épilepsies et les épileptiques*,[12] and hence appears to be the first such work to discuss "epilepsies" in the plural. Féré distinguished between partial and generalised paroxysms, the latter being complete, incomplete, abnormal, or isolated.[12] For this work, specifically the concept of epilepsies as opposed to epilepsy as a unitary phenomenon, Féré has been noted as an important early contributor to the development of the nosology and classification of epilepsy and epileptic seizures.[13]

Perhaps Féré's most memorable neurological contribution dates to 1903, when he published a paper which introduced the term "fou rire prodromique",[14] sometimes translated as "prodrome of crazy laughter", which was used to describe the symptoms of involuntary laughter, sometimes discordant with subjective affect, seen prior to an apoplectic event, now characterised as stroke. This discovery was reported in the context of nineteenth century views of laughter as a phenomenon regulated by various brain centres and tracts. Cases of fou rire prodromique, though rare, have subsequently been reported in association with brainstem (pontine) or lenticular stroke, carotid artery occlusion or dissection, vertebrobasilar stenosis and anterior choroidal artery infarction. A variant of fou rire prodromique wherein crying rather than laughter precedes a brainstem infarct, which was tentatively labelled "folles larmes prodromiques" as derived from Féré's nomenclature, has also been described.[15]

As his portraits show, Féré was of striking appearance, with a high forehead and long black beard, "large and pensive eyes ... features ... expressive of a gentle melancholy. At first glance he appeared rather rough and cold in manner, but he was truly kind, gentle, and exquisitely sensitive".[7] He was reported to lead a simple life, devoted to the hospital and the laboratory, and sought neither honours nor rewards, which may perhaps go some way to explain why he is little remembered today.

Acknowledgment

Adapted from: Larner AJ. Charles Féré (1852–1907). *J Neurol* 2011;258:524–525.

References

1. Skalski JH. Joseph Jules François Félix Babinski (1857–1932). *J Neurol* 2007;254:1140–1141.
2. Poirier J, Chretien F. Pierre Marie (1853–1940). *J Neurol* 2000;247:983–984.
3. Walusinski O, Bogousslavsky J. Georges Gilles de la Tourette. *J Neurol* 2011;258:166–167.
4. Walusinski O. Keeping the fire burning: Georges Gilles de la Tourette, Paul Richer, Charles Féré and Alfred Binet. In: Bogousslavsky J (ed.). *Following Charcot: a forgotten history of neurology and psychiatry* (Frontiers in Neurology and Neuroscience Volume 29), 2009:71–90 [at 82–86].
5. Finger S. Paul Broca (1824–1880). *J Neurol* 2004;251:769–770.
6. Anonymous. [Untitled]. *BMJ* 1907;1:1281.
7. Semalaigne R. Obituary. Dr Chalres Féré. *J Mental Sci* 1907;53:670–671.
8. Féré C. Report on autoscopic or mirror hallucinations and altruistic hallucinations. 1891. *Epilepsy Behav* 2009;16:214–215.
9. Féré C. Contribution à l'étude de la migraine ophthalmique. *Revue de Médecine Paris* 1881;1:625–649.
10. Lane R, Davies P. *Migraine.* New York: Taylor & Francis, 2006:141.
11. Ramadan NM. Migrainous infarction: the Charcot- Féré syndrome? *Cephalalgia* 1993;13:249–252.
12. Féré C. *Les épilepsies et les épileptiques.* Paris: Bailliere, 1890.
13. Shorvon S, Weiss G, Avanzini G, Engel J, Meinardi H, Moshé S et al. *The International League Against Epilepsy 1909–2009. A Centenary History.* Chichester: Wiley-Blackwell, 2009:132,135.
14. Féré C. Le fou rire prodromique. *Rev Neurol (Paris)* 1903;11:353–358.
15. Larner AJ. Basilar artery occlusion associated with pathological crying: "folles larmes prodromiques"? *Neurology* 1998;51:916–917.

Arthur Conan Doyle (1859–1930): the neurology of Sherlock Holmes

Much has been written and committed to film, both motion picture and television, on the subject of Sherlock Holmes and it is not my intention to weary the reader with a further long exposition on Holmesian methods of deduction, which has been cited as analogous to the narrative structure of medical knowledge[1] and more recently adduced to the service of evidence-based medicine.[2] The purpose of this essay is merely to point out a few possible encounters of the great man with subjects of neurological interest as attested to in the canon.[3]

Of course, some of these accounts of neurological disease may reflect upon the medical experiences of his creator, Dr Arthur Conan Doyle (1869–1930), or his mentor and the so-called forerunner of Sherlock Holmes, Dr Joseph Bell (1837–1911),[4] or even possibly of the writer of the stories, Dr John H. Watson, MD, a veteran of Afghanistan who sometimes observes people with a "surgical eye" (p.1041). Some Holmesian examples of neurological illness have previously been documented by Westmoreland and Key.[5]

Headache and facial pain

Conan Doyle suffered from neuralgia from boyhood, apparently so much so that the editors of his collected letters omit examples for "fear of exhausting the reader's patience".[6] In a fictionalised account of parts of Conan Doyle's life, Julian Barnes portrays Jean Leckie, the woman who was to become Conan Doyle's second wife, as suffering from migraines.[7] It might therefore be anticipated that headache and/or neuralgia would feature in Holmes's experiences, but Westmoreland and Key make no mention of headache, unless it be adumbrated by their category of "simulated condition".[5]

In fact, only four references to headache have been found. In two of these, headache is certainly simulated: in *The Adventure of the Speckled Band*, Holmes advises Miss Stoner to confine herself to her room on the pretence of a headache in order to facilitate giving a nocturnal signal which is material to the apprehension of the criminal (p.269), whilst in *The Adventure of the Retired Colourman* Amberley's wife complains of headache "at the last minute" so cannot go to the Haymarket Theatre (p.1115). Headache seems to be genuine in *The Naval Treaty* when Annie Harrison declines her brother's entreaty to come out into the sunshine on the grounds of a slight headache, preferring a "deliciously cool and soothing" room (p.463). In *The Valley of Fear*, McMurdo develops headache as a consequence of excessive drink (p.839).

Altered states of consciousness

There are plenty of examples of "brain fever" and/or delirium. An episode of the former is central to the plot of *The Naval Treaty*, and an episode also occurs in *The Adventure of the Cardboard Box*. Delirium is mentioned by name on several occasions (e.g. p.56,759,797), not simply the once alluded to by Westmoreland and Key,[5] often in the context of fever. Most celebratedly, Holmes himself feigns delirium, sufficient to deceive even the medical gaze of Watson, to ensnare the criminal in *The Adventure of the Dying Detective* (p.935).

Episodes of loss of consciousness, probably syncope rather than epileptic seizure, are also encountered (e.g. p.929), for example, two in quick succession in *The Adventure of the Devil's Foot*:

> . . . the doctor was as white as a sheet. Indeed, he fell into a chair in a sort of faint . . . (p.959)
>
> She had fainted with horror upon entering the room . . . and seeing that dreadful company around the table (p.959).

Both these phenomena are occasioned by seeing two brothers, "the senses stricken clean out of them" (p.957), and their dead sister. The brothers are described as "demented" (p.957), apparently acutely, necessitating transfer to an asylum (p.959). A toxic cause is eventually found responsible for all these events.

A possible out-of-body experience has been claimed by Dieguez[8] in *The Hound of the Baskervilles*:

> After you left I sent down to Stamford's for the ordnance map of this portion of the moor, and my spirit has hovered over it all day. I flatter myself that I could find my way about.

Movement disorders

In *The Sign of Four*, Thaddeus Sholto is reported thus:

> He writhed his hands together as he stood, and his features were in a perpetual jerk – now smiling, now scowling, but never for an instance in repose (p.100).
>
> Mr Thaddeus Sholto . . . sat twitching on his luxurious settee (p.105).

In addition to these apparently involuntary movements, Sholto has a peculiar physiognomy: he is a "small man with a very high head, a bristle of red hair all round the fringe of it, and a bald shining scalp ... In spite of his obtrusive baldness he gave the impression of youth" (p.100).

It would be interesting to know if his identical twin brother, Bartholomew, had a similar movement disorder, but he is only encountered in death: his "features were set ... in a horrible smile, a fixed and unnatural grin" (p.109). Holmes identifies this as an "extreme contraction, far exceeding the usual rigor mortis" and quizzes Watson as to what "this Hippocratic smile, or *risus sardonicus*" might suggest about the cause of death.

In *The Greek Interpreter*, a character called Wilson Kemp has involuntary movements:

> ...his lips and eyelids were continually twitching like a man with St. Vitus's dance. I could not help thinking that his strange, catchy little laugh was also a symptom of some nervous malady (p.441).

As with Sholto, I leave it to movement disorders experts to diagnose the case! With Kemp, the account seems to raise the possibility of both motor and vocal tics.

Catalepsy

Perhaps the most celebrated neurological episode in the Holmes canon occurs in *The Resident Patient*, which features a "Russian Nobleman" reported to have catalepsy who visits Dr Percy Trevelyan who has a particular interest in this condition. An attack occurs during their consultation, which Trevelyan describes thus to Holmes and Watson:

> Suddenly, however, as I sat writing, he ceased to give any answer at all to my inquiries, and on my turning towards him I was shocked to see that he was sitting bolt upright in his chair, staring at me with a perfectly blank and rigid face. He was again in the grip of his mysterious malady (p.427).

Holmes is unimpressed, later telling Watson: "It is a very easy complaint to imitate. I have done it myself" (p.430).

Two very distinguished neurologists, Robin Howard and Hugh Willison, have already written a seminal paper on this topic[9] which renders all further comment superfluous, in which they suggest that the model for Dr Percy Trevelyan was in fact Sir William Gowers (1845–1915), one of the most famous of Queen Square neurologists.[10] Andrew Lees has also suggested that Gowers may be the source for *The Resident Patient.*[11]

Conclusion

To my reading, it seems that Conan Doyle uses neurological illness in the Sherlock Holmes stories as no more than a convenient literary device. Detailed clinical description, which one might have supposed to be at Conan Doyle's disposal based on his clinical experience, is not in evidence, precluding detailed retrospective clinical diagnosis (perhaps just as well, some might think).

As for the suggestion of Holmes *qua* neurologist,[12,13] one imagines he would be easily capable of acquiring the detailed knowledge required (we know from Watson's account in *A Study in Scarlet* that Holmes is "well up in belladonna, opium, and poisons generally" and that his knowledge of anatomy is "accurate, but unsystematic"), but I fear that, being a man of his (Victorian) age, he wouldn't pass the first hurdle into medical school today, based on statements such as this one:

> It is of the first importance not to allow your judgement to be biased by personal qualities. A client to me is a mere unit, a factor in a problem. The emotional qualities are antagonistic to clear reasoning (p.96).

Acknowledgment

Adapted from: Larner AJ. "Neurological literature": Sherlock Holmes and neurology. *Adv Clin Neurosci Rehabil* 2011;11(1):20,22.

References

1. Hunter KM. *Doctors' stories. The narrative structure of medical knowledge.* Princeton: Princeton University Press, 1991.
2. Nordenstrom J. *Evidence-based medicine in Sherlock Holmes' footsteps.* Oxford: Blackwell, 2007.
3. Conan Doyle A. *The Penguin complete Sherlock Holmes.* London: Penguin, 2009 [All page references are to this edition].
4. Godbee DC. Joseph Bell (1837–1911): a clinician's literary legacy. *J Med Biogr* 1999;7:166–170.
5. Westmoreland BF, Key JD. Arthur Conan Doyle, Joseph Bell, and Sherlock Holmes. A neurologic connection. *Arch Neurol* 1991;48:325–329.
6. Lellenberg J, Stashower D, Foley C (eds.). *Arthur Conan Doyle. A life in letters.* London: Harper, 2007:14,31,68–69,195.
7. Barnes J. *Arthur & George.* London: Vintage, 2006:239,242,263,365.
8. Dieguez S. Doubles everywhere: literary contributions to the study of the bodily self. In: Bogousslavsky J, Dieguez S (eds.). *Literary medicine: brain disease and doctors in novels, theater, and film* (Frontiers of Neurology and

Neuroscience Volume 31). Basel: Karger, 2013:77–115 [at 104].
9. Howard R, Willison H. The nature of catalepsy and the model for Percy Trevelyan. *The Sherlock Holmes Journal* 1992;20(4):128–130.
10. Tyler KL. William Richard Gowers (1845–1915). *J Neurol* 2003;250:1012–1013.
11. Lees AJ. The strange case of Dr. William Gowers and Mr. Sherlock Holmes. *Brain* 2015;138:2103–2108.
12. Cherington M. Sherlock Holmes: neurologist. *Neurology* 1987;37:824–825.
13. Kempster PA. Looking for clues. *J Clin Neurosci* 2006;13:178–180.

Anton Chekhov (1860–1904): neurological disorders

Dr Anton Pavlovich Chekhov (1860–1904) is best known for his plays in the realist genre.[1] He also performed significant medical work, not least his 1890 visit to the island of Sakhalin whence he reported on the social and medical conditions of the penal colonies located there.[2]

Chekhov's plays and stories often feature a doctor,[3] and in most there is also a character who looks forward to a bright future destined not for himself but for the generations to come. It has been suggested that Doctor Astrov in the play *Uncle Vania* (first performed in 1899) voices some of Chekhov's personal thoughts.[4,5] Although Chekhov once famously stated that "medicine is my lawful wife"[6] and that he never regretted his choice of career, nonetheless Astrov states of medicine:

> The life itself is tedious, stupid, squalid ... This sort of life drags you down. You're surrounded by queer people – they're a queer lot, all of them – and after you've lived with them for a year or two, you gradually become queer yourself, without noticing it. That's inevitable.

A century on, Chekhov might be interested to see what remarkable progress has been made in medical life.

An analysis of all Chekhov's plays[4] and some of his short stories[7] looking for possible accounts of neurological disorders was undertaken.

Headache

A number of Chekhov's characters profess, or are reported to be suffering from, headaches, a condition he was certainly familiar with in his clinical practice.[8] For example, in the plays:

- Ivanov (*Ivanov*, 1887). Lyebedev suggests that Ivanov's headache is because he thinks too much (a paraphrase of Caesar's comment on Cassius in Shakespeare's *Julius Caesar*, I:ii:194?).
- Olga (*Three Sisters*, 1901), supposes that she gets a continual headache (tension-type?) "because I have to go to school every day and go on teaching right into the evening".
- Shipoochin (*The Jubilee*). specifically "a migraine".[9]

Headache is also encountered in the short stories:

- Kiryak (*Peasants*): "a terrible hangover . . . shaking his splitting head".
- Bishop Peter (*The Bishop*): "he had the same headache as yesterday .."; "he had a splitting headache". These are part of a febrile illness which is eventually diagnosed as typhoid.

Obstructive sleep apnoea

In *The Cherry Orchard* (1903), Boris Borisovich Simeonov-Pishchik, a landowner, "drops asleep and snores" in the midst of speaking, only to wake again "at once" and continue what he was saying. Later, he reports that he has high blood pressure and has had a stroke twice already, which makes dancing difficult, before again falling asleep, snoring, and waking almost at once. These clinical features and the associated hypertension suggest a possible diagnosis of obstructive sleep apnoea.

Agnosia

With his medical training, Chekhov was perhaps alert to defects in human cognitive function. In the short story *The Kiss*, first published in 1887, this passage appears:

> When he first entered the dining room and sat down to tea, he found it impossible to concentrate on any one face or object. All those faces, dresses, cut-glass decanters, steaming glasses, moulded cornices, merged into one composite sensation, making Ryabovich feel ill-at-ease, and he longed to bury his head somewhere. Like a lecturer at his first appearance in public, he could see everything in front of him well enough, but at the same time he could make little sense of it (physicians call this condition, when someone sees without understanding, "psychic blindness").

Although when we consider the history of agnosia, we typically think of Lissauer's distinction of apperceptive and associative types, drawn in 1890, he in fact talked of *Seelenblindheit*,[10] literally "soul-blindness" but technically "psychic blindness" (a term also used by Munk in 1877).[11] It was not until the following year that Sigmund Freud, previously a pupil of Charcot, coined the term "agnosia" ("not knowing" or "without knowledge").[12] There were other, earlier, descriptions relevant to these phenomena which Chekhov might possibly have been aware of: Bastian described "visual perceptive centres" in 1869, Finkelnburg "asymbolia" in 1870, and Hughlings Jackson "imperceptions" in 1876.[11]

Acknowledgments

Adapted from: Larner AJ. Jane Austen on memory; Anton Chekhov on agnosia. *Adv Clin Neurosci Rehabil* 2005;5(2):14; and Ford SF, Larner AJ. Neurological disorders reported by Dr Anton Chekhov (1860–1904). *Eur J Neurol* 2010;17(Suppl3):545.

References

1. Rayfield D. *Anton Chekhov: a life.* London: Harper Collins, 1997.
2. Reeve B (trans.). *Anton Chekhov. A journey to Sakhalin.* Cambridge: Ian Faulkner, 1993.
3. Crommelynck I. Doctor Chekhov's doctors. In: Bogousslavsky J, Dieguez S (eds.). *Literary medicine: brain disease and doctors in novels, theater, and film* (Frontiers of Neurology and Neuroscience Volume 31). Basel: Karger, 2013:236–244.
4. Fen E (trans.). *Chekhov Plays.* Harmondsworth: Penguin, 1954:33,188.
5. Coope J. *Doctor Chekhov: A study in literature and medicine.* Chale: Cross Publishing, 1997.
6. Schwartz RS. "Medicine is my lawful wife" – Anton Chekhov, 1860–1904. *N Engl J Med* 2004;351:213–214.
7. Wilks R (trans.). *Chekhov. The Kiss and other stories.* Harmondsworth: Penguin, 1982.
8. Coope, 1997:109.
9. Fen, 1959:86,250,449.
10. Lissauer H. Ein Fall von Seelenblindheit nebst einem Beitrag zure Theorie derselben. *Archiv fur Psychiatrie und Nervenkrankheiten* 1890;21:222–270 [abridged translation by M Jackson in *Cogn Neuropsychol* 1988;5:157–192].
11. Meyer A. The frontal lobe syndrome, the aphasias and related conditions. *Brain* 1974;97:565–600 [at 571–572].
12. Freud S. *Zur Auffassung der Aphasien, eine Kritische Studie.* Leipzig: Deuticke, 1891.

Charles Thurstan Holland (1863–1941): a genealogical note

Visitors to the Gallery at the Liverpool Medical Institution may be familiar with the Copnall portrait of Charles Thurstan Holland (1863–1941) which hangs there. (The disconcerting mismatch between the name on the portrait, Thurstan, and the name on the adjacent blurb, Thurston, needs correction, as does the incorrect date of death, 1940, but the former is forgivable, since at least one obituary was also in error as regards the final vowel;[1] the blurb errors almost certainly stem from Shepherd, in his history of the LMI.[2])

Many will also be familiar, in no small measure due to the writings of Austin Carty,[3,4] with Charles Thurstan Holland's contributions to the development of radiology in Liverpool, beginning in the 1890s.[5,6] He was present on the occasion of the radiological localisation of a bullet in a boy's wrist, described in *The Lancet* in February 1896 by Sir Robert Jones and Oliver Lodge,[7,8] and is remembered in Egyptology circles for his radiograph of a mummy bird in October 1896, initiating the application of radiological studies to ancient antiquities.[9] He produced over 100 publications during his career.[2] In addition to the portrait at LMI, there is a plaque at 43 Rodney Street commemorating Thurstan Holland, and he is buried in Toxteth Park Cemetery.

All this is well known, at least in Liverpool. The purpose of this article is to explore a little of Charles Thurstan Holland's genealogy. Looking at his portrait, I have wondered, stimulated by my interests[10,11] in a quite different sphere, whether he might be related to the novelist Elizabeth Gaskell (1810–1865), perhaps best known for her final novel, *Wives and Daughters* (1866). What possible link could there be, it might be reasonably asked, between a novelist resident in and associated with Manchester for much of her adult life, and a radiologist in Liverpool, whose lives overlapped by only 2 years?

Reading the collected letters of Mrs Gaskell,[12,13] there are many references to the Holland family. The maiden name of Elizabeth Gaskell's mother, Elizabeth (1764–1812), was Holland. This extensive family produced a number of doctors, most eminent amongst whom was her cousin Henry Holland (1788–1873), later Sir Henry Holland, 1st Baronet.[14] There are several medical characters in Gaskell's works, perhaps most notably Dr Gibson in *Wives and Daughters*, some of whom may possibly owe something to these medical relatives.

To be sure, Holland is a common enough surname, so this might not provoke much interest in a possible link, until it is noted that other Gaskell relatives bore the name "Thurstan Holland", namely Henry Thurstan Holland (1825–1914), one of the sons of the aforementioned Sir Henry Holland; and Edward Thurstan Holland (1836–1884), son of Elizabeth's cousin Edward Holland (1806–1875). Edward Thurstan Holland eventually married Elizabeth Gaskell's eldest daughter, Marianne (1834–1920). A character named Thurstan Benson appears in Elizabeth Gaskell's novel *Ruth*.

Knowing of these Gaskell relatives named "Thurstan Holland", my question now became: how could Charles Thurstan Holland *not* be related to Elizabeth Gaskell? That said, tracing the link did not prove straightforward (for me, at least; a professional genealogist may have worked it out in a much shorter time! Two websites, www.geni.com and www.clement-jones.com, proved particularly helpful in tracing the links in the chain).

Charles Thurstan Holland was born in Bridgwater, Somerset, the son of William Thomas Holland (1834–1899). One website states that "William's great-great-grandfather was the great-great-uncle on her mother's side of Elizabeth Cleghorn Stevenson (1810–1865) who became famous as the 'Manchester novelist' Elizabeth Gaskell". To cut a long story short, it would appear that Charles Thurstan Holland and Elizabeth Gaskell share a common ancestor, one John Holland of Mobberley (1656–1712/3). He was the father of sons, John and Thomas, both born in 1690 and possibly twins. John Holland (1690–1770) was the father of Samuel Holland (1734–1816), who was Elizabeth Gaskell's maternal grandfather. Thomas Holland (1690–1753) initiated a line of Thomas Hollands (born 1725/6, 1760, and 1794), the latter being Thomas Crompton Holland (1794–1861), the father of William Thomas Holland.

Whether Charles Thurstan Holland was ever aware of this distant relationship with an eminent novelist is not, to my knowledge, recorded. Why he should have been named Thurstan is also unknown to me, but it may suggest that the various ramifications of the family remained aware of one another and hence this family name persisted into another generation. The Thurstan name may have been in the Holland family as far back as the 13th century (see www.clement-jones.com).

Acknowledgements

The author would like to thank Dr Nick Clitherow and Dr Austin Carty for comments on this article. Adapted from: Larner AJ. Charles Thurstan Holland: a genealogical note. *Medical Historian (Journal of the Liverpool Medical History Society)* 2015;25:31–33; and Larner AJ. Elizabeth Gaskell and Charles Thurstan Holland – another Liverpool connection. *Gaskell Society Newsletter* 2015;Issue 59:7–8.

References

1. Anonymous. Charles Thurston [*sic*] Holland. *Radiology* 1941;36:382.
2. Shepherd JA. *A history of the Liverpool Medical Institution.* Liverpool: LMI, 1979:passim.
3. Carty AT. X-ray centenary 1895–1995. Roentgen's Big Bang: Liverpool's echo. *LMI Transactions and Report* 1995–6:18–30.
4. Carty A. Charles Thurstan Holland: Pioneer of Liverpool Radiology. *The Invisible Light. The Journal of The Radiology History and Heritage Charitable Trust* 2001;15:18–21.
5. Whitaker PH. The birth and growth of radiology. *LMI Transactions and Report* 1961;21–35.
6. Cope R. Radiologic history exhibit. Charles Thurstan Holland, 1863–1941. *Radiographics* 1995;15:481–8 [Erratum: 1995;15:640].
7. Edwards D. Oliver Lodge and the first medical uses of X-rays. *Medical Historian* 1989;231–40 [at 34].
8. Rowlands P. Oliver Lodge and the birth of Liverpool radiology. *Medical Historian* 2015;25:3–15 [at 9].
9. Holland CT. X-rays in 1896. In: Bruwer AJ (ed.) *Classic descriptions in diagnostic Roentgenology. Volume 1.* Springfield, Ill.: Charles C Thomas, 1964:70–84.
10. Larner AJ. "A habit of headaches": the neurological case of Elizabeth Gaskell. *Gaskell Journal* 2011;25: 97–103.
11. Larner AJ. Headache in the writings of Elizabeth Gaskell (1810–65). *J Med Biogr* 2015;23:191–196.
12. Chapple JAV, Pollard A (eds.) *The letters of Mrs Gaskell.* Manchester: Manchester University Press, [1966] 1997.
13. Chapple J, Shelston A (eds.) *Further letters of Mrs Gaskell.* Manchester: Manchester University Press, [2000] 2003.
14. Hill B. "More fashionable than scientific". Sir Henry Holland, Bt, M.D., F.R.C.P., F.R.S. (1788–1873). *Practitioner* 1974;211:548–552.
15. http://charlesduval.org/william_thomas_holland (accessed 15/11/2014).

Alois Alzheimer (1864–1915): the 100th anniversary of his first case

At the 37th Conference of the South-West German Psychiatrists in Tübingen on 3rd-4th November 1906, Dr Alois Alzheimer presented his clinical and neuropathological findings in the case of a patient, Auguste D., who suffered cognitive decline and behavioural changes in the presenium. The presentation, entitled "On a peculiar disease process of the cerebral cortex", apparently prompted no comments or reaction from the audience. The first case of "Alzheimer's disease" had been reported, although the condition was not to bear this eponym until Emil Kraepelin used it in the 8th edition of his psychiatry textbook published in 1910.[1,2]

Alzheimer's lecture was published in the following year in the *Allgemeine Zeitschrift fur Psychiatrie und Psychisch-Gerichtlich Medizine*[3] (English translations are available[4–6]). It detailed the clinical observations Alzheimer and his colleagues in Frankfurt had made on Auguste Deter from the time of her admission in 1901, aged 51, until her death in 1906, and also Alzheimer's neuropathological findings (by this time he had moved to Munich, via Heidelberg), including peculiar changes in the neuronal neurofibrils visualised with the Bielschowsky silver stain, later to be called neurofibrillary tangles, and miliary foci of extracellular material, corresponding to senile plaques. Both the case file[7] and the pathological slides[8] of Auguste D have been rediscovered and re-reported, confirming that Auguste D did indeed have Alzheimer's disease as we now understand it. Furthermore analysis of archived brain material has suggested that Auguste Deter may have harboured a point mutation in the presenilin-1 gene (p.Phe176Leu);[9] mutations in this gene are now recognised to be the most common cause of autosomal dominant Alzheimer's disease.

In a later contribution[10] (also available in English[11]), Alzheimer described a further personally examined case, Johann F., and three other pathological cases, and linked the neuropathological substrate of neurofibrillary pathology to the clinical correlate of dementia. The pathology of this second patient has also been re-examined:[12] apparently it showed numerous senile plaques but no neurofibrillary tangles in the cerebral cortex. More recently, the kindred of Johann F. has been extensively investigated through the historical records, suggesting an autosomal dominant disorder with variable penetrance and with age of onset between the 30s and mid 60s.[13] The index case was negative for amyloid precursor protein (APP) gene mutations,[12] but was not investigated for presenilin-1 gene mutations.

The 100th anniversary of the first description of Alzheimer's disease has been marked by a publication documenting some of the clinical and scientific progress which has been made over the ensuing century, the vast majority of it within the last 40 years.[14] Although much has been learned about disease aetiology and pathogenesis, the ultimate goal of disease-modifying treatment for AD remains elusive, although it does not seem unreasonable to hope for new therapeutic developments in the foreseeable future.

It is also worth noting that Alzheimer might be commemorated for two other cognitive disorders. The term "Pick's disease" was applied to the syndrome of focal lobar degeneration of the frontal and temporal lobes of the brain causing respectively behavioural and linguistic phenotypes described by Arnold Pick, based on the neuropathological findings made by Alzheimer of ballooned achromatic neurones (Pick cells) and neuronal inclusions (Pick bodies) in some, but not all, cases of lobar degeneration. Alzheimer also produced an early, if not the earliest, account of dementia in motor neurone disease.[15]

Acknowledgment

Adapted from: Larner AJ. Alzheimer 100. *Adv Clin Neurosci Rehabil* 2006;6(5):24.

References

1. Hoff P. Alzheimer and his time. In: Berrios GE, Freeman HL (eds.) *Alzheimer and the dementias.* London: Royal Society of Medicine, 1991:29–55.
2. Bick KL. The early story of Alzheimer disease. In: Terry RD, Katzman R, Bick KL (eds.). *Alzheimer disease.* New York: Raven, 1994:1–8.
3. Alzheimer A. Über eine eigenartige Erkrankung der Hirnrinde. *Allgemeine Zeitschrift fur Psychiatrie und Psychisch-Gerichtlich Medizine* 1907;64:146–148.
4. Wilkins RH, Brody LA. Alzheimer's disease. *Arch Neurol* 1969;21:109–110.
5. Jarvik L, Greenson H. About a peculiar disease of the cerebral cortex. *Alzheimer Dis Assoc Disord* 1987;1:7–8.
6. Stelzmann RA, Schintzlein HN, Murtagh FR. An English translation of Alzheimer's 1907 paper, Über eine eigenartige Erkrankung der Hirnrinde. *Clin Anat* 1995;8:429–431.
7. Maurer K, Volk S, Gerbaldo H. Auguste D and Alzheimer's disease. *Lancet* 1997;349:1546–1549.
8. Graeber MB, Kösel S, Grasbon-Frodl E, Möller HJ, Mehraein P. Histopathology and APOE genotype of the first Alzheimer disease patient, Auguste D. *Neurogenetics* 1998;1:223–228.
9. Müller U, Winter P, Graeber MB. A presenilin 1 mutation in the first case of Alzheimer's disease. *Lancet Neurol* 2013;13:129–130.

10. Alzheimer A. Über eigenartige Krankheitsfalle des sapteren Alters. *Zeitschrift fur die gesamte Neurologie und Psychiatrie* 1911;4:356–385.
11. Förstl H, Levy R. On certain peculiar diseases of old age. *Hist Psychiatry* 1991;2:71–101.
12. Graeber MB, Kösel S, Egensperger R et al. Rediscovery of the case described by Alois Alzheimer in 1911: historical, histological and molecular genetic analysis. *Neurogenetics* 1997;1:73–80.
13. Klünemann HH, Fronhöfer W, Wurster H, Fischer W, Ibach B, Klein HE. Alzheimer's second patient: Johann F. and his family. *Ann Neurol* 2002;52:520–523.
14. Perry G, Avila J, Kinoshita J, Smith MA (eds.). *Alzheimer's disease: a century of scientific and clinical research.* Amsterdam: IOS Press, 2006.
15. Alzheimer A. On a case of spinal progressive muscle atrophy with accessory disease of bulbar nuclei and the cortex [in German]. *Archiv fur Psychiatrie* 1891;23:459–485.

Solomon Carter Fuller (1872–1953): early accounts of Alzheimer's disease

Whilst the name of Alois Alzheimer (1864–1915) is familiar to every neurologist, if not every schoolboy, and the 100th anniversary of his seminal publications[1,2] on the disease which came to bear his name, courtesy of Kraepelin's systematizing, attracted much attention,[3–5] it is unlikely that the name of Dr Solomon Carter Fuller will be known to any but a handful of Alzheimer's disease (AD) cognoscenti. This obscurity prevails despite the fact that Fuller published what was probably the first paper on AD to appear in the English language.

Fuller's distinguished biography, beginning in Liberia as the grandson of a freed slave and culminating as the first African-American to practice as a psychiatrist in the United States of America, for many years at the Westborough Insane Hospital and at Boston University School of Medicine, has been well documented.[6–8] He was granted leave of absence from his post at Westborough for postgraduate studies with Emil Kraepelin (1856–1926) in Munich for two semesters in 1904–5, and here he was one of only five "privalesmus" admitted to the course run by Alzheimer, his acceptance perhaps facilitated by his prior experience in histology and his working knowledge of the German language.[8]

Little is known about Fuller's work in Alzheimer's laboratory, for example it is not clear if he knew of "Alzheimer's first case", Auguste D. Nevertheless, it is evident from his subsequent work that Fuller took an interest in Alzheimer's publications, not surprisingly. The purpose of this article is to look again at Fuller's major publications related to AD and its pathology which appeared in the *American Journal of Insanity* and the *Journal of Nervous and Mental Disease* between 1907 and 1912.[9–12]

Fuller's 1907 *American Journal of Insanity* paper[9] was a histological study of neurofibrils in various disorders, including three cases of "dementia senilis" as well as cases of dementia paralytica and chronic alcoholism, using the Bielschowsky silver impregnation method. At the outset (416), Fuller acknowledged his "indebtedness to Prof. Kraepelin for his kind permission to use the facilities of the Munich Psychiatric Clinic, where the most of our preliminary work was done, and also to Dr. Alzheimer, of the same institution, under whose direction we began the study of the neurofibrils". The three patients reported (cases VIII, IX, and X; 444–447) were all elderly males (8th decade). Macroscopic atrophy of the cerebral convolutions was noted in two cases.

Diffuse alterations in neurofibrils in the cerebral cortex were noted in all cases: "The cells present a somewhat shrunken appearance and fragmentation, granulation and disappearance of the fibrils are common" (447). Fuller concluded that "diffuse destruction of intercellular [*sic*] fibrils ... is the rule in dementia senilis" (460) and that silver impregnation for neurofibrils might be used to differentiate dementia paralytica "from a disease with a dystrophic substratum such as dementia senilis" (461). There is no account or illustration (Figures 16 and 21, not 20 as reported in the text) which resembles or could be recognised as the neurofibrillary tangle which had been delineated by Alzheimer in his first case, and no mention of Alzheimer's first papers.[1,2] It may be that at this time Fuller was not aware of these publications.

In his 1912 paper (in two parts) in the *Journal of Nervous and Mental Disease*,[10,11] Fuller used the term Alzheimer's disease, acknowledging: "The first published case presenting the combination of clinical and microscopical changes discussed in this paper was reported by Alzheimer in 1906" (440). Fuller cited Alzheimer's 1907 paper[2] (incorrectly as 1906) and included a translation of this case (452–454), as well as material from 11 other papers in the literature reporting similar cases, including Alzheimer's 1911 publication (541–543), the "second case" of Johann F.[13,14] Fuller's patient was a man in his 50s with symptoms which, with hindsight, seem consistent with amnesia, aphasia without anomia, apraxia and possibly agnosia. At autopsy he was noted to have "regional atrophies of cerebrum" (444). With the Bielschowsky method "easily the most characteristic findings are the presence of a great number of plaques" (448) which are illustrated (Figures 1, 2, and 4, the latter with surrounding neuritic change, described as "Alzheimer degeneration", 449). Furthermore, "many ganglion cells ... exhibit the Alzheimer type of degeneration. This degeneration consists of a tangled mass of thick, darkly staining snarls and whirls of the intracellular fibrils" (451), the illustration of which (Figure 3, 448) is typical of neurofibrillary tangles. Glial proliferation was also reported (454). Of note, Fuller used the term "senium praecox" for this case (which he believed to be the 8th recorded case of Alzheimer's disease[12]) and the other cases from the literature which he reviewed, this term apparently synonymous with "Alzheimer's disease" (440,452), presumably to distinguish these cases from "dementia senilis".

Some fifty years later, Allison[15] claimed that in this paper Fuller noted convulsive fits in a confirmed case of Alzheimer's disease in the later stages, if so a most interesting observation in view of current interest in the occurrence of epileptic seizures in AD.[16,17] Reading Fuller's lengthy case report,[10] I can only presume that Allison was referring to the "short periods of unconsciousness or dream-like states" which occurred in the two years before the patient's "final breakdown" (441), but no account of convulsion has been found. However, in his summary of previously published cases,[11] Fuller noted that "In a few of the cases motor disturbances have been noted as residua of epileptiform convulsions. Convulsions with loss of consciousness, however, have not been observed, save in the terminal stage, epileptiform attacks and muscular twitchings being recorded "(554). It is now well-recognised that epileptic seizures and myoclonus become more evident with progression of AD.[16] In Fuller's review, most patients showed evidence of brain atrophy, either general or regional, all but one had evidence of plaques, and all but one had "peculiar basket-like alterations due to the presence of thick, darkly staining intracellular fibrils arranged in whorls or in a tangled mass" (555), the exception being Alzheimer's second case.[13]

With his colleague Henry Klopp, Fuller reported in the *American Journal of Insanity* in 1912 a second personally examined case believed to be an example of Alzheimer's disease.[12] This judgement was based on the clinical history and autopsy findings of plaques but "the Alzheimer degeneration of intracellular neurofibrils ... was not exhibited" (24), as in Alzheimer's second case,[13] and differing from the first Westborough case.[10] The nosological position of "Alzheimer's disease" vis-a-vis senile dementia was discussed, the former being conceived of as an "atypical form of senile dementia" (26).

Fuller's diligence, industry and skill are readily apparent from his papers. Evidently he was in the right place at the right time and possessed the right skills to contribute to the contemporaneous debate on the new diagnostic entity of Alzheimer's disease. In retrospect it is puzzling that he reported nothing resembling neurofibrillary tangles in the brains of patients with "dementia senilis" in his 1907 paper. One may surmise that his views evolved between 1906 and 1912, perhaps as a result of his ongoing studies and his reading of Alzheimer's papers.[1,2,13] Fuller's position as a pioneer of Alzheimer's disease studies in the English language is unquestionable and he deserves to be more widely known.

Acknowledgment

Adapted from: Larner AJ. Solomon Carter Fuller (1872–1953) and the early history of Alzheimer's disease. *Adv Clin Neurosci Rehabil* 2013;12(6):21–22.

References

1. Alzheimer A. Über den Abbau des Nervengewebes. *Centralblatt fur Nervenheilkunde und Psychiatrie* 1906;29:526–528.
2. Alzheimer A. Über eine eigenartige Erkrankung der Hirnrinde. *Allgemeine Zeitschrift fur Psychiatrie und Psychisch-Gerichtlich Medizine* 1907;64:146–148.

3. Hodges JR. Alzheimer's centennial legacy: origins, landmarks and the current status of knowledge concerning cognitive aspects. *Brain* 2006;129:2811–2822.
4. Perry G, Avila J, Kinoshita J, Smith M (eds.). *Alzheimer's disease. A century of scientific and clinical research.* Amsterdam: IOS Press, 2006.
5. Larner AJ. Alzheimer 100. *Adv Clin Neurosci Rehabil* 2006;6(5):24.
6. Cobb WM. Solomon Carter Fuller, 1872–1953. *J Natl Med Assoc* 1954;46:370–372.
7. Kaplan M, Henderson AR. Solomon Carter Fuller, M.D. (1872–1953): American pioneer in Alzheimer's disease research. *J Hist Neurosci* 2000;9:250–261.
8. Kaplan M. *Solomon Carter Fuller. Where my caravan has rested.* Lanham: University Press of America, 2005.
9 Fuller SC. A study of the neurofibrils in dementia paralytica, dementia senilis, chronic alcoholism, cerebral lues and microcephalic idiocy. *Am J Insanity* 1907;63:415–468.
10. Fuller SC. Alzheimer's disease (senium praecox): the report of a case and review of published cases. *J Nerv Ment Dis* 1912;39:440–455.
11. Fuller SC. Alzheimer's disease (senium praecox): the report of a case and review of published cases. *J Nerv Ment Dis* 1912;39:536–557.
12. Fuller SC, Klopp HI. Further observations on Alzheimer's disease. *Am J Insanity* 1912;69:17–29.
13. Alzheimer A. Über eigenartige Krankheitsfalle des spateren Alters. *Zeitschrift fur die gesamte Neurologie und Psychiatrie* 1911;4:356–385.
14. Klünemann HH, Fronhöfer W, Wurster H, Fischer W, Ibach B, Klein HE. Alzheimer's second patient: Johann F. and his family. *Ann Neurol* 2002;52:520–523.
15. Allison RS. *The senile brain. A clinical study.* London: Edward Arnold, 1962:118.
16. Larner AJ. Epileptic seizures in AD patients. *Neuromolecular Med* 2010;12:71–77.
17. Friedman D, Honig LS, Scarmeas N. Seizures and epilepsy in Alzheimer's disease. *CNS Neurosci Ther* 2012;18:285–294.

Howard Knox (1885–1949): a pioneer of neuropsychological testing

Many visitors to New York City will take the brief ferry trip from Battery Park to Liberty Island to see the Statue of Liberty (or "Liberty Enlightening the World" as Frédéric Auguste Bartholdi's monumental sculpture was originally called), and may then travel on to Ellis Island where many immigrants to the United States of America first arrived in the early 20th century.

Viewing the exhibits in the Ellis Island Immigration Museum, the visitor, particularly if from a neuroscience background, may be startled to come across early 20th century photographs of newly arrived immigrants being subjected to neuropsychological testing, and thus may encounter for the first time the work of the physician Howard Andrew Knox (1885–1949). This may prompt the curious visitor to seek more information on this little known and largely neglected figure in the history of neuropsychology, neglected that is until the work of John Richardson to which we are indebted for a vivid portrayal of the man, his work, and times.[1,2]

Knox worked as an assistant surgeon for the US Public Health Service at Ellis Island for just 4 years (May 1912–May1916). Then (as now) anxieties about immigration were prevalent, particularly the risk of large numbers of immigrants with "mental deficiency" being unable to work and hence becoming dependent on the public purse, along with the concerns of the eugenics movement that this would impoverish the racial stock of the country (mental deficiency was viewed at this time as a largely inherited trait). Ellis Island represented a front line for the identification of such immigrants, and their deportation back to their countries of origin (mostly in eastern and southern Europe). But how could such individuals be reliably identified among the mass of people arriving on a daily basis in the voluminous Ellis Island "hall of judgement"?

Along with colleagues at Ellis Island, Knox developed and popularized a number of tests which may be characterized as tests of performance or overt non-verbal behaviour. Tests existing at that time, such as the scale of Binet and Simon, assumed a particular culture and language which rendered them entirely unsuitable for use with the immigrants arriving at Ellis Island. It was recognized that new tests should as far as possible eliminate the language element and cultural knowledge, or in other words should be culture-free or, since this may not be possible, culture-fair. Richardson (ref 2, p.256) identifies Knox as the first proponent of such culture-fair tests.

Knox developed over a dozen tests over a short period of time, such as the Cube Imitation Test and the Feature Profile Test, as well as dabbling with ink blots (Inkblot Imagination Test) independently of Rohrschach, with whom they are more commonly associated. Knox popularized his tests in over a dozen publications, including high profile journals such as the *Journal of the American Medical Association*[3] and *Scientific American*.[4] He believed these constituted a graduated system of accurately standardized performance tests of increasing complexity suited to patient age, education and previous environment.

Although none of Knox's tests remains in use today, performance testing is still an integral part of neuropsychological assessment, as enshrined in the performance IQ component of test batteries, for example that originally designed by Wechsler and its subsequent iterations.

Besides the nature of the tests themselves, Knox was also alert to the issue of the test environment. Imagine that you have left your home, travelled thousands of miles by ship over a period of 10 days or so, perhaps in cramped and unsanitary conditions, with inadequate food and sleep, and upon arrival at your destination you are then required to undertake some form of testing procedure which is entirely alien to the way of life and habits of thought which are familiar to you. Will your performance on such tests be optimal? Almost certainly not. Knox recognized the need for rest, adequate nutrition, sleep, a quiet and well-ventilated testing room, freedom from other distractions, as well as a sympathetic examiner and interpreter, for optimal test performance.[4]

Some of the issues which Knox tried to address remain with us today, specifically issues around language and culture, and test environment. Testing individuals in the cognitive clinic may be difficult if English is not their first language, hence the need for translations of many commonly used cognitive screening instruments, such as the Addenbrooke's Cognitive Examination and its iterations and the Montreal Cognitive Assessment, into different languages. A number of cognitive screening instruments are claimed, sometimes on the basis of cultural modification and cross-cultural testing, to be culture-fair, such as the Clock Drawing Test, the Mini-Cog, the 7–minute screening battery, and the Time and Change test.[5] As for test environment, clinic rooms pervaded by extraneous noise (radio, television) and liable to interruption (passing outpatient department assistants, medical students) are still inappropriately assigned for cognitive clinics, sometimes for lack of more suitable accommodation. The problems which Knox faced 100 years ago are still likely to be with us in future years.

Acknowledgment

Adapted from: Kelly T, Larner AJ. Howard Knox (1885–1949): a pioneer of neuropsychological testing. *Adv Clin Neurosci Rehabil* 2014;14(5):30–31.

References

1. Richardson JT. Howard Andrew Knox and the origins of performance testing on Ellis Island, 1912–1916. *Hist Psychol* 2003;6:143–170.
2. Richardson JT. *Howard Andrew Knox: pioneer of intelligence testing at Ellis Island*. New York: Columbia University Press, 2011.
3. Knox HA. A scale, based on the work at Ellis Island, for estimating mental defect. *JAMA* 1914;62:741–747.
4. Knox HA. Measuring human intelligence. A progressive series of standardized tests used by the Public Health Service to protect our racial stock. *Sci Am* 1915;Jan 9:52–53,57–58.
5. Parker C, Philp I. Screening for cognitive impairment among older people in black and minority ethnic groups. *Age Ageing* 2004;33:447–452.

Diseases

Shakespeare and epilepsy: has Iago deceived again?

Kenneth W Heaton has made a comprehensive review of faints, fits and fatalities in Shakespeare's canon,[1] diligent efforts which demand acknowledgement. I hope it will not be seen as nit-picking if, as a neurologist, I suggest one possible modification to his conclusions.

To my knowledge the only use of the word "epilepsy" in the Shakespearean canon occurs in *Othello, The Moor of Venice* (1604), spoken by Iago (IV;i:50). However, considering the circumstances of Othello's collapse, shortly after being goaded by Iago into the belief that Desdemona has been unfaithful, and his rapid recovery to continue his argument with Iago, I would suggest on clinical grounds that this was more likely to have been a syncope, rather than an epileptic event.

Could it be that Iago's boldly stated diagnosis of epilepsy has succeeded in deceiving his auditors and readers? 'Twas ever thus! Lawson's publication in 1880 on the epilepsy of Othello seemed happy to accept Iago's account that the Moor "has fallen into an epilepsy".[2]

Acknowledgment

Adapted from: Larner AJ. Has Shakespeare's Iago deceived again? http://bmj.com/cgi/eletters/333/7582/1335, 2 January 2007.

References

1. Heaton KW. Faints, fits and fatalities from emotion in Shakespeare's characters: survey of the canon. *BMJ* 2006;333:1335–1338.
2. Lawson R. The epilepsy of Othello. *J Mental Sci* 1880;26:1–11.

Synaesthesia in Swift's *Gulliver's Travels* (1726)

Synaesthesia may be defined as "multisensory perception from single sensory stimulation"[1] or "a permanent involuntary spillover of sensory impressions such that stimulation of one sensory channel leads to a perception in another one or more than one".[2] Examples include the evocation of colours on hearing sounds or geometrical shapes on tasting flavours. Interest in synaesthesia has escalated in recent years[3–6] not least because of the possible insights the condition gives to the mechanisms of human consciousness.[7]

From investigations of the historical record, it has been suggested that the first medical reference to a case of synaesthesia is that by the English ophthalmologist, Thomas Woodhouse, who around 1710 reported a blind man who perceived sound-induced coloured visions.[3,8] Although there are possible earlier accounts, the first full description is ascribed to Sachs in 1812.[5] There are difficulties in identifying cases of synaesthesia from historical records, not least because of the commitment of scientific orthodoxy to the idea of five distinct senses, following Aristotle, with each modality having its characteristic sensory quality, following Muller.[9] I present a further possible case of synaesthesia dating from the mid-seventeenth century, hence predating Woodhouse.

In his book *Gulliver's Travels*, first published in 1726, Dean Jonathan Swift (1667–1745) reported on the fictional travels of a ship's surgeon, Lemuel Gulliver. Amongst his various peregrinnations, Gulliver undertook a Voyage to Laputa, which included (chapters 5 and 6) a visit to the Academy of Lagado. Among the many strange and wonderful things encountered therein,[10] Gulliver included the following account:

> There was a Man born blind, who has several Apprentices in his own Condition: Their Employment was to mix Colours for Painters, which their master taught them to distinguish by feeling and smelling.

A similar account, but without mention of a blind man, appears in *The Memoirs of Martin Scriblerus*, a work contributed to by Swift, Alexander Pope (1688–1744) and John Arbuthnot (1667–1735), first published in Pope's *Prose Works* of 1741, but possibly dating to before 1715:[11]

> He [Martin Scriblerus] it was that first found out the Palpability of Colours; and by the delicacy of his Touch, could distinguish the different Vibrations of the heterogeneous Rays of Light.

Although Gulliver's visit to the Academy of Lagado has been described as "farcical low comedy",[12] Nicholson and Mohler argued in their analysis of the Voyage to Laputa that the sources for nearly all of the ideas and episodes in that part of *Gulliver's Travels* were to be found in the work of Swift's contemporary scientists, particularly members of the Royal Society, of which the Academy of Lagado was a thinly disguised parody.[13] (Scriblerus also "address'd ... Accounts to the Royal Society".[11]) This also holds true for the blind man who could distinguish colours.

Swift's immediate source was the distinguished seventeenth century virtuoso and Fellow of the Royal Society, Robert Boyle (1627–1691), who was also the proximate stimulus for Swift's parody *A Meditation upon a Broom-stick*.[11] *The Philosophical Works of the Honourable Robert Boyle, Abridged, methodized and disposed* by Peter Shaw had appeared in 1725,[14] and was probably the proximate source for much of Swift's information for Gulliver.[13] However, Boyle's report of a man able to distinguish colours by feeling had appeared earlier, in *Experiments and Considerations Touching Colours. First occasionally Written, among some other Essays, to a Friend; and now suffer'd to come abroad as the Beginning of an Experimental History of Colours*, which was published in 1664.[14,15] This may have been Swift's source for *Scriblerus*.

Boyle had learned of the case from Sir John Finch (1626–1682), a Padua-trained physician (MD 1657) and Fellow of the Royal Society (1663), who spent most of his life in Italy and was later an ambassador to Constantinople.[16,17] A gentleman scientist or virtuoso, Finch had a special interest in the anatomy of the brain.[17] Boyle reports (*Experimental History of Colours*, chapter 3):

> Meeting casually the other Day with the deservedly Famous Dr J Finch ... and enquiring of this Ingenious Person, what might be the chief Rarity he had seen in his late return out of Italy into England, he told me, it was a Man at Maestricht, in the Low Countrys, who at certain times can distinguish Colours by the touch with his fingers.[15]

Naturally sceptical, and proposing various scruples, Boyle requested Finch to look out his notes on the encounter. Boyle's subsequent account reads:

> ... the Doctor [Finch] having been inform'd at Utrecht, that there lived one at some miles distance from Maestricht, who could distinguish Colours by the Touch, when he came to the last nam'd Town, he sent a Messenger for him, and having Examin'd him, was told upon Enquiry these Particulars:
>
> That the Man's name was John Vermaasen, at that time about 33 years of Age; that when he was but two years Old, he had the Small Pox, which

> rendred [*sic*] him absolutely Blind; That at this present he is an Organist, and serves that Office in a publick Choir.
>
> That the Doctor discoursing with him over Night, the Blind man affirm'd, that he could distinguish Colours by Touch, but that he could not do it, unless he were Fasting; Any quantity of Drink taking from him that Exquisiteness of Touch, which is requisite to so Nice a Sensation.
>
> That hereupon the Doctor provided against the next Morning seven pieces of Ribbon, of these seven Colours, Black, White, Red, Blew, Green, Yellow, and Gray, but as for mingled Colours, this Vermaasen would not undertake to discern them, though if offer'd, he would tell that they were Mixed.
>
> That to discern the Colour of the Ribbon, he places it betwixt the Thumb and the Fore-finger, but his most exquisite perception was in his Thumb, and much better in the right Thumb than in the left.
>
> That after the Blind man had four or five times told the Doctor the several Colours, (though Blinded with a Napkin for fear he might have some Sight) the Doctor found he was twice mistaken, for he called the White Black, and the Red Blew, but still, he, before his Errour, would lay them by in Pairs, saying, that though he could easily distinguish them from all others, yet those two Pairs were not easily distinguish'd amongst themselves, whereupon the Doctor desir'd to be told by him what kind of Discrimination he had of Colours by his Touch, to which he gave a reply ... That all the difference was more or less Asperity, for says he, (I give you the Doctor's own words) Black feels as if you were feeling Needles points, or some harsh Sand, and Red feels very Smooth.
>
> That the Doctor having desir'd him to tell in Order the difference of Colours to his Touch, he did as follows:
>
> Black and White are the most asperous or unequal of all Colours, and so like, that 'tis very hard to distinguish them, but Black is the most Rough of the two, Green is next in Asperity, Gray next to Green in Asperity, Yellow is the fifth in degree of Asperity, Red and Blew are so like, that they are as hard to distinguish as Black and White, but Red is somewhat more Asperous than Blew, so that Red has the sixth place, and Blew the seventh in Asperity[15] (slightly different wording is found in ref. 13).

Boyle wondered whether Vermaasen might not have been distinguishing the colours by smell, based on the ingredients used in the dyes which coloured the ribbons, rather than touch, hence perhaps explaining the need to do the test fasting, a point picked up by Swift in his account in *Gulliver's Travels.*

This is not, of course, a systematic account; all clinicians will empathize with Boyle's confession that "I would gladly have had the Opportunity of Examining this Man my self, and of Questioning him about divers particulars which I do not find to have been yet thought upon." Nonetheless, there are reasons for considering it a possible report of synaesthesia. Cross-modal activation, or "breakdown of modularity",[18] is clearly implied in the account. Coloured touch and/or coloured odour are well-recognised, albeit relatively rare, types of synaesthesia (4% and 6.8% respectively, in the Synaesthesia List [http://home.comcast.net/˜sean.day/html/types.htm], accessed 08/06/2005). Blind patients "seeing" Braille characters as coloured dots when they were touched has been reported.[19,20] Sensing colours by touch would not be an expected consequence of the recognised augmentation of tactile faculties in response to other sensory deprivation, such as blindness (hyperpilaphesie).

The description also includes many of the characteristics ascribed to synaesthetic experience:[3,5] it was involuntary or automatic; consistent (at least over four or five trials); and generic or categorical ("Needles points, ... harsh Sand, ... Smooth"). It is not, however, clear if the experience was affect-laden. Furthermore, synaesthesia is known to be more common in blind individuals.[3,19] The narrow sensory receptive field, with greatest sensitivity attributed to the thumb (presumably of the dominant hand) with its large cortical representation, is of interest, suggesting the faculty may be related to a particular, somatotopic, neural pathway. Impairment of the faculty by a cerebral depressant, alcohol (the staple drink of the age), is also suggestive of a neurally-mediated mechanism. Cross-modal leakage between somatosensory and primary visual areas might be postulated. The opposite pattern, of the visual perception of touch eliciting conscious tactile experience, has been reported.[21] Finally, if one may indulge in speculation, Vermaasen's role as an organist might possibly reflect the possession of perfect pitch, which appears to be associated with synaesthesia.

Although all such accounts are necessarily limited by the frame of historical evidence, nonetheless these considerations lead me to suggest that, courtesy of Dean Jonathan Swift, the Honourable Robert Boyle, and Sir John Finch, this may be an early report of synaesthesia.

This formulation of colour-touch synaesthesia has been challenged by Brugger and Weiss, who suggest that Boyle's account of Finch's patient is in fact an example of dermo-optical perception or fingertip sight.[22] Occasional individuals have been described over the years who can apparently read print, describe pictures, and recognise colours purely by way of touch, perhaps the most celebrated being Rosa Kuleshova from Russia.[23,24] Other forms of paroptic vision have also been described, for example though the nose. Experiments, mostly dating from the 1960s, have suggested that in some cases fingertip sight for colours may be due to minute differences in surface texture or reflected heat, but correct identification of colours through a glass plate by some subjects would seem to rule out these mechanisms. Moreover, it is not clear to me whether subtle differences in reflected heat (emissivity) related exclusively to the different wavelengths of coloured light would be sufficient to reach the threshold for sensory detection defined by the Weber-Fechner law. I am not aware of any patient with fingertip sight having been subjected to modern neuroscientific research methods, so the underlying mechanisms remain to be defined, whereas much is now understood about the cortical mechanisms underlying synaesthesia.

Acknowledgements

Thanks to David Aprahamian Liddle for directing my attention to the work of his father Donald Liddle on fingertip sight. Adapted from Larner AJ. A possible account of synaesthesia dating from the seventeenth century. *J Hist Neurosci* 2006;15:245–249; and Larner AJ, Fisher CAH. Amazing brains: Questions arising from the neurological histories of two blind organists. *Organists' Review* 2009; November:38–39.

References

1. Loring DW (ed.). *INS dictionary of neuropsychology.* New York: Oxford University Press, 1999:155.
2. Pryse-Phillips W. *Companion to clinical neurology* (2nd edition). New York, Oxford University Press, 2003:915.
3. Cytowic RE. *The man who tasted shapes.* Cambridge: MIT Press, [1993] 2003.
4. Baron-Cohen S, Harrison JE. *Synaesthesia: classic and contemporary readings.* Oxford: Blackwell, 1997.
5. Dann KT. *Bright colors falsely seen: synaesthesia and the search for transcendental knowledge.* New Haven and London: Yale University Press, 1998.
6. Ward J. *The frog who croaked blue. Synesthesia and the mixing of the senses.* Hove: Routledge, 2008.
7. Ramachandran VS, Hubbard EM. Synaesthesia – a window into perception, thought and language. *Journal of Consciousness Studies* 2001;8:3–34.
8. Marks LE. On colored-hearing synesthesia: cross-modal translations of sensory dimensions. *Psychol Bull* 1975;82:303–331.
9. Ione A, Tyler C. Synesthesia: is F-sharp colored violet? *J Hist Neurosci* 2004;13:58–65.
10. Larner AJ, Barker RA. An early account of brain transplantation. *Adv Clin Neurosci Rehabil* 2005;5(2):26.
11. Eddy WA. *Satires and Personal Writings by Jonathan Swift.* London: Oxford University Press, 1932:135.
12. Probyn C. Swift, Jonathan (1667–1745). http://www.oxforddnb.com/view/article/26833, (accessed 23/06/2005).
13. Nicholson M, Mohler NM. The scientific background of Swift's "Voyage to Laputa". *Annals of Science* 1937;2:299–334.
14. Fulton JF. *A bibliography of the Honourable Robert Boyle, Fellow of the Royal Society* (2nd edition). Oxford: Clarendon Press, 1961.

15. Hunter M, Davis EB. *The works of Robert Boyle. Volume 4: Colours and Cold, 1664–5.* London, Pickering & Chatto, 1999:40–42.
16. Abbott GF. *Under the Turk in Constantinople. A record of Sir John Finch's embassy 1674–1681.* London: Macmillan, 1920.
17. Hutton S. Finch, Sir John (1626–1682). http://www.oxforddnb.com/view/article/9439, (accessed 23/06/2005).
18. Baron-Cohen S, Harrison J, Goldstein LH, Wyke M. Colored speech perception: is synaesthesia what happens when modularity breaks down? *Perception* 1993;22:419–426.
19. Steven MS, Blakemore C. Visual synaesthesia in the blind. *Perception* 2004;33:855–868.
20. Cytowic RE, Eagleman DM. *Wednesday is indigo blue. Discovering the brain of synesthesia.* Cambridge: MIT Press, 2011:44–45.
21. Blakemore S-J, Bristow D, Bird G, Frith C, Ward J. Somatosensory activations during the observation of touch and a case of vision-touch synaesthesia. *Brain* 2005;128:1571–1583.
22. Brugger P, Weiss PH. Dermo-optical perception: the non-synesthetic "palpability of colors" a comment on Larner (2006). *J Hist Neurosci* 2008;17:253–255.
23. Liddle D. Fingertip sight: fact or fiction. *Discovery* 1964;September:22–26.
24. Critchley M. *The citadel of the senses and other essays.* New York: Raven Press, 1986:196.

An early account of brain transplantation

The accounts with which the surgeon Lemuel Gulliver returned from his various travels in the late 17th and early 18th century were often treated with considerable scepticism if not frank incredulity and ridicule. Nonetheless, as someone with some medical training, we should perhaps look carefully at his reports of his experiences and the medical practice in other lands. Amongst these may be the first report of Lilliputian hallucinations (micropsia).[1] There also appears to be an early account of brain transplantation surgery, originating from the Academy at Lagado on the island of Balnibarbi:

> When Parties in a State are violent, [the Ingenious Doctor] offered a wonderful Contrivance to reconcile them. The Method is this. You take an Hundred Leaders of each Party, you dispose them into Couples of such whose Heads are nearest of a size; then let two nice Operators saw off the *Occiput* of each Couple at the same time, in such a manner that the Brain may be equally divided. Let the Occiputs thus cut off be interchanged, applying each to the head of his opposite Party-man. It seems indeed to be a Work that requireth some exactness, but the Professor assured us, that if it were dextrously performed, the Cure would be infallible. For he argued thus; that the two half Brains being left to debate the Matter between themselves within the space of one Skull, would soon come to a good Understanding, and produce that Moderation as well as Regularity of thinking, so much to be wished for in the Heads of those, who imagine they come into the World only to watch and govern its Motion.

Dean Jonathan Swift (1667–1745), Gulliver's creator, suffered from cognitive decline probably due to a dementing disorder, possibly Alzheimer's disease, in later life.[2,3] In this context, it is perhaps ironic that attempts to transplant brain tissue have been explored for the treatment of dementing disorders such as Alzheimer's disease.[4]

Acknowledgment

Adapted from: Larner AJ, Barker RA. An early account of brain transplantation. *Adv Clin Neurosci Rehabil* 2005;5(2):26.

References

1. Leroy R. Les hallucinations lilliputiennes. *Ann Med Psychol* 1909:279–289.
2. Bewley TH. The health of Jonathan Swift. *J R Soc Med* 1998;91:602–605.
3. Lewis JM. Jonathan Swift and Alzheimer's disease. *Lancet* 1993;342:504.
4. Barker RA, Dunnett SB. *Neural repair, transplantation and rehabilitation.* Hove: Psychology Press, 1999:157–174.

Some accounts of Tourette syndrome and obsessive compulsive disorder

Surely no neurologist today can be unaware of the diagnosis of Tourette's syndrome or disorder. However, this familiarity was not always so. Although the eponymous description was published in 1885, the first full description has been accredited to Itard in 1825, and a possible case dating back to the fifteenth century (the *Malleus Maleficarum* of 1486) has also been found.[1] Herein, four accounts suggestive of individuals suffering from Tourette's syndrome are presented, dating from the eighteenth, nineteenth, and twentieth centuries, two predating Tourette's publication. The sources are a biography and three novels, one of the latter supplemented by an autobiography.

CASE 1: *Dr Samuel Johnson (1709–1784)*

The great English writer, critic, lexicographer and moralist was noted by many of his contemporaries to have involuntary movements. For example, in his biography, *Life of Johnson*, published in 1791, James Boswell (1740–1795) writes:

> That the most minute singularities which belonged to him, and made very observable parts of his appearance and manner, may not be omitted, it is requisite to mention, that while talking or even musing as he sat in his chair, he commonly held his head to one side towards his right shoulder, and shook it in a tremulous manner, moving his body backwards and forwards, and rubbing his left knee in the same direction, with the palm of his hand. In the intervals of articulating he made various sounds with his mouth, sometimes as if ruminating, or what is called chewing the cud, sometimes giving a half whistle, sometimes making his tongue play backwards from the roof of his mouth, as if clucking like a hen, and sometimes protruding it against his upper gums in front, as if pronouncing quickly under his breath, *too, too, too* … Generally when he had concluded a period, in the course of a dispute, by which time he was a good deal exhausted by violence and vociferation, he used to blow out his breath like a whale.

The illustrator William Hogarth (1697–1764) also noted Johnson's movements:

> Mr Hogarth came one day to see Richardson [the author of *Clarissa*] ... While he was talking he perceived a person standing at a window in the room, shaking his head, and rolling himself about in a strange ridiculous manner. He concluded that he was an ideot [*sic*], whom his relations had put under the care of Mr Richardson, as a very good man.

The diarist Fanny Burney (later Madame d'Arblay; 1752–1840) describes Johnson thus:

> I have so true a veneration for him, that the very sight of him inspires me with delight and reverence, notwithstanding the cruel infirmities to which he is subject; for he has almost perpetual convulsive movements, either of his hands, lips, feet or knees, and sometimes of all together.

All these excerpts suggest the presence of motor and vocal tics. Accounts suggestive of obsessive-compulsive behaviour are also to be found in the biography. For example, Boswell noted:

> He had another particularity, of which none of his friends ever ventured to ask an explanation. It appeared to me some superstitious habit, which he had contracted early, and from which he had never called upon his reason to disentangle him. This was his anxious care to go out or in at a door or passage, by a certain number of steps from a certain point, or at least so as that either his right or his left foot, (I am not certain which,) should constantly make the first actual movement when he came close to the door or passage. Thus I conjecture, for I have, upon innumerable occasions, observed him suddenly stop, and then seem to count his steps with a deep earnestness; and when he had neglected or gone wrong in this sort of magical movement, I have seen him go back again, put himself in a proper posture to begin the ceremony, and, having gone through it, walk briskly on ...

Mr S Whyte used his opera glass to observe Johnson approaching along a London street:

> I perceived him at a good distance walking along with a peculiar solemnity of deportment, and an awkward sort of measured step ... Upon every post as he passed along, I could observe he deliberately laid his hand; but missing one of them, when he had got at some distance, he seemed suddenly to recollect himself, and immediately returning back, carefully performed the accustomed ceremony, and resumed his former course, not

> omitting one until he gained the crossing. This ... was his constant practice.

What explanations for these features were contemplated by Johnson's contemporaries?

Boswell stated:

> The infirmity... appeared to me... to be of the convulsive kind, and of the nature of that distemper called St Vitus's dance; and in this opinion I am confirmed by the description which Sydenham gives of that disease. "It manifests itself by halting or unsteadiness of one of the legs which the patient draws after him like an ideot [*sic*]. If the hand of the same side be applied to the breast, or any other part of the body, he cannot keep it a moment in the same posture, but it will be drawn into a different one by a convulsion, notwithstanding all his efforts to the contrary."

It is interesting that Boswell, no medical man, should have been familiar with the works of Thomas Sydenham (1624–1689). As we have seen, Fanny Burney was also of the opinion that the movements were convulsive, as was the writer Alexander Pope (1688–1744):

> [Johnson] has an infirmity of the convulsive kind that attacks him sometimes, so as to make him a sad spectacle.

However, the painter Sir Joshua Reynolds (1723–1792) took a different view

> Those motions or tricks of Dr Johnson are improperly called convulsions. He could sit motionless, when he was told to do so, as well as any other man; my opinion is that it proceeded from a habit which he had indulged himself in, of accompanying his thoughts with certain untoward actions.

This suggests that the movements were suppressible (perhaps a portrait painter was particularly adept at getting people to sit still). However, Boswell counters by stating:

> I still however think that these gestures were involuntary; for surely had that not been the case, he would have restrained them in the publick [*sic*] streets.

The neurologist Lord (Russell) Brain (1895–1966) was a devoted Johnsonian and wrote about his movements,[2] but ascribed them a psychological origin. His failure to mention Tourette's syndrome may perhaps reflect general neurological unawareness of the condition at the time of writing. It was left to later authors to suggest that this was Johnson's diagnosis.[3–5]

CASE 2: "*Mr Pancks" (1857)*

The novelist Charles Dickens (1812–1870) was an author of fecund imagination but also with an acute eye for human oddity or idiosyncrasy. Many subsequent readers have thought they could detect particular neurological conditions in his characters.[6] One such is Mr Pancks, from the 1857 novel *Little Dorrit*:

> he ... snorted and sniffed and puffed and blew, like a little labouring steam-engine.
>
> Mr Pancks here made a singular and startling noise, produced by a strong blowing effort in the region of the nose, unattended by any result but that acoustic one.
>
> ... Mr Pancks, snorting and blowing in a more and more portentous manner as he became more interested, listened with great attention ...

Clear as these descriptions of vocal tics are, there are fewer suggestions of motor tics, although Pancks is described as "darting about in eccentric directions" and of stirring up his hair. Obsessive-compulsive behaviour is suggested by his keeping a notebook in "dictionary order" and by descriptions of his tendency to nail-biting:

> ... snorted Pancks, taking one of his dirty hands ... to bite his nails, if he could find any ...
>
> ...with the fingers of his right hand in his mouth that he might bite the nails ...

Furthermore, Pancks has another behavioural feature which may fall within the spectrum of obsessive-compulsive behaviour: trichotillomania:

> Mr Pancks took hold of himself by the hair of his head, and tore it in desperation ...
>
> All the time, [he] was tearing at his tough hair in a most pitiless and cruel manner.
>
> [He] took hold of his hair again, and gave it such a wrench that he pulled out several prongs of it.

The suggestion that all these symptoms reflected a diagnosis of Tourette's syndrome was first made by Cosnett.[7]

CASE 3: *Pozdnyshev (1889)*

Leo Tolstoy's (1828–1910) novella *The Kreutzer Sonata* of 1889 is a second hand account of the actions of Pozdnyshev. On first encountering him on a train, the unnamed narrator tells us that his "movements were nervous and jerky". Also:

> Another peculiar thing about this man was that every now and again he uttered strange sounds, as if he were clearing his throat or beginning to laugh, but breaking off in silence.

There are further references to him making his peculiar noises, "his peculiar nasal sound".[8] As well as these vocal tics, Pozdnyshev's response to his wife and her music teacher might be construed as having an obsessive-compulsive nature.

CASE 4: *Captain Lancaster (1975), Captain Hardcastle (1984)*

The popular children's author Roald Dahl (1916–1990) included in his 1975 work *Danny the Champion of the World* a schoolmaster named Captain Lancaster:

> ... he would make queer snuffling grunts through his nose, like some dog sniffing round a rabbit hole.
>
> ... I could hear him snorting and snuffling through his nose like a dog outside a rabbit hole.

Knowing Dahl's oeuvre, it would not be difficult to see this strange character as entirely fictional, a product of the author's fecund imagination. However, in his autobiographical work *Boy. Tales of childhood*, published in 1984, Dahl recalled a schoolmaster, a veteran of the first World War, whom he encountered when he was 9 years old (1925–6):

> We called them masters in those days, not teachers, and ... the one I feared most of all ... was Captain Hardcastle.
>
> Captain Hardcastle was never still. His orange head twitched and jerked perpetually from side to side in the most alarming fashion, and each twitch was accompanied by a little grunt that came out of the nostrils.
>
> Prep was in progress. Captain Hardcastle was ... twitching his head and grunting through his nose. ... The only noises to be heard were Captain Hardcastle's little snorting grunts ...

What explanation did the boys have for these movements and sounds?

> Rumour had it that the constant twitching and jerking and snorting was caused by something called shell-shock, but we were not quite sure what that was. We took it to mean that an explosive object had gone off very close to him with such an enormous bang that it had made him jump high in the air and he hadn't stopped jumping since.

It may be that the actual schoolmaster Captain Hardcastle was the template for the fictional Captain Lancaster.

Conclusion

Considering the striking clinical features of Tourette syndrome, it is perhaps not surprising that the condition should have attracted the attention of creative writers, as well as neurologists. Acute observers of nature, including writers and painters may, without the benefit of specific medical training, record medical conditions, sometimes prior to their description by members of the medical professions. The cases reported here may contradict the assertion of one neurologist to have found only one example (the *Malleus Maleficarum* of 1486) which might fulfil the criteria for Tourette's.[9]

Acknowledgment

Adapted from: Larner AJ. Three historical accounts of Gilles de la Tourette syndrome. *Adv Clin Neurosci Rehabil* 2003;3(5):26–27

References

1. Goetz CG, Chmura TA, Lanska DJ. History of tic disorders and Gilles de la Tourette syndrome: Part 5 of the MDS-sponsored history of movement disorders exhibit, Barcelona, June 2000. *Mov Disord* 2001;16:346–349.
2. Brain R. The great convulsionary. In: *Some reflections on genius and other essays.* London: Pitman Medical, 1960:69–91.
3. McHenry LC. Samuel Johnson's tics and gesticulations. *J Hist Med Allied Sci* 1967;22:152–168.
4. Murray TJ. Dr Samuel Johnson's movement disorder. *BMJ* 1979;1:1610–1614.
5. Pearce JMS. Dr Samuel Johnson: a victim of Gilles de la Tourtette syndrome. *J R Soc Med* 1994;87:396–399.
6. Larner AJ. Charles Dickens, *qua* neurologist. *Adv Clin Neurosci Rehabil* 2002;2(1):22.
7. Cosnett JE. Dickens, dystonia and dyskinesia. *J Neurol Neurosurg Psychiatry* 1991;54:184.

8. Tolstoy L. *The Kreutzer Sonata*. London: Penguin, [1889] 2007:3,80,86,100.
9. Perkin GD. Some movement disorders. In: Bogousslavsky J, Dieguez S (eds.). *Literary medicine: brain disease and doctors in novels, theater, and film* (Frontiers of Neurology and Neuroscience Volume 31). Basel: Karger, 2013:188–194 [at 191–192].

Headache in the works of Jane Austen (1775–1817)

Since headache is experienced by over 70% of individuals at one time or another during their lifetime, one may fairly say that this is an almost inevitable feature of the human condition.[1,2] Hence, references to characters with headache in novels, poems or plays may not necessarily be deemed worthy of remark. However, of the canonical writers in the English language none seems to mention headache more frequently than Jane Austen (1775–1817). This has been noted in a critical reading of the novels which analyses them in the light of medical thinking about illness and the body,[3] and also on occasion by clinical neurologists.[4,5] However, to my knowledge, no extended examination of Jane Austen's references to headache has previously been undertaken. The purpose of this article, therefore, is to catalogue all references to headache in the Austen canon including her extant correspondence, and in biographical material written by Austen family members, and to consider them both from the standpoint of clinical neurology and as an authorial narrative device.

"CASE REPORTS"

Love and Freindship [sic] (1790)

In correspondence with Isabel, Laura reports of her friend Sophia:

> [She] complained of a violent pain in her delicate limbs, accompanied with a disagreable Head-ake. She attributed it to a cold caught by her continued faintings in the open Air as the Dew was falling the Evening before.

This progresses to a galloping consumption which carries her off.[6]

Lesley Castle (1792)

In her correspondence with Margaret Lesley, Charlotte Lutterell reports the comment of her sister Eloisa:

> Well Charlotte, I am very glad to find that you have at last left off that ridiculous custom of applauding my Execution on the Harpsichord till you made my head ake, and yourself hoarse.[7]

Sense and Sensibility (1811)

Marianne Dashwood, aged sixteen at the opening of the novel, is reported as having headache on two occasions. The first occurs following the sudden and unanticipated departure of her beau Willoughby from Barton:

> She was awake the whole night ... She got up with an head-ache, was unable to talk, and unwilling to take any nourishment.[8]

The second accompanies Marianne's collapse following the fracture with Willoughby in London, and his return of her letters and lock of hair:

> ... the consequence of all this was felt in an aching head, a weakened stomach, and a general nervous faintness.
>
> ... Elinor saw her lay her aching head on the pillow, and saw her, as she hoped, in a way to get some quiet rest before she left her.[9]

On two other occasions, Elinor uses headache as an excuse for Marianne's behaviour. The arrival of Colonel Brandon at Mrs Jennings's London house shortly after the sisters' arrival there, when Marianne is keenly anticipating a visit from Willoughby, causes Marianne immediately to leave the room in distress. Elinor:

> then talked of head-aches, low spirits, and over fatigues; and of every thing to which she could decently attribute her sister's behaviour.[10]

Later, Marianne avoids a visit from the Miss Steeles, much to their regret, prompting Elinor to remark of Marianne that:

> ... she has been very much plagued lately with nervous head-akes, which make her unfit for company or conversation.[11]

Pride and Prejudice (1813)

The day after Jane Bennet's ride to Netherfield in the rain, at the behest of Mrs Bennet, to see Mr Bingley and his sisters, she writes to Elizabeth of feeling unwell with "sore throat and head-ache", symptoms which worsen after Elizabeth's arrival: "her head ached acutely".[12]

Whilst visiting Charlotte Collins at Hunsford parsonage, Elizabeth Bennet learns from Colonel Fitzwilliam of Darcy's interventions to dissuade Bingley from his attachment to Jane:

> The agitation and tears which the subject occasioned, brought on a headach.

Elizabeth is thus unable to go to tea with Lady Catherine de Bourgh at Rosings, at which time she receives Mr Darcy's unexpected visit and his (even more unexpected) proposal of marriage.[13] Elizabeth's headache, no less than Darcy's perceived ungentleman-like manner, may make her unreceptive to the offer and contribute to her decided refusal.

Following Lydia Bennet's elopement with Wickham, Mrs Bennet is afflicted with many symptoms including, as she reports to Mr Gardiner, "pains in my head".[14]

Mansfield Park (1814)

Fanny Price, aged eighteen, develops a headache after picking roses in the heat.

> "Fanny," said Edmund, after looking at her attentively; "I am sure you have the head-ache?"
>
> She could not deny it, but said it was not very bad.

Mrs Norris opines that "There is nothing so likely to give it [headache] as standing and stooping in a hot sun", which also inclines Lady Bertram to the same view, but Edmund ascribes it to the additional walking twice on an errand to Mrs Norris's house. Fanny, however, reflects that:

> The state of her spirits had probably had its share in her indisposition ... the pain of her mind had been much beyond that in her head.[15]

Returned to her natal home of Portsmouth, following her refusal of Henry Crawford's marriage proposal, Fanny finds that her younger brothers Tom and Charles "had soon burst away from her and slammed the parlour door till her temples ached". As her father ignores her, preferring to read the borrowed newspaper by the light of a candle, Fanny is "glad to have the light screened from her aching head, as she sat in bewildered, broken, sorrowful contemplation". After her sister Susan assists in making the tea, Fanny's "head and heart were soon the better for such well-timed kindness".[16]

Enumerating reasons for not attending divine service to listen to sermons, Mary Crawford states that:

> ... when men and women might lie another ten minutes in bed, when they woke with a head-ache, without danger of reprobation, because chapel was missed, they would have jumped with joy and envy.[17]

Emma (1816)

Emma has been described as a novel concerned with health[18] and some of the instances of headache have been noted in an examination of the role of Mr Perry, the apothecary.[19]

The chief sufferer is Jane Fairfax, who is the same age, 20, as Emma. Although Jane is ill from the time of her arrival in Highbury, the first mention of headache comes shortly after the first departure of Frank Churchill:

> She had been particularly unwell, however, suffering from headache to a degree.[20]

However, it is on the morning after the excursion to Box Hill that she avoids Emma's visit, her aunt Miss Bates reporting that "… she has a dreadful headach just now, writing all the morning", these being the letters to accept the lowly position of governess with Mrs Smallridge, prompted by the belief that her secret engagement to Frank Churchill is over; "… if you were to see what a headach she has".[21] She is visited by Mr Perry, the apothecary, who is reported to find that:

> … she was suffering under severe headachs, and a nervous fever … Her health seemed for the moment completely deranged … Her present home was unfavourable to a nervous disorder.[22]

Isabella Knightley, Emma's sister, reports to her father that "excepting those little nervous head-aches and palpitations which I am never entirely free from any where, I am quite well myself".[23]

Miss Bates fears that Mrs Weston may have headache as a consequence of her work in preparation for the ball at the Crown:

> So afraid you might have a headach! – Seeing you pass by so often, and knowing how much trouble you must have.[24]

Persuasion (1817)

Anne Elliot, aged 27, pleads a headache to avoid a dinner with the Musgroves at which Captain Wentworth will be present.[25]

In the original, discarded, concluding chapters of *Persuasion*, following her reunion with Captain Wentworth at Admiral Croft's Bath lodgings, Anne finds that "It was necessary to stay up half the Night and lie awake the remainder to comprehend with composure her present state, and pay for the overplus of Bliss, by Headake and Fatigue".

Sanditon (1817)

Diana Parker's letter to her brother reports that their sister Susan:

> … has been suffering much from the headache and six leeches a day for ten days together relieved her so little that we thought it right to change our

> measures – and being convinced on examination that much of the evil lay in her gum, I persuaded her to attack the disorder there. She has accordingly had three teeth drawn, and is decidedly better, but her nerves are a good deal deranged. She can only speak in a whisper – and fainted away twice this morning . . .[26]

Later Diana reports that "Susan is to have leeches at one o'clock – which will be a three hours' business",[27] but the specific indication for this treatment is not stated.

I find no direct mention of headache in *Lady Susan*, *Northanger Abbey*, or *The Watsons*, although in the latter Elizabeth Watson notes that her asthmatic and gouty invalid father says that "his head won't bear whist" when cards are being discussed,[28] but whether this is due to a risk of headache is not clear.

Correspondence

In her famous letter to her sister Cassandra, of 29th January 1813 (Letter 79), relating the arrival of the first copy of *Pride and Prejudice* – "my own darling Child" – Jane Austen also mentions, of a recent visit, "I was rather head-achey that day", symptoms which prevented her from eating anything sweet although she did have some jelly.[29] To my knowledge this is the only record of Jane Austen herself having headaches.[30]

There are few further allusions to headache in the extant correspondence, sufficient to indicate that Jane Austen would have been familiar with headache from the experiences of family members, including her mother and her niece Harriet (daughter of Charles Austen), and acquaintances who were afflicted:

Letter 54. To Cassandra Austen, from Godmersham, 26th June 1808:

> Mrs Knight had a sad headache which kept her in bed. She had had too much company the day before.[31]

Letter 88. To Cassandra Austen, from Henrietta Street, 16th September 1813:

> . . . my Mother no more in need of Leeches.[32]

Letter 89. To Cassandra Austen, from Godmersham, 23rd-24th September 1813:

> I told Mrs C[ooke] of my Mother's late oppression in her head.- She says on that subject – "Dear Mrs Austen's is I beleive [sic] an attack frequent at her age [74 years old] & mine. Last year I had for some time the Sensation of a Peck Loaf resting on my head, & they talked of cupping me, but I came off with a dose or two of calomel & have never heard of it since."[33]

Mrs Cooke has been suggested as the source for the afflictions of the Parker family in Sanditon.[34] Mrs Austen herself refers to being "on the Sopha with the head-ache" in May 1814 in a letter sent to Anna Lefroy shortly after the latter's marriage in the autumn of that year.[35,36]

Letter 155. To Fanny Knight, from Chawton, 23rd-25th March 1817:

> Little Harriet's headaches are abated, & Sir Evd is satisfied with the effect of the Mercury, & does not despair of a Cure. The Complaint I find is not considered Incurable nowadays , provided the Patient be young enough not to have the Head hardened. The Water in that case may be drawn off by Mercury. – But though this is a new idea to us, perhaps it may have been long familiar to you . . .[37]

Letter 156. To Caroline Austen, from Chawton, 26th March 1817:

> Harriet headaches were a little releived [sic], & Sir Ev: Hume does not despair of a cure. – He persists in thinking it Water on the Brain, but none of the others are convinced.[38]

Austen's correspondence also indicates that she knew of Caleb Hillier Parry, a fashionable physician in Bath who made contributions in the field of headache as well as other disorders.[39]

Verses

Two of Jane Austen's occasional verses mention headache or pain in the head. Dated 7th February 1811, "Lines on Maria Beckford" (entitled thus in *Minor Works*) runs:

> "I've a pain in my head"
> Said the suffering Beckford;
> To her Doctor so dread.
> "Oh! what shall I take for't?"
>
> Said this Doctor so dread
> Whose name it was Newnham.
> "For this pain in the head
> Ah! What can you do Ma'AM?"
>
> Said Miss Beckford, "Suppose
> If you think there's no risk,
> I take a good Dose
> Of calomel brisk." –

"What a praise worthy Notion."
  Replied Mr. Newnham.
"You shall have such a potion
  And so will I too Ma'am."[40]

Miss Maria Beckford was the spinster sister-in-law who kept house for Mr John Charles Middleton, a widower with six young children, who was the tenant of Chawton Great House from 1808 to 1813. Jane Austen apparently accompanied her in February 1811 to a consultation with Mr Newnham, the apothecary at Alton.[41]

"On a headache" (as entitled in *Minor Works*), apparently dated 27th October 1811, begins:

When stretch'd on one's bed
With a fierce-throbbing head,
Which precludes alike thought or repose,
How little one cares
For the grandest affairs
That may busy the world as it goes!

and ends:

Our own bodily pains
Ev'ry faculty chains;
We can feel on no subject beside.
Tis in health and in ease
We the power must seize
For our friends and our souls to provide.[42]

Though not certain, it is possible that this account is autobiographical.

Other biographical material

Biographical works undertaken by Austen family members who knew Jane Austen and had access to family papers add nothing more.[43] However, from Fanny Knight's diaries we learn that on 18th July 1813: "Aunt Jane confined to the house with a bad face ache in the evening." Matters were worse on 24th July, and the symptoms apparently lingered until 1st or 2nd August: "Aunt Jane's face very indifferent all this week". Lizzy Knight, Fanny's younger sister, recalled seeing her aunt "with head a little to one side, and sometimes a very small cushion pressed against her cheek, if she were suffering from face-ache, as she not unfrequently did in later life".[44] The nature of this ailment is not clear.

Tomalin suggests trigeminal neuralgia, possibly following shingles at a time of immunosuppression such as the beginning of lymphoma,[45] the latter thought to be the cause of her final illness.[46] However, from the clinical standpoint this formulation seems to confuse trigeminal neuralgia with post-herpetic neuralgia.[47] Fanny Knight herself had headaches, and Aunt Jane sat with her on one occasion when she was treated with leeches.[48]

Other headache sufferers noted by or known to Jane Austen include her cousin Eliza de Feuillide,[49] Lady Sondes,[50] Maria Beckford,[40,41] and Anne Sharpe, sometime governess to Fanny Knight.[51]

Discussion

It might be argued that Jane Austen used headache simply as a convenient plot device. The stimulus to do so might have been imitation: in Samuel Richardson's *History of Sir Charles Grandison* (1753), Austen's favourite novel, of which she knew large chunks by heart, Lady G writes to Miss Byron (volume VI, letter xlv) "If these megrims are the effect of Love, thank Heaven, I never knew what it was".[52] Headaches might also be used as a narrative device to "establish a basis of common humanity",[53] as argued, for example, for the headaches of the patriarch in Gabriel Garcia Marquez's novel *The Autumn of the Patriarch* (1978).

This examination of the works of Jane Austen makes clear, however, that headache was something familiar to her, although whether she herself was a frequent sufferer is uncertain. One biographer suggests, a propos the cancelled final chapters of *Persuasion*, that "headache and fatigue she knew well enough"[54] but I find only one unequivocal reference, in her correspondence, to Austen herself having headache.[29,30] The poem "On a headache",[42] however, suggests the possibility that she was more frequently afflicted. Certainly many around her, both relatives and acquaintances, did have headache disorders. Without exception, those mentioned in the various sources are female, and this is mirrored in her fiction. This may be adduced as a further example of the "enabling context" for Austen's work provided by a network female friends and relations.[55] Other sources may have come from her reading: in addition to Johnson, Cowper, Fielding and Richardson, she is said to have read "pedagogical works, books of travel, history, political and *medical pamphlets*" [my italics].[56] As a narrative device, headache appears in both the juvenilia and the mature works (five of the six major novels, the exception being *Northanger Abbey*, as well as in the unfinished fragment of *Sanditon*[5]).

From the biomedical, neurological, standpoint it might be argued that Austen suffered from occasional migraines (the throbbing character of the headache related in her poem is certainly suggestive of this diagnosis).

However, this retrospective diagnosis risks being transcultural and transhistorical. John Wiltshire explores the possibility of somatisation, arguing that headaches are not merely the result of physiological processes but may be psychological as well as social products, Fanny Price's headache whilst cutting roses being envisaged as a bodily reproduction of the social tensions highlighted in the novel.[57] Anna Mae Duane diagnoses Fanny Price with "hysteria", as understood in a Freudian sense,[58] a diagnosis which in more recent times has been re-branded as somatisation.[59] Certainly many of the young women with headache in the novels have some form of acute amatory distress. Illness may therefore be read as "a mode of manners" in relation to social circumstances.[60]

Headache may also reflect Austen's interest in physical experience, being a physical or corporeal aspect of the self acknowledged in the texts. Carol Shields has pointed out the disinclination of Jane Austen to use images of the body, but that the glance may be used as a form of body expressiveness in an age of highly codified behaviour.[61] The same might be true of the headache.[5] It has been suggested by an experienced clinician that migraine provides "some expression of what cannot be expressed".[62]

Acknowledgments

Adapted from: Larner AJ. Jane Austen's (1775–1817) references to headache: fact and fiction. *J Med Biogr* 2010;18:211–215; and Larner AJ. "A transcript of actual life": Jane Austen and headache. *Jane Austen Society (Midlands) Transactions* 2015;Issue 26:6–14.

References

1. Rasmussen BJ, Jensen R, Schroll M, Olesen J. Epidemiology of headache in a general population – a prevalence study. *J Clin Epidemiol* 1991;44:1147–1157.
2. Steiner TJ. Lifting the burden: the global campaign against headache. *Lancet Neurol* 2004;3:204–205.
3. Wiltshire J. *Jane Austen and the body. "The picture of health"*. Cambridge: Cambridge University Press, 1992.
4. Perkin GD. Headache. *J Neurol Neurosurg Psychiatry* 1995;59:632.
5. Larner AJ. "A transcript of actual life": headache in the novels of Jane Austen. *Headache* 2010;50:692–695.
6. Austen, Jane. *Catherine and other writings* (eds. MA Doody, D Murray). Oxford: World's Classics, 1993:98.
7. See reference 6:126.
8. Austen, Jane. *Sense and Sensibility* (ed. R Ballaster). London: Penguin Classics, 2003:83.

9. See reference 8:175,187.
10. See reference 8:155.
11. See reference 8:206.
12. Austen, Jane. *Pride and Prejudice* (ed. V Jones). London: Penguin Classics, 2003:32,34.
13. See reference 12:182.
14. See reference 12:274.
15. Austen, Jane. *Mansfield Park* (ed. K Sutherland). London: Penguin Classics, 2003:68,69,70.
16. See reference 15:354,355,356.
17. See reference 15:82.
18. See reference 3:110.
19. Watson JR. Mr. Perry's patients: a view of Emma. *Essays in Criticism* 1970;20:334–343.
20. Austen, Jane. *Emma* (ed. F Stafford). London: Penguin Classics, 2003:244.
21. See reference 20:354,355
22. See reference 20:365.
23. See reference 20:99.
24. See reference 20:302.
25. Austen, Jane. *Persuasion* (ed. G Beer). London: Penguin Classics, 2003:72.
26. Austen, Jane. *Lady Susan, The Watsons and Sanditon* (ed. M Drabble). London: Penguin Classics, 2003:175–176.
27. See reference 26:209.
28. See reference 26:144.
29. Le Faye D (ed.). *Jane Austen's letters* (3rd edition). Oxford: Oxford University Press, 1995:202.
30. Le Faye D. *Jane Austen. A family record.* London: British Library, 1989:212.
31. See reference 29:134.
32. See reference 29:222,420.
33. See reference 29:228.
34. Edwards A-M. *In the steps of Jane Austen* (3rd edition). Newbury: Countryside Books, 1991:162.
35. See reference 30:196.
36. Shields C. *Jane Austen.* London: Weidenfeld & Nicolson, 2001:123.
37. See reference 29:336.
38. See reference 29:338.
39. See reference 29:221,237–238,248,252,254,260. Also Larner AJ. Caleb Hillier Parry (1755–1822): clinician, scientist, friend of Edward Jenner (1749–1823). *J Med Biogr* 2005;13:189–194; Larner AJ. Neurological contributions of Caleb Hillier Parry. *Adv Clin Neurosci Rehabil* 2004;4(3):38–39.
40. See reference 6:242.
41. See reference 30:155,177–178.
42. See reference 6:243–244.
43. Austen-Leigh JE. *A memoir of Jane Austen and other family recollections.* Oxford: Oxford University Press, 2002.

44. Le Faye D. *Fanny Knight's diaries. Jane Austen through her niece's eyes.* Winchester: Sarsen Press/The Jane Austen Society, 2000:27. Also see reference 29:226.
45. Tomalin C. *Jane Austen. A life.* London: Penguin, 1997:240,290.
46. Upfal A. Jane Austen's lifelong health problems and final illness: new evidence points to a fatal Hodgkin's disease and excludes the widely accepted Addison's. *Journal of Medical Ethics; Medical Humanities* 2005;31:3–11.
47. Barker R, Scolding NJ, Rowe D, Larner AJ. *The A-Z of neurological practice. A guide to clinical neurology.* Cambridge: Cambridge University Press, 2005:418–419,865–866.
48. Honan P. *Jane Austen: her life.* London: Phoenix, 1997:272.
49. See reference 45:60.
50. See reference 29:159.
51. See reference 44:10.
52. Harris J (ed.). *Samuel Richardson. The History of Sir Charles Grandison.* Oxford: Oxford University Press, 1972:III:195.
53. Bell M. *Gabriel Garcia Marquez: solitude and solidarity.* London: MacMillan, 1993:74–75.
54. Nokes D. *Jane Austen. A life.* London: Fourth Estate, 1997:492.
55. Kaplan D. *Jane Austen among women.* Baltimore: Johns Hopkins University Press, 1992:5.
56. Grundy I. Jane Austen and literary traditions. In: Copeland E, McMaster J (eds.). *The Cambridge companion to Jane Austen.* Cambridge: Cambridge University Press, 1997:189–210 [at 200].
57. See reference 3:14,19.
58. Duane AM. Confusions of guilt and complications of evil: hysteria and the high price of love at Mansfield park. *Studies in the Novel* 2001;33:402–415.
59. Trimble M. *Somatoform disorders. A medicolegal guide.* Cambridge: Cambridge University Press, 2004.
60. See reference 3:220.
61. See reference 36:2,57,148–149,150–152.
62. Sacks O. *Migraine* (Revised and expanded). London: Picador, 1992:215.

Headache in the works of Elizabeth Gaskell (1810–1865)

Mrs Elizabeth Cleghorn Gaskell (1810–1865) was a celebrated author of the Victorian era, a friend of both Charles Dickens (1812–1870) and Charlotte Brontë (1816–1855) and the latter's first biographer. She published six major novels between 1848 and 1866 (posthumously) which, as at the time of their first publication, continue to enjoy a high reputation, as well as shorter fiction, some first appearing in serial form in Dickens's popular weekly magazines *Household Words* and *All the Year Round.* She was also a friend of Charlotte Brontë whose biography she was invited to write by Charlotte's father, Patrick Brontë, after his daughter's death. Gaskell's writing was undertaken largely in the interstices of a busy life as the wife of a Unitarian clergyman in Manchester and the mother to four daughters.

Interest in Gaskell's life and work has developed greatly in recent times, facilitated by publication of her extant letters [1–3] and biographical accounts.[4,5] From these it is evident that Elizabeth Gaskell suffered from headaches.[6] Like other 19th century female novelists,[7–9] she also makes use of headaches in her novels. Although a possible reference to mesmerism in one of Mrs Gaskell's letters has been noted,[10] references to medical matters in Gaskell's oeuvre, and to headache in particular,[6] have not attracted significant prior attention, prompting this examination of the major novels and some of the shorter fiction for such references.

References to headache in Mrs Gaskell's six major novels, published between 1848 and 1866, as well as some of her shorter fiction, have been collated in order to examine how the author used headache as a plot device. References have been informed by reading of her extant correspondence,[1–3] supplemented by the biography by Uglow,[4] which is generally acknowledged to be the most comprehensive account available.

"CASE REPORTS": *Novels*

Mary Barton: A Tale of Manchester Life (1848)

George Wilson overhears a conversation when visiting the household of Mr Carson, the mill-owner, to beg for an Infirmary order for a sick mill worker, in which Mrs. Carson, never directly present in the narrative, is reported by a servant, a "semi-upper-housemaid, semi-lady's-maid", to have a "bad headache". Thomas, the Carson's coachman, then replies:

> It's a pity Miss Jenkins is not here to match her. Lord! how she and missis did quarrel which had got the worst headaches; it was that Miss Jenkins left for; she would not give up having bad headaches, and missis could not abide any one to have 'em but herself.[11]

A fuller account of these headaches is given later:

> Mrs Carson was ... sitting upstairs, indulging in the luxury of a headache. ... 'Wind in the head', the servants called it. But it was but the natural consequence of the state of mental and bodily idleness in which she was placed. Without education enough to value the resources of wealth and leisure, she was so circumstanced as to command both. It would have done her more good than all the ether and sal volatile she was daily in the habit of swallowing, if she might have taken the work of one of her own housemaids for a week ... [12]

Mrs Carson's headaches may be contrasted with those of Mary Barton. Having discovered the true identity of the murderer of her erstwhile beau, William Carson, a crime for which her admirer Jem Wilson has been accused, Mary's "head ached with dizzying violence; she must get quit of the pain or it would incapacitate her for thinking and planning". She knew "from experience, how often headaches were caused by long fasting. Then she sought for some water to bathe her throbbing temples ...". Later, Mary has an unsatisfactory interview with a doctor concerning the advisability of Mrs Wilson attending her son Jem's trial in Liverpool, after which "Mary went home. Oh! How her head did ache, and how dizzy her brain was growing!" Again, "her head ached in a terrible manner" as she waits uncertain whether Will Wilson can return to provide Jem with an alibi.[13]

Ruth (1853)

When Ruth Hilton is dismissed from her job by Mrs Mason, and asked to go away by Henry Bellingham:

> Her head ached so much that she could hardly see; even the dusky twilight was a dazzling glare to her poor eyes; and when the daughter of the house brought in the sharp light of the candles ... Ruth hid her face in the soft pillows with a low exclamation of pain.

Shortly before this, it is reported that the "room whirled around before Ruth". Before leaving the inn where she has drunk tea whilst Henry fetches his carriage, the fumes of tobacco from the landlord's pipe "brought back Ruth's sick headache".[14]

In her compromised position, visiting Wales with Henry Bellingham, he tries to teach her card games, after which he reports:

> Do you know, little goose, your blunders have made me laugh myself into one of the worst headaches I have had for years.

Matters progress rapidly to fever and insensibility. A doctor is summoned and a diagnosis of "brain fever" is made.[15]

Discovering by chance the secret of Ruth's true identity, Jemima Bradshaw, her erstwhile friend, "was so oppressed with headache that she had to go to bed directly".[16]

Thurstan Benson speaks to Ruth's son, Leonard, of his mother as "sitting, overcome by headache, in the study for quietness" when the boy learns of their changed circumstances once the secret of Ruth's past and his illegitimacy becomes public knowledge.[17]

When Ruth by chance comes to nurse the sick Henry Bellingham, many years after the end of their relationship, she is "conscious of an oppressive headache".[18]

Cranford (1853)

Miss Matilda (Matty) Jenkyns sends a message to Mary Smith via the maid Martha to tell her to go to dinner alone because she has "one of her bad headaches" shortly after receiving the news of the mortal illness of her former admirer, Thomas Holbrook. Later Miss Matty reports that "a blow of fresh air at the door will do my head good, and it's rather got a trick of aching". Miss Matty is "past middle age", and later said to be "an old lady of fifty-eight".[19]

Encountered veiled and toothless by Mary Smith, Miss Pole "quickly took her departure because, as she said, she had a bad head-ache and did not feel herself up to conversation".[20]

North and South (1855)

When her family's changed circumstances require the major upheaval of moving from the rural South (Helstone) to the industrial North of England (Milton), Margaret Hale develops headaches:

> ... [she] had to remind herself of her father's regard for Mr Thornton, to subdue the irritation of weariness that was stealing over her, and bringing on one of the bad headaches to which she had lately become liable.

Once again in Mr Thornton's presence:

> Margaret's head still ached, as the paleness of her complexion, and her silence might have testified.

Margaret's headaches are also mentioned at other times.[21] Her mother, Mrs Hale, is reported to have suffered from headaches when the family lived in Helstone.[22]

The Hales are not the only family to be troubled with headaches. In the Thornton family, Mrs Thornton is said to have come home with a headache from the jolting of a cab, and Fanny Thornton says that she cannot call on the Hales because she has a headache, although she is prevailed upon by her brother, John Thornton, to go in the horse drawn carriage he has ordered so that his mother will not be discomfited.[23] The night after seeing Margaret with an unidentified young man after dark, John Thornton

> ... had positive bodily pain, – a violent headache, and a throbbing intermittent pulse. He could not bear the noise, the garish light, the continued rumble and movement of the street.[24]

Bessy Higgins thinks her headaches were due to the noise of Thornton's mill in which she worked.[25]

Sylvia's Lovers (1863)

Sylvia Robson states that "my head is aching so" on the day after her mother, Bell Robson, dies and her husband, Philip Hepburn, disappears.[26]

Following a walk with Sylvia, Hester Rose, looks tired:

> ... it's only my headache which is worse to-night. It has been bad all day; but since I came out it has felt just as if there were great guns booming, till I could almost pray 'em to be quiet. I am so weary o' th' sound.[27]

Philip avoids alcohol at the New Year's Fete:

> ... [he] had what was called a weak head, and disliked muddling himself with drink because of the .. consequence ... of a racking headache the next day.[28]

Wives and Daughters: An Every-day Story (1866)

Molly Gibson, visiting the stately Cumnor Towers, finds that "(t)he hot sun told upon her head and it began to ache". She reports this to the unsympathetic Miss Clare, who puts her on her own bed to sleep but then forgets to wake her up, so that Molly is faced with the unwelcome prospect of having to spend the night at the Towers and away from her beloved father. Molly must be eleven or twelve years old at this time, since when she is seventeen the event is recalled as occurring "five or six years ago".[29] The elder of the Miss Brownings, Sally, who escorted Molly to the Towers but then inadvertently left her behind, "fretted herself into a headache" for overlooking the child. She also reports that arguing gives her a headache, as does a surprise visit from Lady Harriet, daughter of Lord Cumnor.[30]

Molly has further symptoms in later years: a weary aching head when Roger Hamley departs to Africa for two years; and also her head ached heavily after caring for Mrs Osborne Hamley.[31]

Mrs Goodenough has a head ache at the Charity Ball when waiting to see the Duchess and her diamonds.[32]

"CASE REPORTS": *The Life Of Charlotte Brontë (1857)*

Charlotte Brontë's letters have many references to headache, suggesting that she may have suffered with migraine,[9] and some of these references are picked up by Elizabeth Gaskell in her biography,[33] no doubt empathising with this particular aspect of her subject consequent upon her own headaches.[6] Gaskell personally witnessed one of Brontë's headaches, as attested to in a letter to an unknown correspondent provisionally dated 25th August 1850.[34]

"CASE REPORTS": *Other Fiction*

In *The Moorland Cottage* (1850) Mrs Browne declares that her head aches when her daughter, Maggie, who has just received a proposal of marriage, answers her questions randomly.[35]

In *Mr Harrison's Confessions* (1851), Mr Will Harrison, a surgeon, wishes he could have had a headache on two occasions, one on arrival in Duncombe when people are inquiring for his health, the other "which should prevent me going to the place I did not care for". He and Mr Morgan call on the Miss Tomkinsons, the younger sister, Caroline, having had a headache and looking very pale according to her elder sister.[36]

In *Morton Hall* (1853), the Sidebotham sisters wonder "how it was that some kinds of pain were genteel and others were not. I said that old families, complaints as high in the body as they could – brain-fevers and headaches had a better sound, and did perhaps belong more to the aristocracy."[37]

In *Half a life-time ago* (1855), the propensity of Cumberland statesmen to go off drinking for days together is blamed for "a dreadful headache the next day". William Dixon, one of these statesmen, complains of head-ache and pains in his limbs one evening and takes to his bed, the next morning he has forgotten all his life since childhood. The doctor from Coniston diagnoses typhus fever. His son, Willie Dixon, is apparently also affected with fever which has "taken away the little wit [he] … ever possessed". Later, his howling cries prompt his sister, Susan Dixon, to say "don't make that noise – it makes my head ache".[38]

In *The Manchester Marriage* (1858), the servant Norah Kennedy, in possession of a dreadful family secret and falsely accused of theft, leaves her home and place of employment, "[h]er poor head aching".[39]

In *The Grey Woman* (1861), the maid of Madame the Baroness de Roeder reports that "she would never let me tie [her beautiful hair] up, saying it made her head ache".[40]

In *A Dark Night's Work* (1863), Ellinor Wilkins's "head ached" after receiving a letter with an unwelcome proposal of marriage from the clergyman, Mr Livingstone. Woken the following morning, after the death of Dunster, by the maid rapping at her door, Ellinor instructs the maid: "in half an hour bring me up a cup of strong tea, for I have a bad headache". At this time Ellinor must be in her late teens, since fifteen years later she is said to be aged thirty-four. Her head also aches after her efforts to secure the release of the faithful servant, Dixon, wrongly accused of the murder of Dunster.[41] Ellinor's father, Mr Wilkins, complains of headache which is reported to have been the consequence of over-indulgence in alcohol, and for which Ellinor puts him down for an hour's rest. Later, he reports that cognac is "a capital thing for the headache; and this nasty lowering weather has given me a racking headache all day". Challenged about Dunster's disappearance, Mr Wilkins explains his shaking as "… nothing, only this headache which shoots through me at times". Ellinor's companion Miss Monro is up late one morning because of a bad headache.[42]

In *Cousin Phillis* (1864), Phillis's mother, Cousin Holman, "has to go to bed with one of her bad headaches" which she later explains: "It's the weather, I think. Some people feel it different to others. It always brings on a headache with me".[43]

Discussion

There is little doubt, based on an analysis of her correspondence,[1–3] that Elizabeth Gaskell had headaches throughout her adult life, presumably migraine, as did three of her four daughters.[6] All of her major novels, with the exception of *Cranford*, feature a young female protagonist who is affected with headache (chronologically Mary Barton, Ruth Hilton, Margaret Hale, Sylvia Robson, and Molly Gibson). As a number of lesser (and usually female) characters also report headache, it seems not unreasonable to infer that Gaskell's experience of headache impinged on her creative impulses.

Some details of headache features are given in the fictional works. Descriptors include throbbing (*North and South*) and booming (*Sylvia's Lovers*), with associated sensory features which might be interpreted as photophobia (*Ruth, North and South*), phonophobia (*North and South*), and osmophobia (*Ruth*), as well as dizziness (*Mary Barton, Ruth*) and pallor (*North and South, Mr Harrison's Confessions*), all recognised as frequent accompaniments of migraine, the condition from which Elizabeth Gaskell probably suffered.[6]

Various possible factors which might predispose to or precipitate headache are alluded to, either by the narrator or her characters. Some of these might be termed physical or sensory, such as a jolting cab (*North and South*), exposure to loud noise (*North and South, Half a life-time ago*), ambient weather conditions (*A Dark Night's Work, Cousin Phillis*) including hot sun (*Wives and Daughters*), missed meals (*Mary Barton*), and alcohol overindulgence (*Sylvia's Lovers, Half a life-time ago, A Dark Night's Work* – all by male characters). Other illnesses may sometimes be associated with headache such as brain fever (*Ruth*) and typhus fever (*Half a life-time ago*), again only reported in men. Other provoking factors might be termed emotional or psychic, such as receipt of unexpected, usually bad, news (*Mary Barton, Cranford*), adverse changes in social circumstances (*North and South*), and bereavement (*Sylvia's Lovers*). Amatory entanglements are central to some of these, such as an unwelcome marriage proposal (*A Dark Night's Work*). John Thornton's headache following his rejection by Margaret Hale (*North and South*) has been ascribed to the "painful effects of passionate love", such that the "experience of powerful emotion results in intense bodily symptoms",[44] a reading which emphasizes the somatic effects of psychic states.

As for headache treatment, options mentioned include quiet and bed rest (*Ruth*), bathing the temples with water (*Mary Barton*), and drinking tea (*A Dark Night's Work*). In *Mary Barton*, Mrs Carson's use of ether and sal volatile is of note as the only reported medicinal treatment of headache. Ether, the first widely used anaesthetic, was also used as a treatment for headache, as shown by other contemporary accounts.[45] Sal volatile, ammonium carbonate smelling salts (also known as hartshorn), which give off ammonia on exposure to air, was suggested as a headache treatment by Gaskell to her friend Harriet Carr in a letter in 1832, in which she also reported that she had "derived great benefit" herself from this treatment.[46]

Aside from such biological analysis, headache might also serve important authorial purposes, particularly metaphorical. As mentioned, many of Gaskell's young female protagonists are afflicted with headache. Jenny Uglow has pointed out that " … emergence from girlhood, … can be a painful experience", this being "… the perilous threshold of adult hood", and that Gaskell is adept at portraying "… young women coming to terms with their sexual power

... finding their own voice and identity".[47] This pain may of course be actual as well as figurative since the onset of migraine in women is common at menarche.

Angus Easson has argued that the use of illness is one way in which Gaskell transforms realism to romanticism, illness being a "marker of crisis not just in the body but also in the mind and the psyche; symptoms and diagnosis are not so important as the significance of sickness".[48] Although headache is not specifically mentioned by Easson, it might be eminently susceptible to such an interpretation, as has also been argued for the use of headache by Jane Austen in her novels.[8]

Acknowledgment

Adapted from: Larner AJ. Headache in the writings of Elizabeth Gaskell (1810–65). *J Med Biogr* 2015;23:191–196.

References

1. Chapple JAV, Pollard A (eds.). *The letters of Mrs Gaskell.* Manchester: Mandolin, [1966] 1997.
2. Chapple JAV, Sharps JG. *Elizabeth Gaskell. A portrait in letters.* Manchester: Manchester University Press/Gaskell Society, [1980] 2003.
3. Chapple J, Shelston A (eds.). *Further letters of Mrs Gaskell.* Manchester: Manchester University Press, [2000] 2003.
4. Uglow J. *Elizabeth Gaskell: a habit of stories.* London: Faber & Faber, 1993.
5. Shelston A. *Brief lives: Elizabeth Gaskell.* London: Hesperus, 2010.
6. Larner AJ. "A habit of headaches": the neurological case of Elizabeth Gaskell. *Gaskell Journal* 2011;25:97–103
7. Larner AJ. "A transcript of actual life": headache in the novels of Jane Austen. *Headache* 2010;50:692–695.
8. Larner AJ. Jane Austen's (1775–1817) references to headache: fact and fiction. *J Med Biogr* 2010;18:211–215.
9. Larner AJ. Charlotte Brontë (1816–1855): migraineur? *Eur J Neurol* 2009;16 (Suppl3):329.
10. Hilton C. Elizabeth Gaskell and mesmerism: an unpublished letter. *Med Hist* 1995;39:219–235.
11. Gaskell E. *Mary Barton: A Tale of Manchester Life* (ed. M. Daly). London: Penguin Classics, 2003:68.
12. See reference 11:201–202.
13. See reference 11:246,274,314.
14. Gaskell E. *Ruth* (ed. A. Easson). London: Penguin Classics, 2004:51,52.
15. See reference 14:65.
16. See reference 14:268.

17. See reference 14:295.
18. See reference 14:364.
19. Gaskell E. *Cranford* (ed. P. Ingham). London: Penguin Classics, 2005:48–49,73,154,155.
20. See reference 19:147.
21. Gaskell E. *North and South* (ed. P. Ingham). London: Penguin Classics, 2003:76,80,189,417.
22. See reference 21:104.
23. See reference 21:94,96.
24. See reference 21:204.
25. See reference 21:101.
26. Gaskell E. *Sylvia's Lovers* (ed. S. Foster). London: Penguin Classics, 2004:361.
27. See reference 26:384.
28. See reference 26:135.
29. Gaskell E. *Wives and Daughters* (ed. M. Roberts). London: Penguin Classics, 2003:15,17,18,103.
30. See reference 29:28,145,149,169,171.
31. See reference 29:376,580.
32. See reference 29:290.
33. Gaskell E. *The Life of Charlotte Brontë* (ed. A. Easson). Oxford: Oxford World's Classics, 1996:353,431,436.
34. See reference 1:127.
35. Gaskell E. *The Moorland Cottage.* London: Hesperus, [1850] 2010:57,58.
36. Gaskell E. *Cranford and other stories.* London: Bloomsbury, 2007:217,257,222.
37. Gaskell E. *Cousin Phillis and other stories* (ed. H. Glen). Oxford: Oxford World's Classics, 2010:63.
38. See reference 37:102,105.
39. See reference 37:152.
40. Gaskell E. *Gothic tales* (ed. L. Kranzler). London: Penguin Classics, 2004:331.
41. Gaskell E. *A Dark Night's Work.* London: Bibliolis, 2010:57,66,133,134,188.
42. See reference 41:101,103,105,113.
43. See reference 37: 223,226.
44. Matus JL. *Mary Barton* and *North and South.* In: Matus JL (ed.). *The Cambridge Companion to Elizabeth Gaskell.* Cambridge: Cambridge University Press, 2007:36,41.
45. Larner AJ. "Neurological literature": headache (part 6). *Adv Clin Neurosci Rehabil* 2010;10(3):38.
46. See reference 3:19.
47. Gaskell E. *Lois the Witch.* London: Hesperus, [1859] 2003:ix.
48. See reference 14:xiv-xv.

Progressive supranuclear palsy described by Dickens

The novels of Charles Dickens have fascinated readers ever since their first publication, not least because of the numerous engaging characters that are described therein.[1] These often minutely-observed figures have prompted later readers to adduce descriptions of specific diseases: the Pickwickian syndrome based on the obese and hypersomnolent "Joe the fat boy" in the *Pickwick Papers* (1837) is a case in point.

Neurologists have been able to detect in Dickens's descriptions various neurological disorders,[2–4] including movement disorders.[5,6] In *David Copperfield* (1850), it has been suggested that Uriah Heep suffers from a generalized dystonia and Mr. Creakle from spasmodic dysphonia;[6] and in *Little Dorrit* (1857) Jeremiah Flintwinch has torticollis and Pancks manifests features of Gilles de la Tourette syndrome,[5] this last account some years before that of the eponymous author (1885). The accuracy of the descriptions, as judged retrospectively, prompts the belief that they are based on the observation of actual patients.[6] Although there are dangers in this type of extrapolation, nonetheless I venture to suggest another possible Dickensian first.

CASE REPORT

In *The Lazy Tour of Two Idle Apprentices*, Dickens and his friend Wilkie Collins (1824–1889), thinly disguised as Francis Goodchild and Thomas Idle, respectively, describe a journey through the north of England from Carlisle to Doncaster undertaken in September 1857. Their account was originally published in instalments, beginning in October 1857, in Dickens's magazine *Household Words*.[7]

In the instalment of 24th October 1857 ("Chapter the Fourth"), the scene is set at an inn in Lancaster where "Mr Goodchild [Dickens] writes the present account of his experience" (p.195), relating an encounter with:

> A chilled, slow, earthy, fixed old man. A cadaverous man of measured speech. An old man who seemed as unable to wink, as if his eyelids had been nailed to his forehead. An old man whose eyes – two spots of fire – had no more motion that [*sic*] if they had been connected with the back of his skull by screws driven through it, and rivetted and bolted outside, among his grey hair.

> He had come in and shut the door, and he now sat down. He did not bend himself to sit, as other people do, but seemed to sink bolt upright, as if in water, until the chair stopped him. (p.194)

Discussion

Read from a neurologist's perspective, these passages suggest the presence of the following clinical features:

- Ophthalmoplegia: "eyes . . . had no motion";
- Lid retraction: "eyelids ... nailed to his forehead"; combined with inability to wink, this hints at the man's staring expression, sometimes known as Stellwag's sign;
- Axial dystonia with rigidity: "fixed"; "he did not . . . bend to sit"; the fact that he sinks "bolt upright" and is stopped by the chair (en bloc sitting) suggests postural instability. This has sometimes been termed the "rocket man sign".

In addition, there are hints of bradykinesia ("slow") and possibly pseudobulbar palsy ("measured speech").

These features are suggestive of the syndrome of progressive supranuclear palsy (PSP) described by Steele and colleagues.[8] The information in Dickens's account, however, is insufficient to fulfil currently accepted clinical diagnostic criteria for PSP:[9,10] significantly, the unsteady gait of PSP is not mentioned, even though the individual is described entering a room. Ankylosing spondylitis might account for the fixed posture that necessitates sinking into a chair bolt upright, but the other neurological features are out with this diagnosis.

In their study, Steele and associates expressed surprise that such a distinctive disorder as PSP had not been previously reported[8] but a number of earlier possible cases have subsequently been identified,[10] dating back to that of the American ophthalmologist Campbell Posey in 1904. If Dickens's account is that of a case of PSP, occurring in the mid-nineteenth century, it predates the eponymous clinical description by more than 100 years.

Acknowledgment

Adapted from: Larner AJ. Did Charles Dickens describe progressive supranuclear palsy in 1857? *Mov Disord* 2002;17:832–833

References

1. Greaves J. *Who's who in Dickens.* London: Hamish Hamilton Elm Tree Books, 1972.
2. Brain R. Dickensian diagnoses. *BMJ* 1955;ii:1553–1556.
3. Perkin GD. Disorders of gait. *J Neurol Neurosurg Psychiatry* 1996;61:199.
4. Cosnett JE. Charles Dickens and sleep disorders. *Dickensian* 1997;93: 200–2004.
5. Cosnett JE. Dickens, dystonia and dyskinesia. *J Neurol Neurosurg Psychiatry* 1991;54:184.
6. Garcia-Ruiz PJ, Gulliksen LL. Movement disorders in David Copperfield [in Spanish]. *Neurologia* 1999;14:359–360.
7. Dickens C, Collins W. The Lazy Tour of Two Idle Apprentices. In: *No through-fare and other stories.* Stroud: Alan Sutton, 1990:128–227. Also in: Slater M (ed.). *Dickens' Journalism. Volume 3. "Gone astray" and other papers from Household Words 1851–59.* London: JM Dent, 1998:420–475 [quotes at 451,452].
8. Steele JC, Richardson JC, Olszewski J. Progressive supranuclear palsy: a heterogeneous degeneration involving the brainstem, basal ganglia and cerebellum with vertical gaze and pseudobulabr palsy, nuchal dystonia, and dementia. *Arch Neurol* 1964;10:333–358.
9. Litvan I, Agid Y, Calne D et al. Clinical research criteria for the diagnosis of progressive supranuclear palsy (Steele-Richardson-Olszewski syndrome): report of the NINDS-SPSP International Workshop. *Neurology* 1996;47:1–9.
10. Lees AJ. The Steele-Richardson-Olszewski syndrome (progressive supranuclear palsy). In: Marsden CD, Fahn S (eds.). *Movement disorders 2.* London: Butterworth, 1987:272–287.

Charles Dickens and epilepsy

As the two hundredth anniversary of the birth of Charles Dickens (1812–1870) is marked, the time is apposite to examine some of his fictional and journalistic portrayals of epilepsy. Further excuse for this undertaking, if needed, comes from Macdonald Critchley's statement that "Both as a stylist, and as a recorder of the *comédie humaine*, Charles Dickens is still insufficiently acclaimed".[1] The current account builds on and extends the observations previously published by Cosnett and others.[2,3] Cosnett referred particularly to three Dickensian characters with epilepsy: Monks, the villainous half-brother of *Oliver Twist* (1838); Bradley Headstone in *Our Mutual Friend* (1865); and Guster in *Bleak House* (1853).

Some Dickensian characters with epilepsy or epileptic seizures

Guster (christened Augusta), Mrs Snagsby's servant, is perhaps the most notable character with epilepsy in the Dickens canon. She is described in *Bleak House* as a child of the workhouse, a subject which Dickens had covered at greater length in *Oliver Twist* (a claim for the discovery of the original for Oliver's workhouse in London's Cleveland Street has recently been made, a building which latterly became the outpatient department of the Middlesex Hospital,[4] and is now the only part thereof not reduced to rubble). Hard though Guster's existence with the Snagsby's is, Dickens's account of *A Walk in a Workhouse*, published in his journal *Household Words* in May 1850, which may possibly have inspired at least in part his account of Guster, suggests that life as a servant may have been a deliverance compared to her possible fate had she remained a workhouse girl:

> In another room, a kind of purgatory or place of transition, six or eight noisy mad-women were gathered together, under the superintendence of one sane attendant. Among them was a girl of two or three and twenty, very prettily dressed, of most respectable appearance, and good manners, who had been brought in from the house where she had lived as domestic servant (having, I suppose, no friends), on account of being subject to epileptic fits, and requiring to be removed under the influence of a very bad one. She was by no means of the same stuff, or the same breeding, or the same experience, or the same state of mind, as those by whom she was surrounded; and she pathetically complained that the daily association and the nightly noise made her worse, and was driving her mad – which was perfectly evident.[5]

It is no wonder that Guster is apprehensive of being returned to the workhouse. She continues to be a model in modern fiction: in Sarah Waters' *The little stranger*, Dr Faraday, the narrator, comments on the ailment of the servant Betty at Hundreds Hall:

> But you can never tell with country girls: they're either hard as nails, wringing chickens necks and so on; or going off into fits, like Guster.[6]

A further account by Dickens, *Wapping Workhouse*, dating from some 10 years later and published in his journal *All the Year Round*, also mentions epilepsy, and suggests little improvement in the care received:

> ... everybody ... in the room had fits, except the wardswoman: an elderly, able-bodied pauperess ... biding her time for catching or holding somebody. This civil personage ... said, "They has 'em continiwal [*sic*], sir. They drops without no more notice than if they was coach-horses dropped from the moon, sir. And, when one drops, another drops, and sometimes there'll be as many as four or five on 'em at once, dear me, a rollin' and a tearin', bless you![7]

The truly dire consequences for epileptics in an age without effective medical treatment, and in which the distinctions between epilepsy and mental subnormality, and indeed criminality, were largely elided,[8,9] is evident in these accounts. The wish to avoid such unenlightened institutionalisation is only too understandable: the poet Emily Dickinson's (1830–1886) withdrawal from public life, and indeed normal social intercourse, may possibly have been occasioned by the onset of epilepsy.[10]

Other accounts of convulsions and seizures may be found in the Dickensian oeuvre. The potential vulnerability of very young children is noted. When Charles Kitterbell asks his uncle Nicodemus Dumps to be godfather to his expected child in *The Bloomsbury Christening* (1834), Dumps states that if the child is a boy it might die before it is christened: "distressing cases frequently occur during the first two or three days of a child's life: fits, I am told, are exceedingly common, and alarming convulsions are almost matters of course".[11] In his diatribe against the genus of untrained and unlicensed midwives (*Births. Mrs Meek, of a Son*: 1851), Mr Meek tells of the various indignities to which his infant son, Augustus George Meek, is subjected, which end with him being "in convulsions".[12] In a piece dating from 1854 lampooning the prime minister, the Earl of Aberdeen (1784–1860) as an old lady ("Abby Dean"), it is stated that he/she "earlier in life had fits, and was much contorted – first on one side and then on the other".[13]

Another possible seizure is described in *The Mystery of Edwin Drood* (1870),

Dickens' final and unfinished novel. John Jasper, taking opium for pain, is witnessed by his nephew Edwin: "Not relaxing his own gaze at the fire, but rather strengthening it with a fierce, firm grip upon his elbow chair", Jasper "sits for a few moments rigid, and then, with thick drops standing on his forehead, and a sharp catch of his breath, becomes as he was before".[14] Although this passage might describe the consequences of acute and severe pain, a partial seizure must enter the differential diagnosis.

Returning to Cosnett's archetypal Dickensian epileptics,[2] the descriptions of the seizure disorder afflicting Monks, real name Edward Leeford, the half-brother of Oliver Twist, are of particular interest. At their first encounter, when Oliver stumbles against him in an inn yard, Monks curses the boy:

> The man shook his fist, and gnashed his teeth, as he uttered these words incoherently, and advancing towards Oliver as if with the intention of aiming a blow at him, fell violently on the ground, writhing and foaming in a fit.
>
> Oliver gazed for a moment at the fearful struggles of the madman, (for such he supposed him to be,) and then darted into the house for help.

The conflation here of epileptic seizure with mental illness, so typical of 19th century conceptions of epilepsy,[8] is of note. Likewise, Dickens suggests a link between epilepsy and facial appearance: when Nancy describes Monks to Mr Brownlow she states:

> His lips are often discoloured and disfigured with the marks of teeth, for he has desperate fits.

At the novel's denouement, when accusing Monks of his evil designs on Oliver, Mr Brownlow speaks of the "hideous disease which has made your face an index even to your mind".[15] The attempt to link facial morphology or physiognomy with criminality and with epilepsy was to culminate in the works of Cesare Lombroso (1835–1909) in the 1880s.[16]

Besides generalised convulsive seizures Monks also has other attacks:

> He remained silent for a few moments, and then removing his hands suddenly from his face, showed ... that it was much distorted, and nearly blank.[17]

That Dickens recognised different types of epileptic seizure may also be evidenced by Guster's falling into a "fit of unusual duration: which she only came out of to go into another, and another, and so on through a chain of fits, with short intervals between".[18] Cosnett suggests this may represent status epilepticus, and that Guster's "staring and vacant state" when listening to the preacher, the Reverend Mr Chadband, might be a complex partial seizure.[2] In addition, there is an account in *David Copperfield* (1850) which has been adduced as a description of the phenomenon of *déjà vu*:[19,20]

> We have all some experience of a feeling which comes over us occasionally, of what we are saying and doing having been said or done before, in a remote time – of our having been surrounded dim ages ago, by the same faces, objects, and circumstances – of our knowing perfectly what will be said next, as if we suddenly remembered it.

However, it has been rightly stated that there is nothing in David Copperfield's history to suggest that this experience of "double consciousness" is a result of epilepsy.[21]

Bradley Headstone, the school master in *Our Mutual Friend*, is first reported to have a fit towards the end of the novel. At a railway station, when he receives the news from Mr Milvey that his beloved Lizzie Hexam has married his rival Eugene Wrayburn, Headstone states "I am accustomed to be seized with giddiness" and is observed by Mr Milvey to "lean against the pillar with his hat in his hand, and to pull at his neckcloth as if he were trying to tear it off". Moments later a station attendant reports to Milvey that Headstone is "in a fit" and was "biting and knocking about him … furiously". Later Headstone's "horrible condition brought on other fits" which are witnessed by his pupils. When Rogue Riderhood arrives in the classroom to accuse Headstone of attacking Eugene Wrayburn, Headstone sits "down on a stool which one of his boys put for him, and he had a passing knowledge that he was in danger of falling, and that his face was becoming distorted. But the fit went off for that time, and he wiped his mouth, and stood up again". After Riderhood's departure, Headstone falls "into the fit which had been long impending".[22]

Despite the extremely limited descriptions of Headstone's fits, Cosnett was of the view that he had complex partial seizures with an aura of giddiness.[2] More recently it has been said that "Bradley Headstone … is perhaps the most developed of Dickens' epileptic characters", the author seemingly willing to accept a category of "epileptic furore" to explain Headstone's homicidal attack on Eugene Wrayburn.[23] I find these contentions hard to accept. Might giddiness and pulling at a neckcloth reflect presyncope with air hunger? In the seminal epilepsy textbook written by William Lennox (1884–1960), one of the leading figures in the study of epilepsy in the 20th century,[24] and his daughter Margaret, it was stated that outbursts of violence were rarely symptoms of epilepsy: "… authors who equate epilepsy with attacks of rage … walk an uncertain and boggy path".[25] There seems to me something rather post hoc about Headstone's seizures, which are only mentioned after his actions turn to the criminal.

Differential diagnosis

In considering Bradley Headstone's first reported fit, the subject of Dickens's awareness of the differential diagnosis of seizures is approached. It is abundantly clear from his writings that Dickens was aware of the difference between syncope and epileptic seizure. For example, Oliver Twist has a "fainting fit" when brought before the magistrate, Mr Fang, falsely accused of pick-pocketing, and also when first encountering the painting in Mr Brownlow's house which eventually transpires to be an image of his dead mother. In the same novel, Nancy faints when restrained by Bill Sikes whilst trying to attack Fagin.[26] The seizure/syncope differential is made manifest in *Our Mutual Friend* when the villagers who witness Betty Higden's blackout tell her that "You have had a faint like ... or a fit". Betty's rapid departure from the scene, alarmed that she may be sent to the workhouse as an indigent pauper, may suggest that a faint is the more likely cause of blackout.[27] It is perhaps of note that, at least in these two novels, faints seem to afflict "good" characters (Oliver, Nancy, Betty Higden) whilst "bad" characters have fits (Monks, Headstone), and moreover that the good characters are women and children whilst the bad are men. This simplistic gender bias has contemporary echoes in cinematic portrayals of epilepsy, male epileptics often being characterised as mad, bad, and dangerous.[28]

Convulsions, seizures, and fits are occasionally used metaphorically by Dickens. Several examples are found in *Nicholas Nickleby* (1839): Mr Lillyvick reports that his niece's mother "instantly falls into strong conwulsions [*sic*]" when the niece announces she is in love; Miss Knag and Madame Mantalini fall into "convulsions of admiration" when examining new bonnets; and, not to be outdone, Mr Mantalini complains to Newman Noggs of the tinkling of a bell being "enough to throw a strong man into blue convulsions".[29] In *Hard Times* (1854), the "seizure of the station with a fit of trembling ... announced the train".[30] In *A Passage in the Life of Mr Watkins Tottle* (1835), it is stated that "a lady would certainly go into convulsions" if the subject of coming together with Mr Watkins Tottle were mentioned.[31] A group of Africans displayed upon the London stage are described by Dickens as "falling into epileptic convulsions".[32] The word "fit" evidently had a broad spectrum of usage in the 19th century (cf. Oliver Twist's "fainting fit") encompassing various sudden and uncontrolled behaviours but not limited to epileptic seizures.

Death in epileptic seizures

Dickens clearly recognised the risk of death from seizures. Monks "sunk under an attack of his old disorder, and died in prison". Individuals with no reported prior history of seizures may also expire in fits. In *Hard Times*, Josiah

Bounderby of Coketown dies "of a fit in the Coketown street".[33] In *Great Expectations* (1860), Joe Gargery tells Pip that his father "went off in a purple leptic [*sic*] fit",[34] its purple nature perhaps suggesting hypoxia and/or petechial haemorrhages. The demise of Anthony Chuzzlewit may be from an epileptic seizure (*Martin Chuzzlewit*, 1844), likewise Little Nell's grandfather in *The Old Curiosity Shop* (1841), and Francis Spenlow, David Copperfield's employer and the father of his wife, Dora.[2,35] "An elderly gentleman who lived in a court of the Temple" in London, one night "had a fit on coming home, and fell and cut his head deep, but partly recovered and groped about in the dark to find the door", but the noise of his stumbling is interpreted as a game of Blindman's Buff by those living in the chamber above, it being Christmas Eve, and the elderly man is found dead the next day.[36] A further example of death in a seizure in a known epileptic, from *No Thoroughfare* (1867), is cited below.

Was Charles Dickens an epileptic?

It has on occasion been suggested that Dickens himself may have suffered from epilepsy. In their seminal epilepsy textbook, the Lennoxes cite Matthew Woods (1848–1916) to the effect that "Charles Dickens ... had convulsions only in childhood".[37,38] (Woods also wrote a book suggesting that St Paul was an epileptic.[39]) GK Chesterton (1874–1936) in his 1906 essay *Charles Dickens* stated (Chapter VI, paragraph 2) that "his excitement was sometimes like an epileptic fit". The notion of an epileptic Dickens may be found repeated online even today[40] but, to my knowledge, no serious biography has advanced any evidence in favour of such a diagnosis. Peter Ackroyd mentions "spasms and seizures", referring to the spasms of pain in his side which Dickens experienced in childhood, including whilst working at the blacking factory, and at stressful times in later life, and conflates these "seizures" with two (unnamed) Dickensian characters, both "marked men" (*ergo* Monks and Headstone?) who, he reports, fall into fits characterised by pallor, sweating, and descent into paroxysm.[41] An earlier biographical work which devoted a chapter to the medical history of Charles Dickens does not mention epilepsy.[42]

A more recent analysis (by a non-neurologist) of Dickens's ailments in later life posits a right parietal or temporoparietal disorder, and mentions that vertiginous attacks have been recorded in seizures of temporoparietal origin.[43] Nevertheless a vascular cause for Dickens's various symptoms seems more likely.[44]

Dickens's death in 1870 was noted in *The Lancet*, which focused on his activities for the amelioration of workhouse infirmaries,[45] whereas the *British Medical Journal* noted his facility in the description of medical disorders.[46] Amongst these was included epilepsy, the example cited being that of Walter

Wilding in *No Thoroughfare*, a work Dickens co-authored with his friend Wilkie Collins (1824–1889). A reading of the published story may occasion some surprise at the *BMJ*'s commendation, since Wilding suffers perhaps only two seizures, coming on with "singing in the head" with momentary confusion.[47] Fits are hardly more evident in the stage adaptation[48] (it was Dickens's most successful drama, running for around 200 performances in London), developed by Collins as a vehicle for the actor Charles Fechter,[49] who played the villain (Obenreizer). In the play, Wilding reports a "strange feeling in my head before it [his first fit] came on" (Act II, scene 2), then is reported to die of a second fit (Act II, scene 3 and Act III, scene 1). I have not found any record of what representation Wilding's fits were given by the actor, John Billington, who played the role. The proximity of the stage production of *No Thoroughfare* (1868) to Dickens's death may have meant it was uppermost in the *BMJ* writer's mind at the time. In retrospect, although it is difficult to see Wilding as a compelling literary account of epilepsy, the portrayal of a partial seizure merits notice, since these are in the minority when compared to accounts of generalised seizures. Interestingly, another Dickens/Collins collaboration, *The Lazy Tour of Two Idle Apprentices* (1857), affords what may be regarded (in hindsight) as a very clear description of a neurological disorder, not hitherto described in the medical literature, namely progressive supranuclear palsy,[50] which was undoubtedly the work of Dickens rather than Collins.[51]

Conclusion

What did Dickens know about epilepsy? He was clearly aware of some of the phenomena of epilepsy, both major convulsion and transient loss of awareness, of the risk of death in seizures, and of the distinction of seizures from other causes of loss of consciousness (syncope). He had certainly encountered people with epilepsy, although they are mentioned only in passing, e.g. the inmates of workhouses;[5,7] Laura Bridgman, a deaf dumb and blind pupil at the Perkins Institution and Massachusetts Asylum for the Blind, who was "subject to severe fits" for the first eighteen months of her life;[52] and in France "a little labourer, who falls into a fit now and then".[53] However, he was certainly less familiar with epilepsy than his near contemporary Dostoevsky (1821–1881), himself an epileptic, who used his knowledge of the disorder in a number of his novels and stories.[54,55]

This lack of familiarity with the disease means that Dickens's construction of epilepsy is somewhat typical of his time, with a formulaic, stereotyped portrayal of adult epileptics as evil, violent, sometimes murderous, individuals (e.g. Monks, Headstone, and possibly John Jasper if one takes the view, as I do, that he is responsible for the mysterious disappearance of Edwin Drood). The taints of criminality, mental abnormality, and degeneration can all be detected in these characters. On the other hand, the portrayal of Guster, although tending to the comic, is not unsympathetic, and clearly Dickens was aware of the potentially dire destiny of epileptics confined to the workhouse system for want of any other resource. Epilepsy is also used by Dickens as a plot device to effect transition (e.g. sudden deaths).

Acknowledgment

Adapted from: Larner AJ. Charles Dickens (1812–1870) and epilepsy. *Epilepsy Behav* 2012;24:422–425.

References

1. Critchley M. *The divine banquet of the brain and other essays.* New York: Raven Press, 1979:136–140.
2. Cosnett JE. Charles Dickens and epilepsy. *Epilepsia* 1994;35:903–905.
3. Jones JM. "The falling sickness" in literature. *South Med J* 2000;93:1169–1172.
4. Richardson R. *Dickens and the Workhouse. Oliver Twist and the London Poor.* Oxford: Oxford University Press, 2012.
5. Slater M (ed.). *Dickens' Journalism. Volume 2. The amusements of the people and other papers: reports, essays and reviews 1834–51.* London: JM Dent, 1996:237.
6. Waters S. *The little stranger.* London: Virago, 2009:15.
7. Slater M, Drew J (eds.). *Dickens' Journalism. Volume 4. "The Uncommercial Traveller" and other papers 1859–70.* London: JM Dent, 2000:46.
8. Shorvon S, Weiss G, Avanzini G, Engel J, Meinardi H, Moshe S, Reynolds E, Wolf P. *International League Against Epilepsy 1909–2009. A centenary history.* Chichester: Wiley-Blackwell, 2009:1–3.
9. Stirling J. *Representing epilepsy. Myth and matter.* Liverpool: Liverpool University Press, 2010:131–177.
10. Gordon L. *Lives like loaded guns: Emily Dickinson and her family's feuds.* London: Virago Press, 2010:114–136.
11. Slater M (ed.). *Dickens' Journalism. Volume 1. Sketches by Boz and other early papers: 1833–39.* London: JM Dent, 1994:450–451.
12. Ref 5:326.
13. Slater M (ed.). *Dickens' Journalism. Volume 3. "Gone astray" and other papers from Household Words 1851–59.* London: JM Dent, 1998:249.
14. Dickens C. *The Mystery of Edwin Drood.* London: Penguin Classics, [1870] 1993:47.
15. Dickens C. *Oliver Twist, or, the Parish Boy's Progress.* London: Penguin Classics, [1838] 2002:270,387,414.
16. Monaco F, Mula M. Cesare Lombroso and epilepsy 100 years later: an unabridged report of his original transactions. *Epilepsia* 2011;52:679–688.

17. Ref 15:309.
18. Dickens C. *Bleak House.* London: Penguin Classics, [1853] 1996:156,179.
19. Lennox WG, Lennox MA. *Epilepsy and related disorders.* London: J&A Churchill, 1960 (2 volumes):275,704.
20. Warren-Gash C, Zeman A. Déjà vu. *Pract Neurol* 2003;3:106–109.
21. Ref 9:110.
22. Dickens C. *Our Mutual Friend.* London: Penguin Classics, [1865] 1997:730–731,771–772,774.
23. Ref 9:106,118,214.
24. Ref 8:26n54.
25. Ref 19:702,703.
26. Ref 15:84,93,133.
27. Ref 22:498–500.
28. Baxendale S. Epilepsy at the movies: possession to presidential assassination. *Lancet Neurol* 2003;2:764–770.
29. Dickens C. *Nicholas Nickleby.* London: Penguin Classics, [1839] 1986:236,295,507.
30. Dickens C. *Hard Times for these times.* London: Penguin Classics, [1854] 1995:213.
31. Ref 11:420.
32. Ref 13:146.
33. Ref 30:296.
34. Dickens C. *Great Expectations.* London: Penguin Classics, [1860] 1996:47.
35. Ref 9:107–108.
36. Ref 7:165.
37. Ref 19:704.
38. Woods M. *In spite of epilepsy. Being a review of the lives of three great epileptics – Julius Caesar, Mohammed, Lord Byron – the founders respectively of an empire, a religion, and a school of poetry.* New York: Cosmopolitan Press, 1913:293.
39. Woods M. *Was the apostle Paul and epileptic?* New York: Cosmopolitan Press, 1913.
40. www.epilepsy.com/epilepsy/famous_writers (accessed 10/04/12).
41. Ackroyd P. *Dickens.* London: Minerva, 1990:87–88,288,460.
42. Bowen WH. *Charles Dickens and his family. A sympathetic study.* Cambridge: WH Heffer & Sons, 1956:134–159.
43. McManus IC. Charles Dickens: a neglected diagnosis. *Lancet* 2001;358:2158–2161.
44. Bateman D. Dickens: an alternative diagnosis. *Lancet* 2002;359:1253.
45. Anon. Charles Dickens. *Lancet* 1870;i:882.
46. Anon. Charles Dickens. *Br Med J* 1870;i:636.
47. Dickens C, Collins W. *No Thoroughfare and other stories.* Stroud: Alan Sutton, 1990:11,21.
48. http://home.earthlink.net/~bsabatini/Inimitable-Boz/etexts/No_Thoroughfare_correct_first_ed.html (accessed 10/04/12)

49. Ref 7:403–409.
50. Larner AJ. Did Charles Dickens describe progressive supranuclear palsy in 1857? *Mov Disord* 2002;17:832–833.
51. Ref 13:447,451,452.
52. Dickens C. *American Notes for General Circulation*. London: Penguin Classics, [1842] 1985: 82.
53. Ref 13:237.
54. Larner AJ. Dostoevsky and epilepsy. *Adv Clin Neurosci Rehabil* 2006;6(1):26.
55. Iniesta I. On the good use of epilepsy by Fedor Dostoevskii. *Clin Med* 2008;8:338–339.

The neurology of Alice, with particular reference to Humpty Dumpty's prosopagnosia

The Reverend Charles Lutwidge Dodgson (1832–1898) has been immortalised as Lewis Carroll, the pseudonym under which he published a number of books, amongst them the two classics *Alice's Adventures in Wonderland* (1865) and *Through the looking-glass and what Alice found there* (1872). These works have been of interest not only to children of all ages but also to neurologists since some of the phenomena they describe, or seem to describe, may be deemed suggestive of neurological conditions, a subject which has been previously discussed.[1]

"Alice in Wonderland" syndrome

The name "Alice in Wonderland" syndrome was coined by Todd in 1955 to describe the phenomena of micro- or macrosomatognosia,[2] *i.e.* altered perceptions of body image, which had first been described by Lippman in the context of migraine some years earlier.[3,4] It has subsequently been suggested that Dodgson's own experience of migraine, recorded in his diaries, may have given rise to his descriptions of Alice's changes in body form, so graphically illustrated in *Alice's Adventures in Wonderland* by Sir John Tenniel. These have been interpreted as somesthetic migrainous auras.[5] However, Blau has challenged this interpretation on chronological grounds, finding no evidence in Dodgson's diaries for the onset of migraine until after he had written the Alice books.[6] Moreover, migraine with somatosensory features is rare, and the diaries have no report of migraine-associated body image hallucinations.[4] Podoll and Robinson have discovered an earlier drawing by Dodgson suggesting that he did in fact suffer migraine aura symptoms before writing the Alice books,[7] but the illustration suggests a right paracentral negative scotoma rather than micro- or macrosomatognosia.

Other conditions may also give rise to the phenomena of micro- or macrosomatognosia, including epilepsy, encephalitis, cerebral mass lesions, schizophrenia, and drug intoxication.[8] It may be speculated that the latter is relevant to Alice since her experiences occur after drinking from a phial (labelled "DRINK ME") and after eating cake (labelled "EAT ME").

Stammering

Dodgson had a developmental stammer. Although ordained a deacon, his unwillingness to preach and to progress to holy orders has been attributed to his speech defect.[9] Carroll parodied this defect in the character of the Dodo ("Do-do-Dodgson") in *Alice's Adventures in Wonderland* (chapters 2 and 3).

Mirror phenomena

Like Leonardo da Vinci, Carroll was a noted mirror writer, penning occasional "looking glass" letters.[10,11] The poem Jabberwocky first appears (*Through the looking-glass*, chapter 1) mirror reversed, in a Looking-glass book; only by holding it up to the mirror is Alice able to read it.

Mirror writing may be associated with stammering, and is much commoner in left handers: Dodgson apparently wrote with his right hand but may have originally been left handed.[10] Gardner states that Dodgson was "handsome and asymmetric – two facts that may have contributed to his interest in mirror reflections. One shoulder was higher than the other, his smile was slightly askew, and the level of his blue eyes not quite the same."[9]

Schott notes that Carroll's mirror letters were written in varying styles, and differed from his normal script, unlike the situation with Leonardo whose two scripts were faithful mirror images,[10] and hence argues that Carroll's letters reflect not an inherent capacity but a contrivance, designed to amuse children who corresponded with him.[10,11] Hence the neural mechanisms of mirror writing, whatever they may be (hypotheses include bilateral cerebral representation of language, motor programmes or visual memory traces or engrams[10,12]), may differ between Carroll and Leonardo. The literary device of mirror letters has been used by other authors when writing for children.[13]

"Mad Hatter syndrome"

The consequences of poisoning with inorganic mercury include a mild sensorimotor peripheral neuropathy, a syndrome which may resemble motor neurone disease, tremor (often circumoral), stomatitis, skin rash, and a neuropsychiatric syndrome characterised by timidity, seclusion, easy blushing, irritability, quarrelsomeness and mood lability (erethism). Hatters were liable to such problems because of the use of mercury in the felt hat industry as a stiffener of rabbit fur, leading to the expression "as mad as a hatter". Hence it might be assumed that Carroll's Mad Hatter is "mad" because of mercury exposure.[14,15] However, as Waldron pointed out,[14] odd though his behaviour certainly is, the Mad Hatter displays none of the typical features of mercury poisoning, either at the mad tea party (*Alice's Adventures in Wonderland*, chapter 7), or during his appearance as the King's Messenger Hatta in *Through the looking-glass* (chapters 5 and 7). Tenniel's illustration of the Mad Hatter/Hatta is said to resemble one Theophilus Carter, a furniture dealer near Oxford, who was known to Dodgson, and known in the locality as the Mad Hatter because he always wore a top hat and was prone to eccentric ideas.[14,16]

Prosopagnosia

Humpty Dumpty, encountered in *Through the looking-glass* (chapter 6), is one of Carroll's most enduring characters, remembered principally for his famous definition of the meaning of a word ("just what I choose it to mean"), and his coining of the term "portmanteau word" ("two meanings packed up into one word").

A re-reading of the encounter between Humpty Dumpty and Alice indicates two passages alluding to facial recognition, the first when Alice makes out that the egg has the face of Humpty Dumpty, and then at parting when Humpty Dumpty, sitting precariously balanced upon a wall, says he would not be able to recognise Alice if they did meet again:

> "Good-bye, till we meet again!" she said as cheerfully as she could.
>
> "I shouldn't know you again if we *did* meet," Humpty Dumpty replied in a discontented tone, giving her one of his fingers to shake: "you're so exactly like other people."
>
> "The face is what one goes by, generally," Alice remarked in a thoughtful tone.
>
> "That's just what I complain of," said Humpty Dumpty. "Your face is the same as everybody else has – the two eyes, so – " (marking their places in the air with his thumb) "nose in the middle, mouth under. It's always the same. Now if you had the two eyes on the same side of the nose, for instance – or the mouth at the top – that would be *some* help."
>
> "It wouldn't look nice," Alice objected.

Humpty Dumpty thus reports an inability to recognise a familiar face, yet is able to recognise eyes, nose, and mouth and their correct positions. Prosopagnosia is a rare form of visual agnosia characterised by impaired recognition of familiar faces (or equivalent stimuli).[17,18] The term was coined by Bodamer in 1947, although Charcot and Hughlings Jackson had recognised the phenomenon toward the end of the nineteenth century.[17] Brief accounts thought to be suggestive of prosopagnosia have been identified in writings from classical antiquity by Thucydides and Seneca.[18] In developmental or congenital prosopagnosia, where the neuropsychological deficit is perhaps most pure, since acquired cases following pathological insults such as cerebrovascular disease may not respect functional boundaries and may be accompanied by additional neurological signs such as visual field defects, there are impairments in face identity matching tasks but the ability to identify gender, age, emotional facial expression and eye gaze direction is preserved.[19,20] As in these cases, Humpty Dumpty's account seems to indicate preserved componential but impaired configural processing. There is also a suggestion that Humpty Dumpty might be able to use extraneous information to assist in facial recognition, his example being two eyes on one side of the nose or the mouth at the top of the face. Prosopagnosics may use extraneous visual cues such as spectacles, facial jewellery, hair colour or style, to aid facial recognition.[18–20]

Whether Dodgson wrote this passage purely from imagination, or may have based it upon observation of a prosopagnosic individual is not known. He did occasionally parody human idiosyncrasies, for example himself as the Dodo on account of his stammer and Theophilus Carter as the Mad Hatter.

Questions for future study?

In *Alice's Adventures in Wonderland*, is the Pool of Tears (chapter 2) a consequence of pathological crying? At the mad tea party (chapter 7), does the dormouse suffer from excessive daytime somnolence, and if so is there an underlying neurological cause? Does the *very* ugly Duchess (chapters 6 and 9) have a dysmorphic syndrome, perhaps with behavioural features to explain her neglectful treatment of her baby?

In *Through the looking-glass*, The Red King (chapter 4) and both the White and Red Queens (chapter 9) snore whilst they are sleeping: might they have obstructive sleep apnoea-hypopnoea syndrome? Does the White Queen's statement that she "can't do subtraction under *any* circumstances" (chapter 9) reflect a selective acalculia?

Acknowledgments

Adapted from: Larner AJ. Lewis Carroll's Humpty Dumpty: an early report of prosopagnosia? *J Neurol Neurosurg Psychiatry* 2004;75:1063; and Larner AJ. The neurology of "Alice". *Adv Clin Neurosci Rehabil* 2005;4(6):35–36.

References

1. Murray TJ. The neurology of Alice in Wonderland. *Can J Neurol Sci* 1982;9:453–457.
2. Todd J. The syndrome of Alice in Wonderland. *Can Med Assoc J* 1955;73:701–704.

3. Lippman CW. Certain hallucinations peculiar to migraine. *J Nerv Ment Dis* 1952;116:346–351.
4. Rolak LA. Literary neurologic syndromes. Alice in Wonderland. *Arch Neurol* 1991;48:649–651.
5. Kew J, Wright A, Halligan PW. Somesthetic aura: the experience of "Alice in Wonderland". *Lancet* 1998;351:1934.
6. Blau JN. Somesthetic aura: the experience of "Alice in Wonderland". *Lancet* 1998;352:582.
7. Podoll K, Robinson D. Lewis Carroll's migraine experiences. *Lancet* 1999;353:1366.
8. Takaoka K, Takata T. "Alice in Wonderland" syndrome and lilliputian hallucinations in a patient with a substance-related disorder. *Psychopathology* 1999;32:47–49.
9. Gardner M (ed.). *The annotated Alice. The definitive edition.* London: Penguin, 2001:xvi-xvii.
10. Schott GD. Mirror writing: Allen's self observations, Lewis Carroll's "looking glass" letters, and Leonardo da Vinci's maps. *Lancet* 1999;354:2158–2161.
11. McManus C. *Right hand, let hand. The origins of asymmetry in brains, bodies, atoms and cultures.* London: Phoenix, 2003:349.
12. Mathewson I. Mirror writing ability is genetic and probably transmitted as a sex-linked dominant trait: it is hypothesised that mirror writers have bilateral language centres with a callosal interconnection. *Med Hypotheses* 2004;62:733–739.
13. Ransome A. *Secret Water.* Harmondsworth: Penguin, 1972 [1939]: 175–176, 255.
14. Waldron HA. Did the Mad Hatter have mercury poisoning? *BMJ* 1983;287:1961.
15. O'Carroll RE, Masterton G, Dougall N, Ebmeier KP, Goodwin GM. The neuropsychiatric sequelae of mercury poisoning: the Mad Hatter's disease revisited. *Br J Psychiatry* 1995;167:95–98.
16. Gardner, *op. cit.* ref. 9:72.
17. Pryse-Phillips W. *Companion to clinical neurology* (2nd edition). Oxford: Oxford University Press, 2003:783.
18. De Haan EHF. Covert recognition and anosognosia in prosopagnosic patients. In: Humphreys GW (ed.) *Case studies in the neuropsychology of vision.* Hove: Psychology Press, 1999:161–180.
19. Nunn JA, Postma P, Pearson R. Developmental prosopagnosia: should it be taken at face value? *Neurocase* 2001;7:15–27.
20. Larner AJ, Downes JJ, Hanley JR, Tsivilis D, Doran M. Developmental prosopagnosia: a clinical and neuropsychological study. *J Neurol* 2003;250(suppl2):II156 (abstract P591).

Some accounts of childhood paraplegia

Reading novels may at first sight seem an unpropitious source for identifying examples of the practice of neurorehabilitation. The novels of Charles Dickens (1812–1870) have a few passages which may give some insights into nineteenth century attempts at neurorehabilitation, rudimentary though these were.[1,2] Prostheses are evidenced by the wooden leg of Silas Wegg (*Our Mutual Friend*, 1865) which proves a significant hindrance when he is climbing the dust heaps in search of Mr Boffin's buried treasure, and Captain Cuttle (*Dombey and Son*, 1848) has "a hook instead of a hand attached to his right wrist" which conveniently doubles as a toasting-fork. A wheeled chair is used by Mr Omer (*David Copperfield*, 1850) to facilitate his failing mobility and which, he claims, "runs as light as a feather, and tracks as true as a mail-coach". Most famously, and of potential relevance to the subject of developmental neurorehabilitation, is the little crutch used by Tiny Tim Cratchitt (*A Christmas Carol*, 1843); his limbs are also supported by an "iron frame". Jenny Wren, the dolls' dressmaker (*Our Mutual Friend*, 1865) also uses a crutch. That an acquired inability to walk may suggest to an author of heightened imagination the dramatic potential for recovery, sometimes miraculous in its rapidity, is illustrated by the example of Mrs Clennam (*Little Dorrit*, 1857).

There are also, as previously noted,[3] some literary examples of children who are unable to walk and who undergo a more or less startling recovery. This article examines four accounts (a case series, if you will) of apparent childhood paraplegia, which date from the late nineteenth and early twentieth centuries, noting particularly the approaches which appear, in the narrative, to facilitate clinical recovery.

CASE 1: Katy Carr *in What Katy Did* (1872) by Susan Coolidge

At the outset of this novel by Susan Coolidge (the pseudonym of Sarah Chauncy Woolsey, 1835–1905), Katy Carr is aged 12 years old and very tall for her age. She is the eldest of six motherless children who are looked after by their stern Aunt Izzie. Katy is headstrong and gets into various scrapes which bring her into conflict with her aunt; her father, a doctor, is seldom present because of his work. Despite being told not to, Katy plays on a swing which is not safe and suffers a fall. Coming to on the sofa in the dining room, she has pain in her back and when she tries to get up she is unable to stand. Examined by a Dr. Alsop, she has little movement in her legs. He advises bed rest and prescribes a rub. Four weeks later, at Katy's behest, her father tries to explain what has happened:

> ... the spine is a bone ... made up of a row of smaller bones – or knobs – and in the middle of it is a sort of rope of nerves called the spinal cord. Nerves, you know, are the things we feel with. Well, this spinal cord is rolled up for safe-keeping in a soft wrapping, called membrane. When you fell out of the swing, you struck against one of these knobs, and bruised the membrane inside, and the nerve inflamed, and gave you a fever in the back.

Now her "once active limbs hung heavy and lifeless" and her legs feel queer, like marble.

As regards treatment, her father advises that "the only cure for such a hurt is time and patience", the hope being that she will outgrow the injury over a period of months. She remains in her darkened room. Eventually a chair is provided, "very large and curious ... with a long-cushioned back, which ended in a footstool", which can tip back so as to be just like a bed, and which allows Katy to sit out and be wheeled across her room to look out of the window. An attempt to go out in her father's carriage brings on too much pain and is not repeated. Later she has a chair with large wheels with which she can roll herself across the room, by which time she has "grown accustomed to her invalid life".

Katy has a relation, invalid Cousin Helen, who cannot walk, possibly due to paraplegia. She advises Katy to be a student in the "School of Pain" where she must learn the lessons of patience, cheerfulness, making the best of things, hopefulness, and neatness. Cousin Helen has tried the "Water Cure" but this option is apparently not considered for Katy.

Following the death of Aunt Izzie from typhoid fever, Katy takes over the running of the household from her room, and becomes a surrogate mother to her younger siblings. Some four years later, Katy summons her sisters to announce "I stood up!". Thereafter she progressively improves, albeit slowly:

> At first she only stood on her feet a few seconds, then a minute, then five minutes, holding tightly all the while by the chair. Next she ventured to let go the chair, and stand alone. After that she began to walk a step at a time, pushing a chair before her ...

Katy returns, fully ambulant, for further adventures in *What Katy Did At School* (1873) and *What Katy Did Next* (1886). It is perhaps ironic that in the former work, the author states, of another character who has recovered from a long illness, "It is only in novels that rheumatic fever sweetens tempers, and makes disagreeable people over into agreeable ones". *Mutatis mutandis*, the same might be said of the fictional character of Katy.

CASE 2: Clara Sessman in *Heidi* (1880) by Johanna Spyri

In this classic tale by Johanna Spyri (1827–1901), Clara Sessman is 12 years old when Heidi, having been effectively abducted by her aunt Dete from her home on the Swiss mountain where she has lived with her grandfather, arrives in Frankfurt as a companion for her. An only daughter, Clara's mother is dead and her father, a businessman, is often away, so she is looked after by the stern lady-housekeeper Fraulein Rottenmeier. Neither the cause nor the duration of Clara's inability to walk is given, but she spends her whole day on an invalid couch "with beautiful red padding" in which she is wheeled from room to room. There are hints that her illness has attacks, and cod liver oil is administered when she is getting weak.

She attends the baths at Ragatz "for the cure" for 6 weeks, after which she visits Heidi, now returned to her grandfather on the mountain. Here Clara eats goats milk, toasted cheese and bread and butter, and for "the first time in her life ... felt the fresh morning breeze, and the pure mountain air". After three weeks, Grandfather, who has to carry her downstairs, asks if she will try to stand for a minute or two; she does so clinging to him and exclaiming that it hurts her feet as they touch the ground, but Grandfather lets her try a little longer each day.

Deprived of Heidi's friendship by the newcomer, Peter the goatherd petulantly pushes Clara's chair down the mountain. Wishing to see the field of flowers, Clara must be carried by Heidi and Peter. She tries to use her feet, but draws them back quickly until encouraged by Heidi to "put your foot down firmly", after which she makes proper steps. Soon she is walking a little way with the grandfather's left arm behind her and right to lean upon. She practices, every day finding walking easier and able to go a longer distance, and is declared cured to the astonishment and delight of her father.

CASE 3: Colin Craven in *The Secret Garden* (1909) by Frances Hodgson Burnett

In this story by Frances Hodgson Burnett (1849–1924), the reclusive Colin Craven is 10 years old when he is "discovered" by his orphaned cousin, Mary Lennox, several months after her arrival at his isolated home of Misselthwaite Manor in Yorkshire. Mary learns that Colin's mother died when he was born, at which time his father, Archibald Craven, a "hunchback", locked up the garden which Colin's mother so loved. Because of his resemblance to his mother, Mr Craven does not like to look at the boy and although he provides for all his material needs he spends most of his time away from home on travels, leaving Colin to be looked after by the servants who must comply with anything he asks for: if contradicted, he has violent tantrums. Always a sickly boy, Colin has to lie down or sit on a sofa, does not walk and rarely goes outside, even in a wheeled chair, in part because he does not like to be looked at. His leg muscles have become atrophied (the author defines this term for the benefit of her readers as "wasted away through want of use"), his legs likened to "drumsticks i' stockin" by the gardener, Ben Weatherstaff. The fear is that, like his father, Colin will develop a hunchback, and die as a consequence. At one time he wore an iron brace to keep his back straight but a "grand doctor came from London" and ordered its removal and prescribed fresh air. Colin continues to fear that a lump will develop on his back, but Mary sees none when she examines him.

By chance Mary discovers the key to the locked garden and with a local boy, Dickon Sowerby, begins to work there. Colin is let into the secret and then taken by the other children to the garden where he can enjoy fresh air away from any grown-ups. Dickon predicts that "Us'll have thee walkin' ... afore long" and even Colin admits of his legs that "Nothing really ails them ... but they are so thin and weak ... I'm afraid to try and stand on them". Ben Weatherstaff chances to see him in the garden, and Colin, angered by being thought a cripple, stands and, with Dickon's support, walks: "his anger and insulted pride ... filled him with power ... an almost unnatural strength".

Now that Colin has made himself believe that he will get well, or, as he puts it, in "the Magic in this garden", progress is swift. He has daily walking exercise, buoyed by a diet of milk, loaf, buns, potatoes, eggs, heather honey, oatcakes and clotted cream, mostly supplied by Mrs Susan Sowerby, Dickon's mother. Dickon also applies to Bob Haworth, a champion wrestler and the strongest man on the moor, for exercises to make muscles "stick out", which he learns by heart and then teaches to Colin. Soon Colin is not only walking but running, eventually running by accident into his father's arms when the latter returns unexpectedly from his travels.

CASE 4: Pollyanna Whittier in *Pollyanna* (1913) by Eleanor H Porter

Pollyanna is 11 years old in the novel by Eleanor H Porter (1868–1920) when she moves to live with her maternal aunt Polly (for whom she is partly named) in Beldingsville, Vermont, following the death of her clergyman father. "On the last day of October" (she arrived in June) she suffers an accident with an automobile as a consequence of which her legs "don't *feel*" and there is a "pitiful motionlessness of the once active little feet and legs". A nurse, Miss Hunt, is employed to help look after her, and sedating pills are prescribed by Dr. Warren, who also suggests a consultation with a "very famous" New York specialist named Dr. Mead (is it purely coincidence that he shares the name of the great 18th century doyen of London medicine, Richard Mead?). Dr. Mead opines that Pollyanna will never walk again, an opinion which the child accidentally overhears to her great distress. Miss Hunt tries to comfort her by pointing out that "all doctors make mistakes sometimes" (plainly the voice of experience!). Dr. Mead prescribes certain (unspecified) treatments and medicines but with almost no hope of their efficacy. Pollyanna is not allowed visitors.

By the following Spring (hence approximately 4 months post accident), and with little change in her condition, Pollyanna is seen by her friend Dr. Thomas Chilton who, as the former beau of Aunt Polly, has been hitherto excluded from the house, despite Dr. Warren's suggestion that his opinion be sought. Chilton believes – "nine chances out of ten" – that Pollyanna can walk again, since he has a college friend who has "been making this sort of thing a special study". Aunt Polly relents, and Pollyanna is sent to the great doctor in "a big house many miles from here made on purpose for just such people as you are", whence she writes, in the novel's concluding chapter, to report that after almost 10 months (hence 14–15 months post accident) that she is able to take a few steps.

Like Katy Carr, Pollyanna also returns, her crippled legs cured, in *Pollyanna Grows Up* (1915), a novel which features a boy called Jamie who cannot walk and is in a wheelchair, and who is not cured.

Discussion

As sources of medical information, all literary accounts must be acknowledged to have profound shortcomings: the "problem of the frame", which vouchsafes only a limited view over the reality of the past. For example, for want of further, more definitive, information such as a clinician might obtain through history, examination and investigation, it might be argued that none of these children had paraplegia, understood to mean damage to or pathology of the spinal cord, even though two (Katy, Pollyanna) have undoubtedly suffered physical trauma. Being only partial accounts, no direct information relevant to aetiology is given for either Clara or Colin, in both of whom somatisation is certainly possible; this may also contribute to the longevity of Katy's illness.

By chance, these same four fictional cases have been discussed by Lois Keith[4] who points out that "drama rather than medical plausibility is the business of the sentimental novelist" who will "ignore medical accuracy in order to allow their characters to walk again". In these books, illness and recovery may be used as metaphors for transformation and renewal, and inability to walk may be symbolic of psychological distress. The fact that one patient (Pollyanna) is an orphan and the other three have all lost their mothers and have fathers who may be (Katy, Clara) or are (Colin) emotionally rather distant might invite speculative psychoanalytic or psychodynamic formulations. Indeed it has been suggested of Katy that her misfortunes unconsciously reflect female ambivalence towards the implications of puberty in the Victorian era, the transition from wild girlhood to ladylike womanhood (www.wikipedia.org/wiki.What_Katy_Did, accessed 06/04/08). Restoration to health is explicitly linked to a moral message: the "long year of schooling had taught her self-control". In similar vein, it has been surmised that Colin never learned to walk for "purely psychological reasons" (www.wikipedia.org/wiki.The_Secret_Garden, accessed 06/04/08).

It may be further argued that the current examples are based far more on authorial imagination rather than any empirical observations. It is unlikely that any of these authors possessed significant medical knowledge: Johanna Spyri's father was a village doctor, and Frances Hodgson Burnett is said to have had extensive dealings with crippled children and adults[4] but I am not aware of any other medical connections, although it is just possible that these authors were aware of accounts of Charcot "curing" paraplegics at the Salpetriere.[5] Another objection may be that rehabilitation of neurological illness as a discipline did not exist before the Second World War. Hence none of these accounts may be suggested to portray an example of developmental neurorehabilitation, as currently understood,[6] and any information vouchsafed concerning efforts at rehabilitation is at best involuntary, unwitting, and anecdotal.

Nonetheless, certain common themes may be identified and inferences may be drawn. In the case of Katy Carr, the approach is entirely passive: no intervention other than the passage of time seems to be applied, and no specialist advice sought. At the end of 4 years of confinement to her room, she simply stands again. This is in contrast to the other children, for whom advice is sought from other doctors, including eminent specialists (Colin, Pollyanna), and other treatments used (baths at Ragatz for Clara, iron brace for Colin).

A change of environment may be significant for recovery: Heidi's mountain home for Clara, the secret garden for Colin. Pollyanna goes to an institution dedicated to treating people with similar problems. Change to a more healthy diet ensuring adequate nutrition may also be relevant: fresh goat's milk and toasted cheese for Clara; Mrs Susan Sowerby's cooking for Colin. A conducive psychological milieu may also be significant: new friends for Clara (Heidi, Grandfather) and Colin (Mary, Dickon, Ben Weatherstaff). Pollyanna's "Glad

Game" – finding something in everything to be glad about – taught to her by her father and based on the 800 "rejoicing texts" in the Bible, might be deemed a form of cognitive behavioural therapy, based as it is on identifying and challenging negative cognitions.

Exercise plays a central role in the "rehabilitation" of these children. Once standing, an informal programme of graded exercise seems evident in the accounts of Katy, Clara and Colin. Katy stands for progressively longer periods, then walks holding on to her chair for support. Clara effectively receives informal physiotherapy which is graded from standing with support, to stepping with the support of two, to walking with the support of one. Likewise Colin who progresses from standing, to walking with support, to undertaking an exercise programme designed to build muscle bulk. Whereas recovery is swift for Katy, Clara and Colin (days to months), for Pollyanna it is many months before even a few steps can be taken.

In conclusion, since little was written on the subject of childhood paraplegia in professional texts of this period,[4] these literary accounts may, despite all their acknowledged shortcomings, give some insights into contemporary lay concepts of neurorehabilitation.

Acknowledgements

Thanks to Elizabeth Larner for reading these novels with me. Adapted from: Larner AJ. Some literary accounts of possible childhood paraplegia and neurorehabilitation. *Dev Neurorehabil* 2009;12:248–252.

References

1. Wainapel SF. Dickens and disability. *Disabil Rehabil* 1996;18:629–632.
2. Larner AJ. Charles Dickens, qua neurologist. *Adv Clin Neurosci Rehabil* 2002;2(1):22.
3. Larner AJ. "Neurological literature": headache. *Adv Clin Neurosci Rehabil* 2006;5(6):23–24.
4. Keith L. *Take up thy bed and walk: death, disability and cure in classic fiction for girls.* London: Routledge, 2001.
5. Ellenberger H. *The discovery of the unconscious.* London: Fontana, 1994.
6. Forsyth R. More than a name change. *Dev Neurorehabil* 2007;10:1–2.

Illusory visual spread described by Margiad Evans

> "Another very sudden psychic experience was seeing the aura of a dog. . . . The dog was a black labrador, fat and glossy. I was walking into the village when suddenly he appeared with a bluish-lilac halo all round him in pure daylight. . . . I was not frightened but . . . strangely delighted . . . and coming back from the shop, was disappointed to see the dog a plain black body again without his incandescent background."[1]

This extract might initially prompt concerns in some readers about the author's mental health. Certainly Margiad Evans (1909–1958) did suffer from epilepsy, symptomatic of an underlying brain tumour, which blighted her creative powers in the last years of her life.[2] However, this description from her book describing her experience of epilepsy may well represent an account of a form of visual perseveration known as illusory visual spread or visuospatial perseveration. Evans was recognised to have a strongly visual imagination.[3]

Critchley noted a number of unusual subjective visual experiences which might fall under the rubric of "visual perseveration", viz.:[4]

- The hallucinatory and recurring appearance of an object after its removal; in other words, palinopsia;
- Visual perseveration *in sensu strictu*, when a disappearing visual stimulus does not fade from view; however, there is no recurrence of the visual image as in palinopsia;
- Illusory visual spread or visuospatial perseveration: the visual stimulus is sensed over an unduly extensive area of environmental space, especially with images of vivid pattern or hue.

The example Critchley gives of illusory visual spread, which is apparently the rarest form of visual perseveration, is of the colour of a bright frock extending to the wearer's face, arms, legs and for a distance beyond. He also reports a case (Case 1) in which this phenomenon occurred at the onset of a migraine. Illusory visual spread has no temporal factor, for when the stimulus is removed the effect disappears.

What mechanism(s) might explain illusory visual spread? My sketchy knowledge of visual neurophysiology is that the brain undertakes parallel processing of various visual attributes (shape, colour, etc), and that some form of "binding" must occur to ensure a coherent, comprehensible visual percept with all these attributes. Perhaps a transient breakdown of this binding process, of colour to shape, might account for the phenomenon of illusory visual spread. Whether this is the same as the "coloured auras around objects" which has been described in emotionally mediated synaesthesia[5] remains to be clarified.

Acknowledgment

Adapted from: Larner AJ. Illusory visual spread or visuospatial perseveration. *Adv Clin Neurosci Rehabil* 2009;9(5):14.

References

1. Evans M. *A ray of darkness.* London: John Calder, 1978 [1952]:162.
2. Larner AJ. "A ray of darkness": Margiad Evans's account of her epilepsy (1952). *Clin Med* 2009; 9:193–194.
3. Larner AJ. Sherlock Holmes as "an exact embodiment of somebody or other". *The Sherlock Holmes Journal* 2017;33:60–61.
4. Critchley M. *The divine banquet of the brain and other essays.* New York: Raven Press, 1979:149–155.
5. Cytowic RE, Eagleman DM. *Wednesday is indigo blue. Discovering the brain of synesthesia.* Cambridge: MIT Press, 2011:10.

Lycanthropy: from Homer to the present day

I had always understood lycanthropy to mean the transformation of a human into a wolf (Greek: lukos-wolf, anthropos-man). Such animal-like behaviour has a long history.[1,2] The mythical werewolves so beloved of the film industry aside, these cases, sometimes labelled "clinical lycanthropy" to emphasize the distinction, usually seem to be associated with psychiatric disorders such as psychosis or depression and have been understood as delusional disorders in the sense of self-identity disorder.[3]

I was somewhat surprised to read in a recent case report the word lycanthropy used to denote conversion to a pig.[4] However, this was simply a reflection of my own ignorance, since in a review of over thirty published cases of clinical lycanthropy only a minority had wolf or dog themes.[3] Hence the "animal-like behaviour" may encompass a broader phenotype than simply that of the wolf: multiple serial lycanthropy encompassing four different animal species during a psychotic illness has been reported.[5] I have seen one patient with behavioural variant frontotemporal dementia who, according to his wife, used to bark like a dog. Perhaps Gregor Samsa's metamorphosis into a gigantic insect in Franz Kafka's story *Metamorphosis* (*Die Verwandlung*, 1915) is therefore also an example?

This broader definition including the pig obviously stimulates a few literary reminiscences, perhaps first to come to mind being George Orwell's *Animal Farm* (1945), wherein the pig Napoleon and his supporters gradually adopt human characteristics, walking on two legs.

Lycanthropy as pig conversion may perhaps be one of the oldest neuropsychiatric syndromes described in literature, not just the medical literature, since a possible example occurs in Homer's *Odyssey* which may date from the 8th century BCE, and be based on even earlier traditions of oral story telling. In Book X, Odysseus and his men encounter the beautiful Circe, "a formidable goddess with a mortal woman's voice", on the island of Aeaea:

> Circe ... prepared them a mixture of cheese, barley-meal, and yellow honey flavoured with Pramnian wine. But into this dish she introduced a noxious drug, to make them lose all memory of their native land. And when they had emptied the bowls which she had handed them, she drove them with blows of a stick into the pigsties. Now they had pigs' heads and bristles, *and they grunted like pigs; but their minds were as humans they had been before.* So, weeping, they were penned in their sties. Then Circe flung

> them some forest nuts, acorns, and cornel-berries – the usual food of pigs that wallow in the mud. [my italics]

Odysseus's men may not be alone, since "Prowling about the place were mountain wolves and lions that Circe had bewitched with her magic drugs".[6]

John Wain's short story *A message from the Pig-man* (1960) may perhaps been seen as within the same tradition, conveying a six year-old child's anxieties about encountering the "Pig-man", whom he imagines to be part man part beast.

As a footnote to this consideration of some of the interrelationships between pigs and men, Ambrose Bierce in his *Devil's Dictionary* (1906) defined trichinosis, infection with the nematode worm *Trichinella spiralis* due to ingestion of undercooked pork containing encysted *T. spiralis* larvae, as "the pig's reply to proponents of porcophagy".

Acknowledgment

Adapted from: Larner AJ. Neurological signs: Lycanthropy. *Adv Clin Neurosci Rehabil* 2010;10(4):50.

References

1. Poulakou-Rebelakou E, Tsiamis C, Panteleakos LG, Ploumpidis D. Lycanthropy in Byzantine times (AD 330–1453). *Hist Psychiatry* 2009;20:468–479.
2. Fahy TA. Lycanthropy: a review. *J R Soc Med* 1989;82:37–39.
3. Garlipp P, Godecke-Koch T, Dietrich DE, Haltenhof H. Lycanthropy – psychopathological and psychodynamical aspects. *Acta Psychiatr Scand* 2004;109:19–22.
4. Grover S, Shah R, Ghosh A. Electroconvulsive therapy for lycanthropy and Cotard syndrome: a case report. *J ECT* 2010;26:280–281.
5. Dening TR, West A. Multiple serial lycanthropy. *Psychopathology* 1989;22:344–347.
6. Rieu EV, Rieu DCH (trans.). *Homer The Odyssey*. London: Penguin Classics, 2003:128–131.

Neurological literature: Headache

1.

A number of physicians and physiologists have given accounts of their migraine over the past 200 years, most particularly the aura, with or without headache: examples include Caleb Hillier Parry,[1] Emil Du Bois-Reymond,[2] Sigmund Freud,[3] Karl Lashley,[4] and, in our own time, C. Miller Fisher[5] and Graeme Hankey.[6] Another notable migraineur was the philosopher Immanuel Kant.[7] It has been questioned whether migraine, most particularly the aura, may have influenced the work of visual artists such as Pablo Picasso (1881–1973)[8] and Giorgio de Chirico (1888–1978).[9]

Such is the prevalence of headache in general and migraine in particular that it might be anticipated that such phenomena may also stimulate accounts from non-medical authors, possibly influencing or occurring in their imaginative works, whether or not they themselves were sufferers. For example, it has been suggested that Charles Lutwidge Dodgson's experience of migraine may (or may not) have contributed to Lewis Carroll's depiction of Alice's strange experiences of expanding and contracting in size (macro- and microsomatognosia) in *Alice's Adventures in Wonderland* (1865), hence the "Alice in Wonderland syndrome".[10] The only direct reference to headache in Carroll's Alice books of which I am aware is in chapter 4 of *Through the looking-glass and what Alice found there* (1872), wherein Tweedledum excuses his lack of bravery, and hence explains his unwillingness to fight Tweedledee, by saying that he has a headache, and Alice agrees that he may look a little pale.

However, just as there is a paucity of neurologists in the UK willing to declare a special interest in headache, despite it being the most prevalent of "neurological" conditions, so literary accounts of headache seemed to me to be few compared, say, to illnesses with more dramatic potential, such as the inability to walk (paraplegia?) which miraculously improves: think of Mrs Clennam in Charles Dickens's *Little Dorrit* (1857); Clara Sessman in Johanna Spyri's *Heidi* (1880); Colin in *The Secret Garden* by Frances Hodgson Burnett (1911); and *Pollyanna* (1913) by Eleanor H Porter. Nonetheless, once the search is begun, literary accounts of headache may readily be found.

Arthur Ransome, famed for the *Swallows and Amazons* series of children's books, gives an account in *We didn't mean to go to sea* (1937) of what sounds (at least to this neurologist) like childhood migraine, apparently induced by seasickness or at least by the motion of the sea:

> ... Titty suddenly clutched the coaming of the cockpit and leant over it.
> "She's being sick," said Roger ...
> "Leave me alone," said Titty, "... It's only one of my heads. I'll be all right if I lie down for a bit."
> ... Down in the fore-cabin Titty scrambled into her bunk. Something was hammering in her head as if to burst it.[11]

In *Northern Lights* (1995), the first book in Philip Pullman's trilogy *His Dark Materials*, the young heroine, Lyra Belacqua, wakes with a "sick headache", ascribed to her proximity to the gas fumes of a boat engine near which she is in hiding.[12]

In L.M. Montgomery's *Anne of Green Gables* (1908), "warnings of a sick headache", presumably migraine, prevent Marilla Cuthbert from escorting Anne Shirley to church shortly after the latter first arrives at Green Gables, with the result that the young orphan indulges her wish to adorn her hat with wayside flowers, much to the astonishment of the other parishioners. The episodic nature of Marilla's headaches later becomes evident, necessitating Anne to attend to the housework whilst Marilla rests. She has to lie down, and their effect is to leave her weak, "tuckered out", and "somewhat sarcastic". She feels they are becoming worse and worse and that she must see a doctor about them. Her local attendant, Dr Spencer, insists she see a specialist, who turns out to be an oculist, whose recommendation is that Marilla should give up reading, sewing, and any kind of work that strains the eyes. If she is careful not to cry, and wears the glasses he gives her, he thinks her eyes may not get any worse and the headaches will be cured; if not, she will be stone blind in six months.[13] Even today, consulting an optician about headaches in the belief they originate from "eye strain" is common, and sometimes suggested by general practitioners,[14] even though refractive errors are rarely a cause of headache.

The social consequences of headache are also noted by the creator of Just William, and arch social critic, Richmal Crompton:

> ... Mrs Jones had a lively sense of her own importance ... there was no doubt at all that people weren't making enough fuss of her, so she rose and said with an air of great dignity:
> "Mrs Hawkins, I am suffering from a headache. May I go into your drawing room and lie down?"
> She had often found that that focused the attention of everyone upon her. It did in this instance. They all leapt to their feet solicitously, fussed about her, escorted her to the drawing room, drew down the blinds and left her well pleased with the stir she had made.[15]

Another archetypal boy hero, JK Rowling's Harry Potter, uses the pretext of headache to escape from Professor Trelawney's divination class at Hogwarts after seeing an apparition of his arch-enemy Voldemort.[16]

Social realism is also to be expected from Anton Chekhov (1860–1904). As a doctor, he was certainly familiar with headache in his clinical practice,[17] and a number of his characters profess, or are reported to be suffering from, headaches: Ivanov (in the play of the same name, 1887), Olga (in *Three Sisters*, 1901), and Shipoochin (specifically "a migraine", in *The Jubilee*). The character Lyebedev suggests that Ivanov's headache is because he thinks too much; Olga supposes that she gets a continual headache (tension-type?) "because I have to go to school every day and go on teaching right into the evening".[18]

Jane Austen, another keen social observer, reports in *Sense and Sensibility* (1811, chapter 16) that Marianne Dashwood, following the departure of her beau, Mr Willoughby, is;

> . . . awake the whole night . . . She got up with an head-ache, was unable to talk, and unwilling to take any nourishment.

Are these simply the consequences of young and unrequited love, or does she have a migraine, perhaps triggered by young and unrequited love? In *Pride and Prejudice* (1813, chapter 7), Jane Bennet develops "sore throat and head-ache" which worsens as her feverish symptoms increase, having ridden (at her mother's suggestion) to Netherfield in the rain to see Mr Bingley; her illness requires the attendance of her sister, Elizabeth Bennet, which brings her into the social orbit of Mr Darcy. Later (chapter 33), Elizabeth has a headache, and hence is unable to go to tea at Rosings, at which time Mr Darcy calls unexpectedly to make his first (unsuccessful) proposal of marriage: obviously Elizabeth's indisposition will not help his case. Jane Austen is also alert to the potential dangers of new (fashionable?) headache treatments, as evinced in her novel *Sanditon*, left unfinished at her death in 1817:

> [Susan] has been suffering much from the headache and six leeches a day for ten days together relieved her so little that we thought it right to change our measures – and being convinced on examination that much of the evil lay in her gum, I persuaded her to attack the disorder there. She has accordingly had three teeth drawn, and is decidedly better, but her nerves are a good deal deranged. She can only speak in a whisper – and fainted away twice this morning . . .

Before we indulge in what the historian EP Thompson called the condescension of posterity after reading this passage, it may be worth considering which current headache treatments might be held up to ridicule in a century or two (acupuncture?[19] botulinum toxin injections?).

Perhaps it is purely a chance observation or selection bias, but readers may note that all the physicians and physiologists who wrote about their migraine and are referred to in this article were men,[1–6] which might be considered unusual since migraine is more prevalent in women, whereas all the literary accounts of migraine or presumed migraine, with the exception of Chekhov's Shipoochin,[18] relate to women.[11–13,15,18] Could it be that literary discourses may sometimes reflect the human condition more accurately than professional medical discourses?

Acknowledgment

Adapted from: Larner AJ. "Neurological literature": Headache. *Adv Clin Neurosci Rehabil* 2006;5(6):23–24.

References

1. Larner AJ. Neurological contributions of Caleb Hillier Parry. *Adv Clin Neurosci Rehabil* 2004;4(3):38–39.
2. Pearce JMS. Historical aspects of migraine. *J Neurol Neurosurg Psychiatry* 1986;49:1097–1103.
3. Pearce JMS. Freud's migraine, and contributions to neurology. In: *Fragments of neurological history*. London: Imperial College Press, 2003:615–621.
4. Lashley KS. Patterns of cerebral integration indicated by the scotomas of migraine. *Arch Neurol Psychiatry* 1941;46:331–339.
5. Fisher CM. Late-life (migrainous) scintillating zigzags without headache: one person's 27–year experience. *Headache* 1999;39:391–397.
6. Hankey GJ. Recurrent migraine aura triggered by coronary angiography. *Pract Neurol* 2004;4:308–309.
7. Podoll K, Hoff P, Sass H. The migraine of Immanuel Kant. *Fortschr Neurol Psychiatr* 2000;68:332–337.
8. Ferrari MD, Haan J. Migraine aura, illusory vertical splitting, and Picasso. *Cephalalgia* 2000;20:686.
9. Fuller GN, Gale MV. Migraine aura as artistic inspiration. *BMJ* 1988; 297: 1670–1672.
10. Larner AJ. The neurology of "Alice". *Adv Clin Neurosci Rehabil* 2005;4(6):35–36.
11. Ransome A. *We didn't mean to go to sea*. Harmondsworth: Puffin, [1937] 1969:135.
12. Pullman P. *Northern lights*. London: Scholastic, 1995:150.
13. Montgomery LM. *Anne of Green Gables*. Godalming: Colour Library, [1908] 1994:125,256–257,345–346,469,473–474.

14. Larner AJ. What role do optometrists currently play in the management of headache? A hospital-based perspective. *Optometry in Practice* 2005;6:173–174.
15. Crompton R. William – the good. In: *The Just William Collection*. London: WH Smith, 1991:193–194.
16. Rowling JK. *Harry Potter and the goblet of fire*. London: Bloomsbury, 2000:501.
17. Coope J. *Doctor Chekhov: a study in literature and medicine*. Chale: Cross Publishing, 1997:109.
18. Fen E (transl.). *Chekhov: Plays*. Harmondsworth: Penguin, 1959:86,250,449.
19. Larner AJ. Acupuncture use for the treatment of headache prior to neurological referral. *J Headache Pain* 2005;6:97–99.

2.

The Oxford English Dictionary defines headache as:

> An ache or continuous pain, more or less deep-seated, in the cranial region of the head.

Compared with the richness and variety of definition to be found in the IHS classification of headache,[1] the OED seems a little prosaic.

Although accounts recognisable as descriptions of migraine may be found in the remaining works of several ancient civilizations,[2] and afflicting greats of antiquity such as Julius Caesar and St Paul,[3] the earliest reference to headache acknowledged in the OED comes from a Saxon document of ca. 1000 AD, followed by a quote from a work of John de Trevisa dated 1398:

> Also heed-ache cometh of grete fastinge and abstynences

The first literary reference to headache mentioned in the OED is from 1581, Sir Philip Sidney's (1554–1586) *An apologie for poetrie*:

> How many head-aches a passionate life bringeth us to

Not mentioned in OED, but perhaps the first literary work devoted to headache is a poem of 1648, entitled *The Head-ake* by Robert Herrick (1591–1674), in his collection *Hesperides* (H-591):

> My head doth ake,
> O Sappho! take
> Thy fillit,
> And bind the paine;
> Or bring some bane
> To kill it.
>
> But lesse that part,
> Then my poore heart,
> Now is sick:
> One kisse from thee
> Will counsell be,
> And Physick.[4]

One wonders whether this might be an example of art imitating life: did the author's experience of headache prompt the writing of the poem? [There is another possible reference in one of Herrick's poems entitled *Upon Love*, H-509: I held Love's head while it did ake;/But so it chanc't to be;/The cruell paine did his forsake,/And forthwith came to me.[4]] A similar question may be addressed to the many writers who have mentioned headache in their works, some of which have already been documented.[5] For example, did Charles Lutwidge Dodgson's headaches influence the pseudonymous Lewis Carroll's depictions of Alice in Wonderland?[6] Seldom can this question be definitively answered, although Vlad Zayas has skilfully traced the possible links between the character Pontius Pilate's headaches in *The Master and Margarita* and the author Bulgakov's (1891–1940) headaches.[7]

Herrick's poem is quoted in full in one of his earliest extant letters (November 1898) by the American writer Jack London (1876–1916).[8] Interestingly, headaches crop up in several of London's books: *The People of the Abyss* (1903; chapter 21, describing the effects of industrial white lead poisoning in the East End of London); *The Sea-Wolf* (1904; chapters 10,13,33); and *The Iron Heel* (1908; chapters 23,24), in both the latter afflicting London's characters. Did London himself suffer from headaches? Only three mentions of headache are to be found amongst the largest published collection of his letters (1557 in all), occurring in the context of other systemic illness (fever, cold) or on a boat in driving wind and snow; in the latter he was "nearly blind with a headache" (is migraine a possibility?).[8] Even in the autobiographical *John Barleycorn or, Alcoholic Memoirs* (1913), there is no mention of headache per se, although following the consumption of wine at the tender age of seven London reports "The alcohol I had drunk was striking my . . . brain like a club".[9]

Another American author aware of headaches was Louisa May Alcott (1832–1888), as exemplified in her best known novel, *Little Women, or Meg, Jo, Beth and Amy* (1868).[10] Alcott herself certainly suffered from headaches, notably in the early months of 1867 when, according to her journal "Did nothing all month but sit in a dark room & ache. Head and eyes full of neuralgia."[11] Whether these headaches were part of, or entirely separate from, a multisystem disorder characterised by later diagnosticians as lupus[12] is not apparent. Three of the four *Little Women* are afflicted at one time or another; only Amy, aged 12, seems unaffected (pre-menarche?). Beth, aged 13, has headaches which force her to lie on the sofa and cuddle her cats; headache is also the first symptom of the scarlet fever from which she becomes delirious. Jo, aged 15, has a headache which is ascribed to reading too much, although of note this occurs when her usual daily routine of looking after a trying elderly relative, Aunt March, comes to an end and the "experiment" of not working is tried. Like London, Alcott also recognises the perils of alcohol: Meg, aged 16, is warned by the girls' neighbour, Laurie, of the risk of "splitting headache" if she drinks too much champagne.[10]

This latter example may fulfil IHS criteria for "Alcohol-induced headache immediate",[1] as may Jack London's boyhood experience with wine. Are young people, perhaps sampling alcohol for the first time, particularly susceptible? Another possible example occurs in *The Amber Spyglass*,[13] the third book in Philip Pullman's trilogy *His Dark Materials*, when young Will Parry is treated to vodka by Semyon Borisovitch. In a short story entitled *The man who liked Dickens* (1933), Evelyn Waugh, himself no stranger to the effects of alcohol, has the character Henty ("a shadowy version of [Waugh] himself") wake with a headache after drinking "piwari", a local South American brew, so missing his chance to escape from the jungle and from McMaster, the man who likes Dickens but who cannot read and hence wishes Henty to remain permanently to read him the novels.[14]

Ian McEwan has made a name for himself in medical circles with his accounts of the life and thought of a neurosurgeon (*Saturday*, 2005) and of De Clerambault's syndrome (erotomania) (*Enduring Love*, 1997). In *Atonement*,[15] the matriarch Emily Tallis suffers from "the beast migraine":

> She was not in pain, not yet, but she was retreating before its threat. There were illuminated points in her vision, little pinpricks, as though the worn fabric of the visible world was being held up against a far brighter light. She felt in the top right corner of her brain a heaviness, the inert body weight of some curled and sleeping animal; but when she touched her

> head and pressed, the presence disappeared from the coordinates of actual space. ... It was important ... not to provoke it; once this lazy creature moved from the peripheries to the centre, then the knifing pains would obliterate all thought ... It bore her no malice, this animal, it was indifferent to her misery.

As for the pain: "At worst, unrestrained, a matching set of sharpened kitchen knives would be drawn across her optic nerve, and then again, with a greater downward pressure, and she would be entirely shut in and alone". This is set in 1935, and no specific treatment is mentioned. But is it purely chance that one of the plants growing in the cracks between the paving stones on the terrace is feverfew, sometimes prescribed as a migraine prophylactic?

As a consequence of her migraine, Emily has developed an "expertise born of a thousand headaches, avoiding all things sudden or harsh", wearing dark glasses before going outside to fetch her daughter, and has "learned her patience through years of side-stepping migraine". Nonetheless, when unforeseen trouble comes, "she rose to the crisis, free of migraine and the need to be alone". The migraines also impact on the family: "As children they claimed to be able to tell from across the far side of the park whenever their mother had a migraine by a certain darkening at the windows." Her daughter avoids troubling her mother, since "nothing but migraine would have come of it". At another time, they see the migraines as "a comic interlude in a light opera".

McEwan is perhaps less secure in a later description, which purports to be of vascular dementia. A seventy-seven year old woman reports:

> My headaches, the sensation of tightness around the temples, have a particular and sinister cause. He [the doctor] pointed out some granular smears across a section of the [brain] scan. ... I was experiencing, he said, a series of tiny, nearly imperceptible strokes. The process will be slow, but my brain, my mind, is closing down. ... I have vascular dementia, the doctor told me ... it's not as bad as Alzheimer's, with its mood swings and aggression.

Yet later she reports, "I fell asleep again and when I woke ... a painful tightness was around my forehead. I took from my handbag three aspirins which I chewed and swallowed with distaste. Which portion of my mind, of my memory, had I lost to a minuscule stroke while I was asleep?"

Surely these are tension type headaches, possibly medication overuse headaches (waking from sleep, excessive analgesic consumption) and the scan appearances entirely incidental and appropriate for age? Has this fictional doctor (or possibly McEwan's source) had any training in the disciplines of headache or cognitive disorders? It is surprising that the careful research done for the historical parts of the book is not matched when it comes to medicine. Artistic licence, no doubt; the need for melodrama, possibly.

Acknowledgment

Adapted from: Larner AJ. "Neurological literature": headache (part 2). *Adv Clin Neurosci Rehabil* 2006;6(2):37–38.

References

1. International Headache Society Classification Subcommittee. The international classification of headache disorders, second edition. *Cephalalgia* 2004;24(suppl1):1–160.
2. Rose FC. The history of migraine from Mesopotamian to Medieval times. *Cephalalgia* 1995;suppl15:1–3.
3. Jones JM. Great pains: famous people with headaches. *Cephalalgia* 1999;19:627–630.
4. Patrick JM (ed.). *The complete poetry of Robert Herrick*. New York: New York University Press, 1963:280,252.
5. Larner AJ. "Neurological literature": headache. *Adv Clin Neurosci Rehabil* 2006;5(6):23–24.
6. Larner AJ. The neurology of "Alice". *Adv Clin Neurosci Rehabil* 2005;4(6):35–36.
7. Zayas V. Sympathy for Pontius Pilate. Hemicrania in M.A. Bulgakov's "The Master and Margarita". *Eur J Neurol* 2005;12(suppl2):296 (abstract P2506).
8. Labor E, Leitz RC, Shepard IM (eds.). *The letters of Jack London* (3 volumes). Stanford: Stanford University Press, 1988:20;54,206,412–413.
9. London J. *John Barleycorn or Alcoholic Memoirs*. New York: Signet Classic, [1913] 1990:31.
10. Alcott LM. *Little Women*. Godalming: Colour Library, [1868] 1994:70–71,346,348; 214;192–193.
11. Reisen H. *Louisa May Alcott. The woman behind Little Women*. New York: Henry Holt & Co., 2009:79,205,210,221,223,242,250.
12. Hirschhorn N, Greaves IA. Louisa May Alcott: her mysterious illness. *Perspect Biol Med* 2007;50:243–259.
13. Pullman P. *The Amber Spyglass*. London: Scholastic, 2000:107.
14. Pasternak Slater A (ed.). *Evelyn Waugh: the complete short stories and selected drawings*. London: Everymans, 1998:xxvii,133.
15. McEwan I. *Atonement*. London: Jonathan Cape, 2001:20,48,63, 66,67,106,109, 148,150,153,175,180,354–355,362.

3.

> English, which can express the thoughts of Hamlet and the tragedy of Lear, has no words for the shiver and the headache. ... let a sufferer try to describe a pain in his head to a doctor and language at once runs dry.[1]

This famous declaration by Virginia Woolf (1882–1941) in her essay *On Being Ill*, first published in 1930, will strike a chord with many neurologists who have sat listening to patients attempting to convey their headache symptoms: "It's difficult to describe" is a common refrain.

Nonetheless, many authors have felt able to use headache in their works, sometimes as a literary device, sometimes with a fuller account of symptoms. David Perkin has identified accounts of headache and migraine in works by George Eliot, Jane Austen, Tolstoy, Trollope, Saki, Arnold Bennett, Thomas Mann, Charlotte Bronte, and Victor Hugo,[2,3] and other examples have been reported by JMS Pearce[4] and in two earlier articles in this series.[5,6] These pieces have not exhausted the fund of literary descriptions of headache; some further observations are offered here.

The spectrum of authors who have incorporated headache in their work is noteworthy, perhaps reflecting the ubiquity of headache disorders. The master dramatist who was able to "express the thoughts of Hamlet and the tragedy of Lear", William Shakespeare (1564–1616), may also be included: he has Juliet's nurse in *Romeo and Juliet* (1595–6), acting as a go-between for the "star-cross'd lovers", say (Act II, scene V: 49–50):

> Lord! How my head aches; what a head have I!
> It beats as it would fall in twenty pieces.

This, of course, is entirely incidental to the plot. However, headache, as one feature of a temporal lobe tumour along with epilepsy, is central to the action of Allan Cubitt's play *The Pool of Bethesda*, in which the central character, a surgeon, has psychic seizures in which he "talks" to William Hogarth as the latter paints the mural of Christ healing the lame man at the pool of Bethesda, still visible at St Bartholomew's Hospital, London.[7]

Fyodor Dostoyevsky (1821–1881) is known for his descriptions of epilepsy, a condition from which he suffered,[8] and it has also been claimed that he described hemifacial spasm.[9] Hence it is perhaps not surprising that headache should also appear in his work. For example, in the short story *Bobok* (1873):

> Something strange is happening to me. My character is changing and my head aches. I am beginning to see and hear some very strange things.

Namely the voices of those buried in the graveyard. Headache also occurs in *The Idiot* (as noted by Perkin[2]) and in Dostoyevsky's master work, the *Brothers Karamazov* (1881: books III, V, VI, IX and XI). Of these, Marfa Ignatyevna's headache following consumption of her herbal remedy for lumbago, which cures Grigory Vassilyevitch (book V), might be "headache induced by acute substance use or exposure", and Madame Hohlakov's presentiment of a nocturnal sick headache following excitement (book IX) might be migraine.

In a previous article,[5] a passage was quoted from one of the novels of Arthur Ransome (1884–1967), *We didn't mean to go to sea* (1937), describing a headache which may well have been childhood migraine. As with other such passages, it may prompt the question as to whether the author was writing from personal experience. Examining the published selection of Ransome's correspondence, his posthumously published autobiography, and the definitive biography of his life, headache is mentioned on various occasions. Features which emerge from these accounts of his headache include its recurrent nature, extreme severity preventing work, apparently accompanied by a desire to move about, and probable periods of remission, leading to the suggestion that he may have suffered from cluster headache or some form of trigeminal autonomic cephalalgia, although no definitive reference to unilaterality of headache was found.[10]

Diaries, as contemporaneous records, may also be of interest. That of the Reverend Francis Kilvert (1840–1879) is well known as a resource for social history in the period 1870–9, but of relevance to this article it seems he was also a sufferer from headaches and facial pains:[11]

> Drunk too much port after dinner . . . last night and a splitting headache all today in revenge. . . . Everything in a daze and dazzle and I could hardly see to read (20th February 1870)

Aside from episodes with obvious triggers, Kilvert also suffered from "face ache", which he sometimes calls "neuralgia", associated with sleep disturbance and restlessness:

> Tossing about with face ache till 3 o'clock this morning (27th February 1871)
>
> Neuralgia very troublesome all the week, no sleep at nights (27th April 1878)

Again the details vouchsafed by the author are insufficient to permit a confident retrospective diagnosis (if that is not a tautology!), but it would seem to lie between cluster headache and trigeminal neuralgia.

Grim though the experience of headache may be, it may also be a subject for wit. Oscar Wilde (1854–1900) has this exchange in Act Two of *The Importance of Being Earnest* (1899):

> CECILY: Miss Prism has just been complaining of a slight headache. I think it would do her so much good to have a short stroll with you in the Park, Dr Chasuble.
> MISS PRISM: Cecily, I have not mentioned anything about a headache.
> CECILY: No, dear Miss Prism, I know that, but I felt instinctively that you had a headache.

After a little further conversation. Miss Prism remarks "I find I have a headache after all, and a walk might do it good". Either Cecily has preternatural diagnostic skills which would be the envy of most neurologists, or Miss Prism is highly suggestible.

The difficulty in finding efficacious treatment for headache may also be reflected in jests, extreme acts, or "sick jokes". St Stephen, the first Christian martyr, was killed by stoning (Acts of the Apostles 7:58–59); because of the manner of his death, in the Middle Ages he was invoked against headaches.[12] Fasting, one of the cornerstones of Christian observance in the Middle Ages, might also be tried: William Tyndale (1494–1536), first translator of most of the Bible into English before he was burned at the stake for his troubles, noted in *The Parable of Wicked Mammon*, published in Antwerp in 1528, that "Some fast ... for the head ache".[13] Charles Dickens, in *A Tale of Two Cities* (1859; Book III, chapter IV, "Calm in Storm"), describes La Guillotine thus: "It was the popular theme for jests; it was the best cure for headaches .. ". Perhaps the National Insitute for Health and Clinical Excellence should submit it to a cost-effectiveness analysis?

Acknowledgment

Adapted from: Larner AJ. "Neurological literature": headache (part 3). *Adv Clin Neurosci Rehabil* 2007;7(1):27–28.

References

1. Woolf V. *Collected Essays (volume IV)*. London: Hogarth Press, 1967:193–203 [at 194].
2. Perkin GD. Migraine. *J Neurol Neurosurg Psychiatry* 1995;59:486.
3. Perkin GD. Headache. *J Neurol Neurosurg Psychiatry* 1995;59:632.
4. Pearce JMS. Migraine. *Eur Neurol* 2005;53:109–110.
5. Larner AJ. "Neurological literature": headache. *Adv Clin Neurosci Rehabil* 2006;5(6):23–24

6. Larner AJ. "Neurological literature": headache (part 2). *Adv Clin Neurosci Rehabil* 2006;6(2):37–38
7. Cubitt A. *The Pool of Bethesda.* London: Warner Chappell, 1992:2,40,44, 47,82,93.
8. Larner AJ. Dostoyevsky and epilepsy. *Adv Clin Neurosci Rehabil* 2006;6(1):26.
9. Perkin GD. Hemifacial spasm. *J Neurol Neurosurg Psychiatry* 1994;57:284.
10. Larner AJ. The headache disorder of Arthur Ransome, author of "Swallows and Amazons". *Eur J Neurol* 2006;13(suppl2):140 (abstract P1382).
11. Plomer W (ed.). *Kilvert's diary 1870–1879. Selections from the diary of the Rev. Francis Kilvert.* London: Cape, 1944:9,38,108,110,111,155,166,262,329,331.
12. Burns P. *Butler's lives of the saints. New concise edition.* London: Burns & Oates, 2003:601.
13. Daniell D. *William Tyndale. A biography.* New Haven & London: Yale University Press, 1994:167.

4.

> "Existence is just an ache in the head" – Margiad Evans, diary entry for 23rd November 1949

That headache has been a feature of the human condition since prehistory may be inferred from the finding of skulls with holes cut in them. Such trepanations date from as far back as the Neolithic era, and have been found in Europe, Asia, the Americas, and north Africa.[1] Although their purpose will be forever obscure to us, the possibility that they were undertaken to relieve headache, perhaps through a perception that such surgery would release malign spirits from inside the head, seems at least plausible. Recourse to such extreme, life-threatening, measures may suggest the presence of severe symptoms.

That no record of headache is to be found, as far as I am aware, in the doings of the numinous, extracorporeal, God of the Jews and Christians is perhaps no surprise. Nor that the domestic soap opera of the Olympian gods of ancient Greece, amounting at times almost to farce (e.g. in the Homeric epics *Iliad* and *Odyssey*), should give an example of something so quotidian as headache, specifically in one of the myths of the birth of Athene, the goddess of wisdom.[2,3] Zeus, ruler of the gods, lusted after Metis the Titaness; she has been identified with the planet Mercury, itself associated with wisdom. Having gained his wicked way with Metis, Zeus was warned by a prophecy that she would bear a son strong enough to depose him, in the same way that Zeus himself had deposed his father Cronos with the assistance of Metis. To avoid this eventuality, Zeus swallowed Metis. However, this was not the end of the matter: "In due process of time, he was seized by a raging headache ... so that his skull seemed about to burst, and he howled for rage until the whole firmament echoed". Hermes divined the cause of Zeus's discomfort and summoned Hephaestus, the blacksmith god, who with his wedge made a breach in Zeus's skull, from which sprang forth Athene, the goddess of wisdom. Hence, our evidence-based conclusion is clear: wisdom is born of headache by way of unsafe sex.

The early Socratic dialogue *Charmides*, named for Plato's maternal uncle, is ostensibly a search for the definition of *sophrosune* (Σωφροσύνη), variously translated as soundness of mind, self-knowledge, or self-control. Internal evidence dates the action of this dialogue to 432 BCE. It begins with Socrates trying to gain the attention of Charmides by means of suggesting a remedy for the headaches Charmides has been having recently on getting up in the morning (155b). The remedy is a leaf and a charm: chanting the charm at the same time as using the leaf will produce a complete cure, but the leaf on its own is no use at all. Socrates learned the secret from a Thracian doctor whilst on military duty (156d). However, before he will disclose it, the discussion of *sophrosune* must be undertaken. The dialogue ends inconclusively, with the characteristic Socratic aporia; we learn neither the definition of *sophrosune*, nor the headache remedy.[4] Perhaps the implicit suggestion is that philosophy is the best treatment for headache.

Socrates also makes a passing reference to headache when discussing the subject of education in Plato's *Republic* (407c):

> If you are always wondering if you've got a headache or are feeling giddy, and blaming your philosophical studies for it, you will always be prevented from exercising and proving your talents.[5]

Charms, with their appeal to the supernatural, may be one of the most ancient forms of headache treatment. John Kirk, medical officer on David Livingstone's expedition to the Zambesi between 1858 and 1863,[6] noted amongst the indigenous people the use of charms, such as fruit, for treatment of, amongst other things, headache.[7]

Unlike Plato's transcendentalism, we may rely on Aristotle for sound empirical observation. In the *Historia animalia*, he reports (Book 5, chapter 31) that those with lousy heads are "less than ordinarily troubled with headache", but sadly proposes no mechanism for this beneficial effect of the humble head louse. Later, he reports (Book 7, chapter 4) that after conception women experience a sensation of headache in front of the eyes and suffer also from heaviness throughout the body and darkness before the eyes, these symptoms occurring as early as the tenth day. A humoral mechanism is adduced ("according as the patient be more or less burthened with superfluous humours").

Saints may perhaps have taken the place of charms in Christian iconography. As mentioned in a previous article,[8] St Stephen, the first Christian martyr, was invoked against headaches because of the manner of his death by stoning. He was not alone: in Brittany, legend has it that there are 7777 local saints, enough to intercede for every eventuality, including Saint Livertin for headaches.[9] In the Koran (Chapter LVI), when the "inevitable" happens, the "foremost" shall enjoy a cup of flowing wine and "no headache shall they feel therefrom, nor shall their wits be dimmed".

The abbess Hildegard of Bingen (1098–1179) was a woman of extraordinary intellectual ability, whose works include volumes dealing with illness and medical treatment, the *Causae et curae* and *Physica.*[10] Throughout her long life she had visions, which she believed to be divinely inspired and which she used to inform and illustrate her theological works (e.g. *Scivias*, *Liber divinorum operum*). Writing on "The visions of Hildegard of Bingen", Charles Singer suggested that "the medical reader or the sufferer from migraine will … easily recognize the symptoms of 'scintillating scotoma'",[11] a theme later taken up by Oliver Sacks who found the visions to be "indisputably migrainous in nature".[12] Indeed, perhaps as a consequence of this, she has attracted the label of "The most distinguished migraine sufferer" (see www.fordham.edu/halsall/med/hildegarde.html).

Acknowledgements

Thanks to Michele Marietta of Oxford University Press for directing my attention to Hildegard of Bingen. Adapted from: Larner AJ. "Neurological literature": headache (part 4). *Adv Clin Neurosci Rehabil* 2008;7(6):17.

References

1. Arnott R, Finger S, Smith CUM (eds.). *Trepanation: history, discovery, theory.* London: Psychology Press, 2003.
2. Graves R. *The Greek myths. Combined edition.* London: Penguin, 1992:46.
3. Jones P. *Ancient and modern.* London: Duckworth, 1999:13.
4. Saunders TJ (ed.). *Early Socratic dialogues.* London: Penguin, 2005.
5. Plato. *The Republic.* London: Penguin, 1987:111.
6. Larner AJ. Charles Meller and John Kirk: medical practitioners and practice on Livingstone's Zambesi expedition, 1858–64. *J Med Biogr* 2002;10:129–134.
7. Foskett R (ed.). *The Zambesi journal and letters of Dr John Kirk, 1858–63.* Edinburgh: Oliver & Boyd, 1965:176,285.
8. Larner AJ. "Neurological literature": headache (part 3). *Adv Clin Neurosci Rehabil* 2007;7(1):27–28.

9. Labounsky A. *Jean Langlais. The man and his music.* Portland, Oregon: Amadeus Press, 2000:18.
10. Bobko J (ed.). *Vision. The life and music of Hildegard von Bingen.* New York: Penguin, 1995:17–21.
11. Singer C. *From magic to science. Essays on the scientific twilight.* London: Ernest Benn, 1928:199–239 [quote at 232].
12. Sacks O. *Migraine.* London: Picador, 1992:53,299–301.

5: Treatment

Previous articles in this series[1–4] have focused on literary descriptions of headache. As in clinical practice, it is now finally time for headache description (relatively easy) to give way to headache treatment (very difficult), specifically literary accounts of therapy for headache. The magnitude of the problem before us is perhaps no better illustrated than by the fact that many great and able individuals have suffered from headache without having specific solutions to their problem. Among famous migraineurs one may note characters as diverse as John Hughlings Jackson (the "father of English neurology")[5] and, possibly, Harry Potter[6] (interestingly, Daniel Radcliffe, the actor who portrayed Harry Potter in all the film versions of JK Rowling's books, has been reported to suffer from cluster headache).

Some possible therapies have been mentioned in previous articles: leeches and dental extractions in Jane Austen's *Sanditon*,[1] eye glasses in LM Montgomery's *Anne of Green Gables*,[1] a kiss in Robert Herrick's poem *The Head-ake*,[2] praying to saints or fasting,[3] and using a leaf and charm by Socrates in Plato's *Charmides*.[4] (The use of the guillotine, reported by Dickens as an effective headache cure,[3] may be discounted because of the invariably unfavourable adverse effect profile.) A further possible example of charms may be the glass balls sold for headaches by Melquiades and his tribe of gypsies to the villagers of Macondo in *One hundred years of solitude* by Gabriel Garcia Marquez. Four generations later in the same village, the adolescent Meme drinks cane liquor with her girl friends, then wakes at midnight with "her head splitting with pain and drowning in vomited gall": could the diagnosis be migraine? Her mother, Fernanda, gives her a vial of castor oil (a purgative), puts compresses on her stomach and ice cubes on her head.[7] Progress!

Other plant products have been recorded as therapeutic for headache. The herb skullcap, which was thought to bear an affinity to the shape of a skull, was once used as a cure for headache,[8] evidently an example of the theory of signatures. Tobacco was apparently a treatment for migraine, amongst other ailments, in Shakespeare's London.[9] Not all plants however are beneficial: OED lists "head-ache" as a rustic name used in the nineteenth century for the wild poppy *Papaver Rhoeas*, since "any one by smelling it for a very short time may convince himself of the propriety of the name". In *What Katy Did* by Susan Coolidge (1872), camphor is suggested for Katy's friend Imogen when she has a headache, and likewise for Aunt Izzie, but the latter turns out to have typhoid fever from which she succumbs.

Thomas Mann's novel *Doctor Faustus* (1947) has been noted to contain accounts of several neurological disorders, including neurosyphilis, meningitis, and stroke, as well as migraine.[10,11] For the latter, the landlady Frau Schweigstill suggests that the victim, Adrian Leverkühn, take "real strong tea, made real sour with lots of lemon". (It is not clear whether Mann himself suffered headaches: his autobiographically inspired work *Tonio Kroger* published in his late twenties [1903] contains no reference.) The efficacy of this (folkloric?) remedy is not recorded, but in Jane Austen's *Mansfield Park* (1814) Fanny Price's headache, one of several instances in which this author mentions headache,[12] improves after drinking tea prepared by her sister Susan, though it may be the "well-timed kindness" rather than caffeine which induces this effect. The efficacy of strong tea in migraine has been emphasized by some authors,[13] for example Elizabeth Garrett Anderson (1836–1917) in her 1870 doctoral thesis emphasized the importance of nutrition, regular meals and regular habits, with attacks treated with medication, rest and great quantities of tea.[14] Others insist on the withdrawal of all tea, as a source of caffeine, itself an analgesic, particularly in chronic migraine. Might the presence or absence of milk be the cause of such diametrically opposed medical advice? "It is a bad thing to give milk to persons having headache" according to Hippocrates (*Aphorisms*, 64), but equally he advises elsewhere that "abstinence is bad in headache" (*Regimen in acute disease*, 8).

Abstinence from what, we might wonder? Could the father of medicine have meant sex, perhaps? No less an authority than John F. Kennedy (1917–1963) is said to have stated, in conversation with Harold Macmillan in Bermuda in 1961, that "If I don't have a woman for three days, I get terrible headaches" (http://en.wikiquote.org/wiki/John_ F_Kennedy). If this were an efficacious form of prophylaxis, one can imagine that many headache patients would be enthusiastic about giving it a try, although of course headache itself may be a consequence (primary headache associated with sexual activity). What about drugs and alcohol? The nineteenth century clergyman Francis Kilvert who suffered from headache and face ache which may have been cluster headache[3,15] reported in his diary trying "laudanum and port wine, but nothing did any good", although on a later occasion he found that "After dinner and four glasses of port I felt better".

Returning to the theme of headache treatment recommended by doctors, rather than laymen, one might consider the case of Roald Dahl (1916–1990). Recovering in Alexandria after a war-time plane crash (he was at that time a fighter pilot in the Royal Air Force) which caused head injuries, Dahl had "such terrific headaches" that he had to lie flat for seven days in darkness doing nothing, followed by a new treatment regime: "... they are going to give me intravenal [sic] saline and pituatory [sic] injections & make me drink gallons of water – its another stunt to get rid of the headaches." Might he have had low pressure headache? The efficacy of this measure is not recorded, but Dahl did return to active service, only to be invalided out later because of "blinding headaches ... when I was flying ... doing very steep turns and making sudden changes of direction".[16]

William Heberden (1710–1801) was one of the most noted physicians of his day, remembered not only for Heberden's nodes but also for one of the first clear descriptions of angina, although he was not aware of its cardiac origin, a discovery ascribed to Edward Jenner. Heberden's approach to headache may be surmised from the correspondence of one of his notable patients, the potter Josiah Wedgwood (1730–1795). Between 1788 and 1790 Wedgwood told correspondents of his "nervous or rheumatic headache" which one physician had ascribed to gout. In 1788, Heberden prescribed for him a "blister", which apparently proved partially successful, and advised a holiday.[17]

Another noted physician of the eighteenth century was Erasmus Darwin (1731–1802), whose contributions to neurology include descriptions of psychiatric illness, neuro-ophthalmology (colour vision, afterimages, the blind spot) and electrical therapy for childhood hemiplegia.[18] Writing to his friend and fellow member of the Lunar Society James Watt (1736–1819) on 19th January 1790, he recommended:

> your headaches ... would recieve [sic] permanent relief from warm bathing I dare say.[19]

The risks of medication in the genesis of headache are, perhaps unwittingly, alluded to by Anthony Horowitz,[20] who says of an accident-prone character in *The blurred man* that "He bought headache pills that actually gave you a headache ...". The possibility of medication (aspirin) overuse headache in a patient labelled, implausibly to my diagnostic eye, as having "vascular dementia" in Ian McEwan's *Atonement* has been previously noted.[2]

Acknowledgment

Adapted from: Larner AJ. "Neurological literature": headache (part 5). *Adv Clin Neurosci Rehabil* 2009;8(6):27–28.

References

1. Larner AJ. "Neurological literature": headache. *Adv Clin Neurosci Rehabil* 2006;5(6):23–24.
2. Larner AJ. "Neurological literature": headache (part 2). *Adv Clin Neurosci Rehabil* 2006;6(2):37–38.
3. Larner AJ. "Neurological literature": headache (part 3). *Adv Clin Neurosci Rehabil* 2007;7(1):27–28.
4. Larner AJ. "Neurological literature": headache (part 4). *Adv Clin Neurosci Rehabil* 2008;7(6):17.
5. Critchley M, Critchley EA. *John Hughlings Jackson. Father of English neurology.* New York: Oxford University Press, 1998:192.
6. Sheftell F, Steiner TJ, Thomas H. Harry Potter and the curse of headache. *Headache* 2007;47:911–916.
7. Garcia Marquez G. *One hundred years of solitude.* London: Picador, [1967] 1978: 15;221,222.
8. Richardson R. *Death, dissection, and the destitute.* London: Routledge & Kegan Paul, 1987:301 n73.
9. Bryson B. *Shakespeare. The world as a stage.* London: Harper, 2007:54–55.
10. Kierulf H. Neurology in Thomas Mann's novels. *Acta Neurol Scand* 2003;107:430.
11. Rot U. Thomas Mann: neurological cases from Doctor Faustus. *Pract Neurol* 2004;4:180–183.
12. Larner AJ. "A transcript of actual life": headache in the novels of Jane Austen. *Headache* 2010;50:692–695.
13. Sacks O. *Migraine* (Revised and expanded). London: Picador, 1992:241,253,254.
14. Wilkinson M, Isler H. The pioneer woman's view of migraine: Elizabeth Garrett Anderson's thesis "Sur la migraine". *Cephalalgia* 1999;19:3–15.
15. Larner AJ. Francis Kilvert (1840–1879): an early self-report of cluster headache? *Cephalalgia* 2008;28:763–766.
16. Dahl R. *Going solo.* London: Puffin, [1986] 2001:116,202.
17. Finer A, Savage G (eds.). *The selected letters of Josiah Wedgwood.* London: Cory, Adams & Mackay, 1965:309,311,312,321–322.
18. Gardner-Thorpe C, Pearn J. Erasmus Darwin (1731–1802). Neurologist. *Neurology* 2006;66:1913–1916.
19. Fara P. *Erasmus Darwin. Sex, science and serendipity.* Oxford: Oxford University Press, 2012:143.
20. Horowitz A. *The blurred man.* London: Walker Books, 2002:61.

6.

> . . . all went to Pitcombe Church this Afternoon. I stayed at home having a little Head-Ache and thinking also that they would be crowded at Church.[1]

Thus the Reverend James Woodforde's diary for 30th July 1786, indicating that the impact of headache on day-to-day occupation is nothing new, although increasingly recognised in recent times.

Further literary historical accounts of the occupational impact of headache may also be given, for example from Dr Oliver Wendell Holmes (1809–1894), speaking of a school mistress, Helen Darley, aged "22 or 23 years old" in 1861:

> She was consequently . . . overworked, and an overworked woman is always a sad sight . . . because she is so much more fertile in capacities of suffering than a man. She has so many varieties of headache, – sometimes as if Jael were driving the nail that killed Sisera into her temples, – sometimes letting her work with half her brain while the other half throbs as if it would go to pieces, – sometimes tightening round the brows as if her cap-band were a ring of iron.[2]

(Those unfamiliar with the Old Testament account of the murder of the Canaanite general Sisera by Jael in the Book of Judges might consult the painting by Artemisia Gentileschi dating from 1620.)

This account by Holmes is quoted, in part, in two books devoted to the history of anaesthesia[3,4] as illustrations of the 19th century willingness to treat pain by means of anaesthetic agents. In this context, it is of interest that both chloroform and ether were at times used to treat headache.[5] For example, in the story *Sur l'eau* (*Afloat*, 1888) by Guy de Maupassant (1850–1893), the narrator breathes ether to relieve migraine. However, anaesthetic agents had adverse effects as well, and sometimes had fatal consequences, for example the case of Miss Mary Duff "Found dead in a bathhouse":

> The charitable construction put upon the terrible tragedy is that young Titus administered to his sweetheart [Miss Mary Duff] a dose of chloroform to dispel a headache, and that she took an overdose that caused her death. In the despair following her death, it is believed that he killed himself.[6]

Christopher Isherwood (1904–1986), enjoying a brief renaissance with the recent popularity of the film *A Single Man* (2009), diverging though it does from his novella of 1964, is perhaps best remembered for *Goodbye to Berlin* (1939), hailed as one of the most popular novels of the 20th century. Besides obliquely chronicling the rise of the Nazis, it also contains some casual examples of headache: Otto Nowak, a working class boy from Berlin, aged 16 or 17, "had a touch of sunstroke, and went to bed early, with a headache" whilst holidaying on Reugen Island in summer 1931. Frau Landauer is reported to have "tairrible [sic] headaches" by her daughter Natalia, such that she cannot be left, but she never has a headache when the narrator proposes going out with Natalia. Interestingly, when he does take Natalia out, to hear Mozart concertos, he finds that "The audience plainly regarded the concert as a religious ceremony. Their taut, devotional enthusiasm oppressed me like a headache".[7] Isherwood was briefly a medical student, as may perhaps be evidenced by the clinical detail in the final pages of *A Single Man*.

The author JD Salinger (1919–2010) is remembered chiefly for his novel *The catcher in the rye*, a paperback copy of which was held, infamously, by Mark Chapman on the night he shot John Lennon. The novel's anti-hero protagonist, Holden Caulfield, at one stage "had a helluva headache all of a sudden", "felt lousy" and "even had a sort of stomach-ache" which felt a little better after coffee but later felt worse. Prior to this, in his peregrinations about New York city, Caulfield had evidently missed sleep and meals, and consumed alcohol. Interestingly Holden's mother also complains of a splitting headache, and is said to get headaches quite frequently. "Take a few aspirins" suggests her 10 year-old daughter Phoebe.[8] Diagnosis: migraine? No other headache reference is found in a collection of Salinger's short stories.[9]

Phoebe Caulfield's suggestion of aspirin is perhaps not an unreasonable one, particularly from a 10 year-old, but it is now recognised that this is not so straightforward a therapeutic avenue as was once thought:

> Years ago ... if you had a headache you would have thought aspirin the best you could hope for, wouldn't you? Now, you would be wrong. Endless shelves of medicine are now common, specific medicines for specific headaches. Is it a sinus headache or a migraine headache? Now, it makes a difference.[10]

Will improved recognition, identification and treatment spell the end of headache as a major neurological problem? A tantalising glimpse into the future, specifically the 26th century, as imagined by Yevgeny Zamyatin (1884–1937) does not seem to augur well:

> After what happened yesterday, my head's been in tight bandages. Or rather, no – it isn't a bandage, but more like a hoop, a merciless hoop made of glass steel and riveted to my head.
>
> Compressed inside the tight hoop, my temples were pounding,
>
> My head was on fire and pounding. I sat up the whole night like this and fell asleep only around seven in the morning
>
> ... my head killing me.[11]

Acknowledgements

Thanks to Thomas Larner for drawing my attention to Yevgeny Zamyatin's novel *We*. Adapted from: Larner AJ. "Neurological literature": headache (part 6). *Adv Clin Neurosci Rehabil* 2010;10(3):38.

References

1. Beresford J (ed.). *The Diary of a Country Parson 1758–1802 James Woodforde*. Oxford: The World's Classics, 1949:276–277. [I am grateful to Professor Neil Scolding of Bristol for bringing this book to my attention.]
2. Holmes OW. *Elsie Venner. A romance of destiny*. Edinburgh: William Paterson, [1861] 1883:61.
3. Pernick MS. *A calculus of suffering. Pain, professionalism, and anesthesia in nineteenth-century America*. New York: Columbia University Press, 1985:149.
4. Snow SJ. *Blessed days of anaesthesia. How anaesthetics changed the world*. Oxford: Oxford University Press, 2008:64.
5. Ibid., 128,164.
6. *New York Times*, 19 October 1894:2. See also *The chloroform habit as described by one of its victims*. Detroit Lancet 1884–1885;8:251–254.
7. Isherwood C. *Goodbye to Berlin*. London: Vintage Books, [1939] 1998:102,181,184.
8. Salinger JD. *The catcher in the rye*. London: Penguin, [1945–46] 1994:160,165,166,168,175.
9. Salinger JD. *Nine Stories*. New York: Little, Brown & Co., 1953.
10. Block SM. *The story of forgetting*. London: Faber & Faber, 2008:116.
11. Zamyatin, YI. *We*. London: Penguin, [1924] 1993:198,201,218,219.

7: Megrim

A Google search for megrim will reveal several definitions, including a species of left-eyed flatfish (the whiff, or *Lepidorhombus whiffiagonis*), although neurologists will recall that this word is also an archaic (some would say obsolete) word for migraine. (Pubmed contains no references to megrim, as far as I can ascertain.) Other usages of megrim are reported to include:

- a caprice, fancy, whim or fad (often in the plural, megrims); and
- depression, melancholy, low spirits or unhappiness.

An example of the latter usage is said to be from Samuel Richardson's *History of Sir Charles Grandison* (1753) wherein Lady G writes to Miss Byron (volume VI, letter xlv) "If these megrims are the effect of Love, thank Heaven, I never knew what it was".[1] It remains possible, however, that this could equally well refer to headaches. *Sir Charles Grandison* was the favourite novel of Jane Austen (1775–1817), large passages of which she apparently knew by heart, and it may have been one stimulus, specifically imitation, for her use of headache as a plot device in several of her novels, as well as in other written work.[2]

Lane and Davies explain in their book on migraine that Galen's term "hemicrania" was translated into low Latin as "hemigranea", and that through successive transliterations and abbreviations this evolved by the 16th century into megrim in English, denoting sick headache, blind headache and bilious headache[3] (the latter term was still in common usage in the mid-twentieth century, used for example by my maternal grandmother[4]). The Oxford English Dictionary has its earliest references to megrim in the sense of headache dating to the mid-fifteenth century, hence postdating the earliest recorded use of headache (*ca.* 1000AD) by more than four centuries.[5] A seventeenth century translation of the *Chirurgical Works* of the French surgeon Ambroise Paré (1510–1590) includes the statement:

> The Megrim is properly a disease affecting the one side of the head, right or left.

Perhaps most famously in the neurological context, the word megrim was used by Edward Liveing in the title of his 1873 work, one of the seminal works in the history of headache, *On Megrim, Sick-Headache, And Some Allied Disorders: A Contribution To The Pathology Of Nerve-Storms*[6] which addressed his ideas on the pathophysiology of these headaches.[7] The following year Sydney Ringer wrote in the *BMJ* on the action of hydrate of croton-chloral on megrim.[8]

Some literary uses of megrim may also be noted here, some almost contemporaneous with its aforementioned uses in the 19th century medical literature. The word was certainly known to George Eliot, pseudonym of Marian Evans (1819–1880). In *Adam Bede* (1859), her first major novel, it is said of one female character:

> ... it was a pity she should take such megrims into her head, when she might ha' stayed wi' us all summer, and eaten twice as much as she wanted, and it 'ud niver ha' been missed.

In *Felix Holt, the Radical* (1866), a character asks:

> Can't one work for sheer truth as hard as for megrims?

OED records this as an example of megrims in the sense of a whim, fancy or fad. Another example may be Dr Tertius Lydgate in *Middlemarch* (1871–2) who is reported to be:

> ... abrupt but not irritable, taking little notice of megrims in healthy people.

Eliot's contemporary Wilkie Collins (1824–1889) was also familiar with the word. For example in *Armadale* (1866), one character asks of another:

> How did you manage to clear your head of those confounded megrims?

The context suggests that this may refer to either fancies or low spirits, but in *The Moonstone* (1868), possibly Collins's best known work, the use of the word certainly suggests the possibility of headaches:

> This was the first attack of the megrims that I remembered in my mistress since the time when she was a young girl.

Moving to a more contemporary literary use of the word megrim, two examples may be found in the oeuvre of Stephen King (born 1947). In *Gerald's Game* (1992) it is used in the sense of fancy, whim, freak, caprice:

> No, she thought her imagination had more than earned its right to a few hallucinatory megrims, but it remained important for her to remember she'd been alone that night.

In *Desperation* (1996), it is used in the sense of low spirits, unhappiness:

> He was turning around, zipping his fly, talking mostly to keep the megrims away (they had been gathering like vultures just lately, those megrims), and now he stopped doing everything at once.

One can understand how this word may perhaps appeal to King's sensibilities.

On a musical note, the composer Barry Ferguson uses megrim in his song *The Ruined Maid* (1997), again in the sense of melancholy, from a cycle of songs written for Catherine King.

Lardreau has traced the multiple meanings of the word megrim in both veterinary and clinical medicine of the 19th century, which included both hemicrania and vertigo and may therefore imply an overlap in the usages to encompass both these features,[9] perhaps akin to the modern terminology of "migrainous vertigo". However, in addition to such usages, ophthalmologists and neurologists have long recognised that megrim may be used to refer to the visual symptoms associated with migraine headache. For example, the Franco-Polish ophthalmologist Xavier Galezowski (1832–1907)[10] used the term "ophthalmic megrim" to denote visual symptoms associated with headache in a presentation given to the Congress of Genoa in 1877.[11] Two years later, Edward Nettleship (1879) published an article in the *British Medical Journal* in which he noted that:

> It is well known that certain of the subjects of megrim are liable to a very peculiar affection of sight, in which a part of the field of vision becomes obscured by a flickering or waving cloud, the edges of which in many persons are sharply defined, serrated and brilliantly coloured.[12]

These visual phenomena, falling within the contemporary clinical rubric of megrim, would now be recognised as the visual aura of migraine. These publications suggest that the term megrim cannot be defined as "headache with vertigo" as argued by Lardreau.[9] It was used as a synonym for migraine,[7,8,11–15] sometimes with additional visual or vertiginous symptoms.

Acknowledgements

Adapted from: Larner AJ. "Neurological literature": headache (part 7): Megrim. *Adv Clin Neurosci Rehabil* 2010;10(5):16; and Grzybowski A, Larner AJ. Letter to the editor and author's response: megrim does not mean migrainous vertigo – a comment on Lardreau (2012). *J Hist Neurosci* 2013;22:425–426.

References

1. Harris J (ed.). *Samuel Richardson. The History of Sir Charles Grandison.* Oxford: Oxford University Press, 1972:III:195.
2. Larner AJ. Jane Austen's (1775–1817) references to headache: fact and fiction. *J Med Biogr* 2010;18:211–215.
3. Lane R, Davies P. *Migraine.* Taylor & Francis: New York, 2006:8.
4. Larner AJ. Familial migraine without aura with perimenopausal onset. *Int J Clin Pract* 2010;64:128–129.
5. Larner AJ. "Neurological literature": headache (part 2). *Adv Clin Neurosci Rehabil* 2006;6(2):37–38.
6. Liveing E. Observations on megrim or sick-headache. *BMJ* 1872;1:364–366.
7. Pearce JMS. Edward Living's (1832–1919) theory of nerve-storms in migraine. In: Rose FC (ed.). *A short history of neurology. The British contribution 1660–1910.* Oxford: Butterworth Heinemann, 1999:192–203.
8. Ringer S. Remarks on the action of hydrate of croton-chloral on megrim. *BMJ* 1874;2:637.
9. Lardreau E. A curiosity in the history of sciences: the words "megrim" and "migraine". *J Hist Neurosci* 2012;21:31–40.

10. Amalric PM. The Galezowski tradition in Paris. *Doc Ophthalmol* 1999;98:105–113.
11. Galezowski X. Ophthalmic megrim. *Lancet* 1882:1:176–177.
12. Nettleship E. Repeated paroxysmal failure of sight in connection with heart-disease. *BMJ* 1879;1:889–891.
13. Wadsworth OF. A case of recurrent paralysis of the motor oculi. *Trans Am Ophthalmol Soc* 1887;4:460–470 [at 465,466].
14. Moritz S. The causes, symptoms, and complications of the diseases of the nasal accessory sinuses in their relation to general diseases, ophthalmology, and neurology. *BMJ* 1905;1:174–177 [at 175].
15. Mott FW. The reproductive organs in relation to mental disorders. *BMJ* 1922;1:463–466 [at 463].

8.

The Master and Margarita, the posthumously published masterpiece of the Russian author Mikhail Bulgakov (1891–1940), depicts Pontius Pilate as suffering from:

> ... the invincible, terrible illness ... hemicrania, when half of the head aches ... there's no remedy for it, no escape ... I'll try not to move my head.

Thus afflicted, Pilate interrogates the prisoner, Yeshua Ha-Nozri, who assures him "your suffering will soon be over, your headache will go away", but "a dull, slightly aching reminder of the morning's infernal pain" still lingers later in the day following the execution of the prisoner. Other characters in the novel also are affected, or nearly so, with headaches: Margarita has an ache like a needle in her temple all evening; Woland almost has a migraine from the roaring in the bar; and both the Master and Margarita have a slight ache in the left temple following Satan's ball.[1] Zayas has argued that Pilate's hemicrania reflects Bulgakov's personal experience of migraine, based on the evidence of his diaries.[2] Since Bulgakov was a qualified doctor, it might also be reasonably assumed that he encountered headache in practice, some corroboration for which may be found in his semi-fictional accounts published as *A Country Doctor's Notebook*. In *Black as Egypt's Night*, a miller from Dultsevo reports to young Dr Bulgakov that "Every day at twelve o'clock my head starts to ache, then I seem to get hot all over. ... It makes me shiver for a couple of hours or so and then it goes", leading the doctor to diagnose malaria. In *Morphine*, an account of morphine addiction, an "absurd, hysterical letter" from the addict provokes a migraine in the recipient (Bulgakov).[3]

Another Bulgakov, Valentin Fedorovich (1886–1966), acted as secretary to Leo Tolstoy (1828–1910) in the last year of the novelist's life, and subsequently published his diary for that year, which in turn became the starting point for Jay Parini's novel *The Last Station*, the motion picture of which was strangely neglected by mainstream cinemas in 2010. The story is told from several viewpoints, including that of Tolstoy's wife, Sofya Andreyevna, who on several occasions reports herself afflicted with headache, e.g.:

> I've been lying in bed with a headache, watching the snow fall, drinking tea. I cannot read. My head is tight as a drum, pounding. And I do not have the gramophone in my bedroom.[4]

Parini's novel is based on the diaries kept by those in Tolstoy's inner circle. The edited diary of Sofia Tolstoy, covering the period 1862 to 1919,[5] attests not only to her headaches, but also to those of Tolstoy himself, and other family members including their youngest daughter, Sasha (born 1884):

> *21st June 1897.* Sasha ... was looking very pale and said she felt sick and had a headache. ... Then she vomited and had to lie down. She often gets migraines, like her father.

Reading the diaries, I cannot escape the conclusion that Sofia's portrayal in the film of *The Last Station* is not entirely fair. Indeed, some might gauge that her character has been impudently traduced, or, at the very least, that she was perhaps more sinned against that sinning. However, the tradition of cinematographic misrepresentation of Tolstoy's last days is a long one, dating to 1912 (*The Flight of a Great Old Man*, described by Sofia as a lampoon of her), and at least *The Last Station* secured for Helen Mirren an (obligatory?) Oscar nomination for her portrayal of Sofia. Parenthetically, one may note that two figures in the history of neurology appear transiently, as offstage figures, in Sofia Tolstoy's diary. Kozhevnikov, later credited with the earliest description of what has come to be known as Rasmussen's encephalitis,[6] was apparently consulted by Tolstoy's son Lyova in 1895; and on 24th November 1900 Tolstoy "went to a musical evening at the lunatic asylum", namely the psychiatric clinic of Professor SS Korsakov.

Chekhov was one of Leo Tolstoy's many occasional visitors, both at Yasnaya Polyana and in Yalta. Previous examples of headache in Chekov's plays have been cited,[7] and they may also be found in some of his short stories.[8] For example, in *Peasants*, Kiryak has "a terrible hangover ... shaking his splitting head". In *The Bishop*, Bishop Peter "had the same headache as yesterday ..", and later "he had a splitting headache". This is one symptom of a febrile illness which is eventually diagnosed as typhoid.

Whilst headache is an incidental finding in all the aforementioned works, occasional pieces proclaim this to be their subject matter: one thinks of Robert

Herrick's 1648 poem *The Head-ake.*[9] Another is example is the short story entitled *Migraine* by Tobias Wolff, from the collection *The night in question.* The story begins:

> It began while she was at work.

(Although the nature of this work is not made explicit, the fact that she, Joyce, works at a keyboard, with lab reports, and with cubicles around her from which the "steady click of other keyboards" is heard, suggests the possibility of a medical secretary.) It transpires that this headache is occurring in the context of a relationship which is breaking up. At home Joyce tries herbal tea, which "helped. Not much, really …", and kneading her temples, and she has apparently tried other remedies in the past including getting drunk and stoned, but it is head massages from her (soon to depart) partner which help most. Her symptoms include dizziness and:

> … at the worst moment she went suddenly deaf, as if someone had pushed her head underwater …

a symptom which recurs later. Of note, headache also crops up in another of Wolff's stories, *Flyboys*:

> … handsome families … it was clear, did not … come down with migraines.
>
> The sound grew larger and louder and emptier, the sound of emptiness itself, emptiness throbbing like a headache.[10]

Acknowledgements

Adapted from: Larner AJ. "Neurological literature": headache (part 8). *Adv Clin Neurosci Rehabil* 2011;11(2):21.

References

1. Bulgakov M. *The Master and Margarita.* London: Penguin, [1966–67] 2003:19–24,310 (Pilate); 231 (Margarita); 277 (Woland); 364 (Master and Margarita).
2. Zayas V. Sympathy for Pontius Pilate. Hemicrania in M.A. Bulgakov's "The Master and Margarita". *Eur J Neurol* 2005;12(suppl2):296 (abstract P2506).
3. Bulgakov M. *A Country Doctor's Notebook.* London: Harvill Press, [1925–27] 1975:47;119–120.
4. Parini J. *The last station. A novel of Tolstoy's final year.* New York: Anchor Books, [1990] 2009:60; also 152,160,224 ("temples throbbed"); Bulgakov

complains of a mild headache at 109, and Sasha, Tolstoy's daughter, reports at 139 that her "head no longer throbbed".

5. Porter C (trans.). *The diaries of Sofia Tolstoy*. London: Alma Books, 2009: xxiv,6,8,14,26(x2),55,125,146,155,163,210,263,277,312,357(x2),364,382,389, 392,395,401,404; "neuralgia" 73,132,211,255,264,277; Lev Nikolaevich Tolstoy's headaches 13,26,222,250,400,518,520; Tatyana (Tanya) Tolstaya 92; Alexandra (Sasha) Tolstaya 161; Maria (Masha) Tolstaya 242. Kozhevnikov 148, Koraskov 278,554.
6. Andermann F (ed.). *Chronic encephalitis and epilepsy. Rasmussen's syndrome.* Boston: Butterworth-Heinemann, 1991:245–261.
7. Larner AJ. "Neurological literature": headache. *Adv Clin Neurosci Rehabil* 2006;5(6):23–24.
8. Ford SF, Larner AJ. Neurological disorders reported by Dr Anton Chekhov (1860–1904). *Eur J Neurol* 2010;17(suppl 3):545 (abstract P2530).
9. Larner AJ. "Neurological literature": headache (part 2). *Adv Clin Neurosci Rehabil* 2006;6(2):37–38.
10. Wolff T. *The night in question*. London: Bloomsbury, 1996: *Migraine* 120–130; *Flyboys* 57–73 [at 57,64].

9.

It is some years since the previous article in this series presenting accounts of headache encountered in literary or biographical material,[1] and, astonishingly, almost a decade since the first.[2] I hope readers will indulge me by accepting this further offering.

As neurologists, we now draw a clear clinical distinction between "headache" and "neuralgia", as enshrined in diagnostic criteria.[3] However, our clinical experience indicates that this distinction may not be evident to patients (or even sometimes primary care physicians) who may use the terms interchangeably. The author W Somerset Maugham (1874–1965) was a medical student at St Thomas' Hospital, London, in the 1890s,[4] during which time he attended, according to his own account, 63 confinements in 3 weeks in houses in Lambeth, experience of the labouring poor which provided the source material for his first novel, *Liza of Lambeth* (1897). The heroine's mother, Mrs Kemp speaks to her daughter:

> 'Oo, my 'ead!' she was saying, as she pressed her hands on each side of her forehead. 'I've got the neuralgy again; wot shall I do? I dunno 'ow it is, but it always comes on Sunday mornings'.

Later in the novel, apparently neglected by her daughter one day, she complains on her return:

> 'I've 'ad the neuralgy all the mornin', and my 'ead's been simply splittin', so thet I thought the bones 'ud come apart and all my brains go streamin' on the floor.'

The good lady's drinking habits may give us an all too transparent a clue to the timing of her headaches.[5]

Like Mrs Kemp, "neuralgia" as a description of head pains, sometimes apparently interchangeably with headache and even migraine, may be encountered elsewhere, for example in the writings of Elizabeth Gaskell (1810–1865),[6] Louisa May Alcott (1832–1888),[7] and Francis Kilvert (1840–1879).[8] I suppose it may be possible that this reflects the usage of the term in the nineteenth century.

In none of these individuals, with the exception of Mrs Kemp, did headache appear to stifle creativity, although it might interrupt for a time social and occupational functions. Hence it is unsurprising to note that the possessors of very disparate talents may also be afflicted by headache, ranging from the levity of the comedian Peter Kay, who reports:

> Nowadays I get a blinding migraine if I stay up until the end of *News at Ten* and I have to have a siesta the following day.[9]

to the gravitas of Thomas Henry Huxley (1825–1895), Darwin's "bulldog". In Adrian Desmond's biography, Huxley is reported to be "crushed by headaches after lecturing". Developing his interests in fossils, he "started another course for his students but it took the inevitable toll. Headaches plagued him". Both references relate to the mid-1850s, when Huxley was in his late 20s or early 30s, and still trying to establish himself, this being in the midst of what Desmond chooses to call the "Lost in Wilderness Years (1850–1858)".[10] One might wonder whether Huxley's "dyspepsia", accounted one of his "Town afflictions", might also be ultimately migrainous in origin.

Although a "plague", might headaches ever enhance, facilitate or stimulate creativity, perhaps by affording new insights, or granting different mind states, which may then be translated to the non-headache state? On the extremely rare occasions that I have had a migraine-type headache I have been subjectively aware that I am seeing things or thinking about things differently from my usual non-headache state.

There is of course a considerable literature addressing these possibilities, from which only a few examples are mentioned here. One relates to the suggestion that Pablo Picasso may have been a migraineur, the cubist style being in part a response to the fragmentation and distortion of visual images experienced in migraine aura. It is a fascinating idea, but one currently still without any definite evidence to prove or refute.[11]

Acknowledgements

Adapted from: Larner AJ. "Neurological literature": headache (part 9). *Adv Clin Neurosci Rehabil* 2016;16 (2):17.

References

1. Larner AJ. "Neurological literature": headache (part 8). Adv Clin Neurosci Rehabil 2011;11(2):21.
2. Larner AJ. "Neurological literature": Headache. *Adv Clin Neurosci Rehabil* 2006;5(6):23–24.
3. Headache Classification Committee of the International Headache Society (IHS). The International Classification of Headache Disorders, 3rd edition (beta version). *Cephalalgia* 2013;33:629–808.
4. O'Mahony S. W Somerset Maugham (1874–1965) and St Thomas's Hospital: Medical School and the making of a writer. *J Med Biogr* 2014;22:56–60.
5. Maugham WS. *Liza of Lambeth.* London: Vintage Books, 2000 [1897]:19,80.
6. Larner AJ. "A habit of headaches": the neurological case of Elizabeth Gaskell. *Gaskell Journal* 2011;25:97–103.
7. Larner AJ. Louisa May Alcott and headache. *Adv Clin Neurosci Rehabil* 2014;14(2):20.
8. Larner AJ. Francis Kilvert (1840–1879): an early self-report of cluster headache? *Cephalalgia* 2008;28:763–766.
9. Kay P. *The sound of laughter.* London: Century, 2006:151.
10. Desmond A. *Huxley. The devil's disciple.* London: Michael Joseph, 1994:217,232.
11. Haan J, Ferrari MD. Picasso's migraine: illusory cubist splitting or illusion? *Cephalalgia* 2011;31:1057–1060.

Neurological literature: Epilepsy

A classic account of epilepsy as the "falling sickness" is given in William Shakespeare's *Julius Caesar* (1599; Act I, scene ii, lines 253–256):

> CASCA: He fell down in the market-place, and foamed at mouth, and was speechless.
> BRUTUS: 'Tis very like: he hath the falling-sickness.

However, the only use of the word "epilepsy" in the Shakespearean canon, to my knowledge, occurs in *Othello, The Moor of Venice* (1604), spoken by Iago shortly after Othello has collapsed, having been goaded by Iago into the belief that Desdemona has been unfaithful (Act IV, scene I, lines 51–56):

> IAGO: My lord is fallen into an epilepsy;
> This is his second fit; he had one yesterday.
> CASSIO: Rub him about the temples.
> IAGO: No, forbear;
> The lethargy must have his quiet course,
> If not he foams at mouth, and by and by
> Breaks out to savage madness.

Considering the circumstances of the event, and Othello's rapid recovery to continue the argument with Iago, I would suggest that this was more likely to be syncope, rather than an epileptic event. However, in his comprehensive recording of faints and fits in Shakespeare's works, Kenneth Heaton seems ready to accept Iago's diagnosis.[1]

An episode of impaired consciousness is central to the plot of *Silas Marner, the weaver of Raveloe* (1861) by George Eliot (1819–1880), occasioning the exile of the protagonist to Raveloe, where the locals observe further attacks:

> ... he saw that Marner's eyes were set like a dead man's, and he spoke to him, and shook him, and his limbs were stiff ... just as he had made up his mind that the weaver was dead, he came all right again ... and said "Good-night", and walked off.

The locals are uncertain as to the cause of these events:

> Some said Marner must have been in a "fit", a word which seemed to explain things otherwise incredible; but ... Mr Macey ... asked if anybody

> was ever known to go off in a fit and not fall down. A fit was a stroke, wasn't it?

What influence may epilepsy have on creative endeavour? It was once thought that Vincent van Gogh suffered from temporal lobe epilepsy but in recent times there seems to have been some movement away from this idea to suggestions of borderline personality disorder[2] and bipolar affective disorder.[3] It is well known that Fyodor Dostoyevsky (1821–1881) suffered from epilepsy, and that a number of characters in his oeuvre are epileptics, their fictional experiences likely based on the author's own.[4]

"Dostoëffsky" is mentioned, in passing, in *A ray of darkness*[5] (p.14,19,170), a work devoted to epilepsy by the Anglo-Welsh author Margiad Evans (1909–1958).[6] An acclaimed novelist of the 1930s, Evans was first diagnosed with epilepsy at the age of 42 whilst living in Gloucestershire. Her experiences prompted her to write "the story of my epilepsy ... an adventure of body and mind" (p.12). Her first major seizure occurred on the evening of 11th May 1950 whilst she was alone in her cottage, and is described thus (p.78):

> [I] looked up at the clock .. saw that it was ten minutes past eleven. The next thing I was still looking up at the clock and the hands stood at five and twenty minutes past midnight. I had fallen through Time, Continuity and Being.

In the immediate aftermath, recalled later, her brain "worked ... like an engine misfiring and unsteered" (p.80). She found herself to have been incontinent of urine (p.81) and later found a cut at the base of her head at the back (p.86).

> ... in one moment, I realised the incredible, impossible and ghastly truth – I had had an epileptic fit. (p.81).

She rebutted the suggestions of relatives that it was simply a faint (p.98) and that she had just passed out, showing a clear understanding of the different symptoms of syncope:

> I had been close enough to it to be absolutely sure that one did not faint as I had fallen. There was a sinking away, a sick feeling, and a remembrance of it afterwards. (p.99)

Retrospectively, she recalled "moments of separation from my consciousness" dating back to childhood, lasting a few seconds, which had been more frequent in the previous year (p.38,39), episodes which might possibly have been complex partial seizures.

Seen by her general practitioner the day following the first major seizure, he immediately prescribed luminal (p.85) (phenobarbital) and arranged for an appointment with Professor T, "a man of international reputation" (p.104), who, following an EEG, confirmed the diagnosis of epilepsy when he saw Margiad on 8th June 1950 (i.e. 4 weeks after the first major seizure): "he thought that I must have a slight scar on the brain from an old injury" (p.106).

Two problems which are still grappled with in epilepsy management today presently became apparent: pregnancy, and impaired cognitive function.[7,8] After commencing the luminal, "I was never so tired in my life", and by 29th September 1950 Evans reported that she was "4 months gone with child" (p.111).

> Epilepsy and pregnancy. The shock of waking every morning to such a grim problem of life (p.125).

Concerns that epilepsy might be hereditary (although there was no family history; p.37,105) were finally overcome, by her general practitioner

> . . . reading . . . a passage from *Nervous Diseases* by the Professor of Neurology at London University, which he said was the last and most up-to-date work on epilepsy. . . . there was in reality only the very slightest danger of its being hereditary. (p.128)

Her baby daughter was born uneventfully, but after a post partum fit "I was never again able to feed my child" (p.153).

The other major issue was the effect of anti-epileptic medications ("luminal and epinutin" [*sic*], p.108) on a creative writer:

> since taking drugs I cannot keep awake for those free quiet hours which were my most creative. True my power of concentration is lost also (p.19)
>
> . . . the drugs I have to take . . . make me apathetic, have faded and dulled and dimmed the powers of imagination and concentration (p.189)

In her final years, an exploratory operation revealed a brain tumour to have been the cause of her epilepsy (ref. 6:55).

Acknowledgements

Adapted from: Larner AJ. "Neurological literature": epilepsy. *Adv Clin Neurosci Rehabil* 2007;7(3):16.

References

1. Heaton KW. Faints, fits, and fatalities from emotion in Shakespeare's characters: survey of the canon. *BMJ* 2006;333:1335–1338.
2. Van Meekeren E. *Starry starry night: life and psychiatric history of Vincent van Gogh.* Amsterdam: Benecke, 2003.
3. Carota A, Iaria G, Berney A, Bogousslavsky J. Understanding van Gogh's night: bipolar disorder. In: Bogousslavsky J, Boller F (eds.). *Neurological disorders in famous artists.* Basel: Karger, 2005:121–131.
4. Larner AJ. Dostoevsky and epilepsy. *Adv Clin Neurosci Rehabil* 2006;6(1):26.
5. Evans M. *A ray of darkness.* London: John Calder, [1952] 1978.
6. Prys-Williams B. *Twentieth-century autobiography. Writing Wales in English.* Cardiff: University of Wales Press, 2004:32–57 [at 50–57].
7. O'Brien MD, Gilmour-White SK. Management of epilepsy in women. *Postgrad Med J* 2005;81:278–285.
8. Brookes JA, Baker GA. Epilepsy and memory. *Epilepsy Professional* 2006;1(2):21–23.

Neurological literature: Cognitive disorders

Cognitive disorders may not perhaps lend themselves well to literary description, in the way that, for example, headache disorders, as almost purely subjective states, do. Nonetheless, attempts have been made, some examples of which are reviewed here.

Amnesia

Many authors have been fascinated by memory, indeed it has been argued that novels are all about memory.[1] One example is Jane Austen in *Mansfield Park*:[2,3]

> If any one faculty of our nature may be called more wonderful than the rest, I do think it is memory. There seems something more speakingly incomprehensible in the powers, the failures, the inequalities of memory, than in any other of our intelligences. The memory is sometimes so retentive, so serviceable, so obedient – at others, so bewildered and so weak – and at others again, so tyrannic, so beyond controul [sic]!
>
> ... our powers of recollecting and of forgetting, do seem peculiarly past finding out.

As pointed out by Papanicolaou in his textbook on amnesia,[4] the villagers of Macondo in *One hundred years of solitude* by Gabriel Garcia Marquez (1927–2014) suffer loss of memory for object names following an "insomnia plague", in response to which they paste labels to objects bearing their names and functions.[5] Poor sleep quality is of course not an uncommon accompaniment, and of probable aetiological significance, in memory clinic attenders complaining of poor memory, although in the case of Marquez the trope is probably symbolic rather than naturalistic.[6] Others have seen these villagers as suffering from semantic dementia.[7]

Memory problems are also the defining characteristic of *Mr Forgetful*, number 14 in the *Mister Men* series of children's books by Roger Hargreaves: entrusted with a message, Mr Forgetful forgets it, inasmuch as he is only able to pass on a garbled version, only to recall the correct message later, suggesting his problem is one of retrieval rather than encoding and storage. In JK Rowling's *Harry Potter and the Chamber of Secrets*, Gilderoy Lockhart, Hogwarts' Defence Against the Dark Arts teacher, threatens Harry and Ron with a "Memory Charm" after admitting he was not in fact the perpetrator of the heroic deeds described in his books, but he is "impaled upon his own sword", according to Dumbledore, when the charm backfires on the threshold of the Chamber of Secrets.[8]

Amnesia is, of course, a staple of Hollywood hokum (see Box; film buffs will surely be able to recall more examples); it is perhaps as popular a theme as the maverick cop or the wrongly accused. Loss of personal identity is a frequent aspect of these formulaic screen episodes of amnesia, and recovery an inevitable part of the filmic denouement, both features suggestive of psychogenic amnesia, transient psychological amnesia, or fugue. These features have attracted criticism as unrepresentative of most episodes of clinical amnesia.[9] In connection with loss of personal identity, boys of a certain vintage will recall that this is the fate which befell the quintessential toy doll action hero Action Man, sadly without recovery.

It has been suggested that *Memento* (2000), wherein Shelby (Guy Pearce) suffers from a kind of memory loss whereby he remembers life before the murder of his wife but is unable since then to recall anything for more than a few minutes, was inspired by the classic case of HM (Henry Molaison, 1926–2008) who developed profound anterograde amnesia after bilateral anterior temporal lobe resection, including parts of the hippocampi, for an intractable seizure disorder. Viewing the film, however, is little substitute for reading the many reports on HM.[10,11] Shelby is never happy, in contrast with HMs apparent contentment. SJ Watson's novel *Before I go to sleep* (now also a film) also portrays anterograde amnesia with acknowledgements to HM and to Clive Wearing,[12] an account of whose amnesia has also been published.[13]

Amnesia as a feature of dementia or Alzheimer's disease (AD) has attracted screen portrayals such as Mia Farrow in *Forget Me Never* (1999), Michael Caine in *Is Anybody There?*(2008), and perhaps most famously Judi Dench in *Iris* (2001), based on John Bayley's memoir of his wife Iris Murdoch's illness, the linguistic consequences of which have also been chronicled, more objectively, through analysis of novels written at three stages of the author's career.[14] In *Away From Her* (2006), Fiona (Julie Christie) and Gordon are an aging couple whose lives are affected by AD. *Time Out* is perhaps stretching credibility when stating that "the most compelling element ... is the suggestion that Fiona's AD is in part Gordon's cross to bear for his past misdemeanours [infidelity]"! The film is a "rare if difficult pleasure", for which Christie was Oscar nominated. In *The Notebook* (2004), Duke reads to Allie from a storybook about the relationship of two ill-fated young lovers. *Time Out* spots the glaring inconsistency: "Apparently Allie can no longer recognise her husband or children, but has retained enough short-term memory and powers of concentration to follow Duke's romantic narrative from day to day". Similar qualms may be voiced about *Cortex* (2008) in which a police inspector with AD solves a murder mystery in a clinic treating neurodegenerative disorders. Early-onset familial

AD linked to chromosome 14 has also become a subject for fiction,[15] albeit not mentioning mutations in the presenilin 1 gene which are responsible for this condition.

An "amnesia drug" given as a "shot" is available at the Supreme Headquarters of the Alien Defence Organisation (SHADO) in the 1970s Gerry and Sylvia Anderson serial *UFO*, to be administered to individuals who unwittingly come into contact with aliens or SHADO. In the US TV serial *Monk*, about the detective Adrian Monk who has obsessive-compulsive disorder, the protagonist develops memory problems and goes missing after a head injury (season four: *Mr Monk Bumps His Head*). The police surmise amnesia (= loss of identity), but Monk's psychiatrist Dr Kroger states that what they suggest is very rare and thinks some kind of dissociative state more likely. Although Monk is apparently unaware of his identity, nonetheless his obsessive-compulsive traits persist, which allows him to solve a murder despite not knowing that he is a detective. Post-traumatic amnesia also afflicts Professor Calculus in the *Destination Moon* episode of Herge's adventures of Tintin.[16]

Aphasia

Wings by Arthur Kopit,[17] initially conceived as a radioplay and later adapted for the stage, portrays a woman with post-stroke aphasia. Kopit was prompted to examine this issue when his father suffered a stroke, although the author describes the piece as "speculation informed by fact" (xv) and not a case study. The central character, Emily Stilson, is in her 70s when she suffers a stroke. She has what appears to be a fluent aphasia with paraphasias and neologisms, which the author describes, evidently advisedly from the material contained in his introduction, as jargon (p.42). We hear her words from both her own and her medical auditors point of view, indicating the patient's lack of self-monitoring of verbal output. These phenomena are the result of a "left cerebral infarction" (p.66), although interestingly the patient is left handed (p.57) which may complicate any simple interpretation. Mrs Stilson also seems to have an "out of body experience" near the end of the play (p.74).

Kopit's work is also mentioned in the context of a (non-fictional) case of global aphasia characterised by recurrent utterances, sometimes also known as verbal stereotypies, stereotyped aphasia, or monophasia.[18] This of course differs from the total anarthria of the locked-in syndrome reported from the inside, as it were, by Bauby.[19]

Apraxia

David Perkin identified a possible case of "dressing apraxia" in Arnold Bennett's novel *Clayhanger* (1910) in the character of Darius Clayhanger, a portrait perhaps based on the illness suffered by the author's father, Enoch Bennett. Perkin suggests a pathological diagnosis of Pick's disease confined to the parietal lobes in Bennett *père*, based on analogy with a case described by Lhermitte.[20] Certainly a corticobasal degeneration syndrome with the neuropathological substrate of tau-positive Pick body Pick's disease has been described on occasion.[21] However, the symptom of dressing apraxia is now regarded as a disorder of visuoperceptual function rather than an apraxia *per se*.

Difficulty dressing is one feature manifested by a character in the short story *No one's guilty* by the Argentinian author Julio Cortázar (1914–1984), which has been interpreted as an example of ideomotor apraxia. Other symptoms mentioned may be thought representative of alien hand, dystonia, myoclonus and postural instability, which together have been suggested to constitute the gestalt of corticobasal degeneration.[22]

Agnosia

Previous articles have alluded to possible cases of agnosia, specifically visual object agnosia in Anton Chekhov's short story *The Kiss* (1887),[3] and prosopagnosia afflicting Lewis Carroll's Humpty Dumpty in *Through the looking-glass and what Alice found there* (1872).[23]

Acknowledgements

Adapted from: Larner AJ. "Neurological literature": cognitive disorders. *dv Clin Neurosci Rehabil* 2008;8(2):20.

References

1. Dieguez S, Annoni J-M. Stranger than fiction: literary and clinical amnesia. In: Bogousslavsky J, Dieguez S (eds.). *Literary medicine: brain disease and doctors in novels, theater, and film* (Frontiers of Neurology and Neuroscience Volume 31). Basel: Karger, 2013:137–168 [at 137].
2. Harris J. *Jane Austen's art of memory.* Cambridge: Cambridge University Press, 1989.
3. Larner AJ. Jane Austen on memory; Anton Chekhov on agnosia. *Adv Clin Neurosci Rehabil* 2005;5(2):14.
4. Papanicolaou AC (ed.). *The amnesias: a clinical textbook of memory disorders.* Oxford: Oxford University Press, 2006:129,240.

5. Garcia Marquez G. *One hundred years of solitude.* London: Picador, [1967] 1978:43,45–47.
6. Bell M. *Gabriel Garcia Marquez: solitude and solidarity.* London: MacMillan, 1993:43–52.
7. Rascovsky K, Growdon ME, Pardo IR, Grossman S, Miller BL. "The quicksand of forgetfulness": semantic dementia in *One hundred years of solitude. Brain* 2009;132:2609–2616.
8. Rowling JK. *Harry Potter and the Chamber of Secrets.* London: Bloomsbury, 1998:220,224,244.
9. Baxendale S. Memories aren't made of these: amnesia at the movies. *BMJ* 2004;329:1480–1483.
10. Moscovitch M. Memory before and after H.M.: an impressionistic historical perspective. In: Zeman A, Kapur N, Jones-Gotman M (eds.). *Epilepsy and memory.* Oxford: Oxford University Press, 2012:19–50.
11. Corkin S. *Permanent present tense. The man with no memory, and what he taught the world.* London: Allen Lane, 2013.
12. Watson SJ. *Before I go to sleep.* London: Doubleday, 2011.
13. Wearing D. *Forever today. A memoir of love and amnesia.* London: Corgi, 2005.
14. Garrard P, Maloney LM, Hodges JR, Patterson K. The effects of very early Alzheimer's disease on the characteristics of writing by a renowned author. *Brain* 2005;128:250–260.
15. Block SM. *The story of forgetting.* London: Faber & Faber, 2008:49,173,241.
16. Medrano J, Malo P, Uriarte JJ, Lopez AP. Stigma and prejudice in Tintin. *BMJ* 2009;339:b5308.
17. Kopit A. *Wings.* London: Eyre Methuen, 1979.
18. Hale S. *The man who lost his language. A case of aphasia* (Revised edition). London: Jessica Kingsley, 2007:31,39–40,64,138,144,201.
19. Bauby J-D. *The diving-bell and the butterfly.* London: Fourth Estate, 1997.
20. Perkin GD. Arnold Bennett and medicine: with particular reference to his description of dressing apraxia. *BMJ* 1981;283:1666–1668.
21. Doran M, du Plessis DG, Enevoldson TP, Fletcher NA, Ghadiali E, Larner AJ. Pathological heterogeneity of clinically diagnosed corticobasal degeneration. *J Neurol Sci* 2003;216:127–134.
22. Merello M. Julio Cortázar quotes on normal and abnormal movements: magic realism or reality? *Mov Disord* 2006;21:1062–1065.
23. Larner AJ. The neurology of "Alice". *Adv Clin Neurosci Rehabil* 2005;4(6):35–36.

Some films featuring characters with amnesia/memory loss

Overboard (1987). Amnesia after fall from yacht

Shattered (1991). Tom Berenger: car crash, coma, memory erased, unfaithful wife, torrid affair, etc, etc ....

The Long Kiss Goodnight (1996). Amnesiac suburban housewife Samantha, aka Charly (Geena Davis), was a ruthless assassin: "Like Charly's alter ego .. you may have trouble remembering what happened once its all over" (*Time Out*).

Time to say goodbye (1997). End of life drama following diagnosis of Alzheimer's disease

Jackie Chan's Who Am I? (1998). Any more explanation required?

Memento (2000). Shelby (Guy Pearce) suffers from a kind of memory loss whereby he remembers life before the murder of his wife but is unable since then to recall anything for more than a few minutes.

Santa Who? (2000). Santa (Leslie Nielsen) suffers amnesia after crashing his sleigh into the car of a Scrooge-like TV reporter.

The Bourne Identity (2002). Amnesiac (Matt Damon) was deadly CIA assassin, now the target of his former employers; memory still troubled in *The Bourne Supremacy* (2004).

Blind Horizon (2003). Amnesiac (Val Kilmer) believes US president in peril.

Finding Nemo (2003). Dory, a friendly but forgetful regal blue tang fish (*sic*); key memory finally triggered by a visual lexical cue.

Gothika (2003). Psychiatrist (Halle Berry) develops amnesia after a car crash, then is incarcerated in her own hospital accused of murdering her husband. An every day tale of psychiatry practice?

50 First Dates (2004). Amnesiac Lucy (Drew Barrymore) must be wooed afresh each day by would-be Don Juan (Adam Sandler).

Unmade beds (2009). Amnesia after alcohol, wakes up in bed with girl etc, etc ...

Trance (2013). Following a head injury, Jimmy McAvoy forgets where he has stashed the painting he has nicked.

Neurological literature: Sleep-related disorders

Sleep-related disorders have progressively achieved a higher profile in neurological practice in recent years, with the inception of more subspecialty clinics, although the UK still lags behind other countries in such provision. As with other neurological conditions, possible accounts of sleep-related disorders are to be found in stories and novels, which may predate clinical recognition.

As is well-known,[1] one sleep-related disorder takes its name from a literary description, viz. the Pickwickian syndrome. In Charles Dickens's *Posthumous Papers of the Pickwick Club* (1837), Joe the fat boy is reported to be obese, with a ruddy complexion, hypersomnolence, and dropsy, features which subsequently prompted use of the term "Pickwickian syndrome" to describe similar cases, a term more recently superseded by obstructive sleep apnoea-hypopnoea syndrome (OSAHS). However, Cosnett, reviewing this case and other possible instances of sleep-related disorders in the works of Dickens,[2] suggests that Joe may in fact have had a diencephalic tumour or possibly suffered the consequences of a head injury. He also identifies Mr Willet in Dickens's *Barnaby Rudge* (1841) as a possible case of OSAHS.

Although only described as such in recent years, OSAHS has in all likelihood been around for centuries, possibly millenia. Dionysius, the obese tyrant of Heracleia on the south coast of the Black Sea in the fourth century BCE, was in danger of choking if he fell deeply asleep, and thus had to be woken with fine needles pricked into his skin.[3]

Another possible account occurs in Anton Chekhov's play *The Cherry Orchard* (1903): Boris Borisovich Simeonov-Pishchik, a landowner, "drops asleep and snores" in the midst of speaking, only to wake again "at once" and continue what he was saying. Later, he reports that he has high blood pressure and has had a stroke twice already, which makes dancing difficult, before again falling asleep, snoring, and waking almost at once.[4] OSAHS may present in the neurological clinic in various guises, including headache, blackout, seizure, stroke, or memory impairment,[5] and may be associated with high blood pressure and be a risk factor for stroke.

Before he undertook his major expeditions in Africa, Dr David Livingstone had his uvula excised in 1852, ostensibly because he suffered from "clergyman's sore throat", a disorder which affected his ability to preach to large numbers of people.[6] However, he comments of the uvula that:

> It sometimes fell down on the opening of the windpipe in sleep & made me start up as if suffocating.[7]

One wonders if perhaps these were episodes of sleep apnoea, although certainly one nowhere has the impression that Livingstone suffered from excessive daytime somnolence. Another possibility is the "sleeping-choking syndrome", a little-described parasomnia.

Of the many recognised parasomnias, sleepwalking is perhaps the most dramatic, and one which artists have been willing to make use of: Bellini devotes an opera to the subject (*La Sonnambula*). In Johanna Spyri's *Heidi* (1880), strange things come to pass when the little girl is residing in the Frankfurt city home of Clara Sessman: each morning the doors are found wide open, despite being closed at night, leading the servants to believe that there is a ghost in the house. Herr Sessman summons his old friend the doctor to sit up with him all night to solve the mystery: Heidi is a sleepwalker. The doctor elicits the history that during her somnambulation Heidi is dreaming of her natal home with her Grandfather in the mountains. The diagnosis is that Heidi is consumed with home-sickness and must be sent back to her native mountain air. "This illness is not one to be cured with pills and powders" the doctor shrewdly advises. Interestingly, it had been previously mentioned that Heidi's deceased mother, Adelheid, was "a sleep-walker, and had fits".[8]

Excessive daytime somnolence often provokes a provisional diagnosis of narcolepsy, but the full syndrome of daytime somnolence, impaired nocturnal sleep, cataplexy, sleep paralysis, and hypnogogic or hypnopompic hallucinations is rather seldom encountered in clinical practice. One possible literary example of a character with sleep paralysis is to be found in *The Subtle Knife*, the second book in Philip Pullman's trilogy *His Dark Materials*: the aeronaut Lee Scoresby finds himself pursued by airborne enemies, who are counter-attacked by the thought commands of his passenger, the shaman Stanislaus Grumman:

> Pinioned in his dream, Lee could neither move nor cry out, and he suffered the terror of the pilot as the man became aware of what was happening to him.[9]

Possible sleep-related disorders have also been identified in another Oxford based classic, the Alice books: the excessively somnolent dormouse at the mad tea party (*Alice's Adventures in Wonderland*, chapter 7), and the snoring of The Red King and the White and Red Queens (*Through the looking-glass*, chapters 4 and 9).[10]

Sleep and its addenda were clearly subjects which fascinated William Shakespeare (1564–1616). Everyone knows "To sleep, perchance to dream" from the famous "To be or not to be" soliloquy in *Hamlet* (Act III, scene i, line 65). In *The Tempest*, Sebastian is clearly ahead of the medical thinking of his time when he remarks to Antonio "Thou dost snore distinctly. There's meaning in thy snores" (II;i:220–221). The many references to sleep in *Macbeth* include "wicked dreams abuse the curtain'd sleep" (II;i:50–51) and "sleep in the affliction of these terrible dreams, that shake us nightly" (III;ii:17–19). Might these possibly be early references to the dream enactment characteristic of rapid eye movement (REM) sleep behaviour disorder?

Acknowledgements

Adapted from: Larner AJ. "Neurological literature": sleep-related disorders. *Adv Clin Neurosci Rehabil* 2007;7(5):22

References

1. Larner AJ. Charles Dickens, *qua* neurologist. *Adv Clin Neurosci Rehabil* 2002;2(1):22.
2. Cosnett J. Charles Dickens and sleep disorders. *Dickensian* 1997;93:200–204.
3. Jones P. *Ancient and modern.* London: Duckworth, 1999:56.
4. Fen E (trans.). *Chekhov: Plays.* Harmondsworth: Penguin, 1959:346–347,370.
5. Larner AJ. Obstructive sleep apnoea syndrome presenting in a neurology outpatient clinic. *Int J Clin Pract* 2003;57:150–152.
6. Larner AJ. David Livingstone's uvulectomy. *J Med Biogr* 2006;14:104–108.
7. Schapera I (ed.). *David Livingstone: family letters 1841–1856* (2 volumes). London: Chatto & Windus, 1959:II.177–178.
8. Spyri J. *Heidi.* Godalming: Colour Library, [1880] 1999:155–165,70.
9. Pullman P. *The subtle knife.* London: Scholastic, 1997:305.
10. Larner AJ. The neurology of "Alice". *Adv Clin Neurosci Rehabil* 2005;4(6):35–36.

Neurological literature: Neurophysiology

Previous articles in this series have focused on literary accounts or narratives of various neurological disorders, including headache, epilepsy, cognitive disorders, and sleep-related disorders. Since these conditions are the very stuff of human experience, and likely to be encountered at either first or second hand by the majority of the population, it is perhaps unsurprising that novelists have on occasion taken such conditions as source material for elaboration in their narratives. Neurological investigations, on the other hand, are perhaps less familiar to the general populace. This brief article looks at some literary references to neurophysiological investigations.

Electroencephalography (EEG)

It is perhaps unsurprising that authors within the genre broadly described as "science fiction" have been attracted by the technological implications of EEG for recording and/or monitoring the human nervous system.

The prolific sci-fi author Philip K Dick (1928–1982) explored the possibilities of EEG in his 1974 novel *Flow, my tears, the policeman said.*[1] (Musicophiles may know that "Flow, my tears" is taken from the title of a lute song composed by John Dowland in the late 16th century; the phrase was also used, almost three centuries later, by Gary Numan, based on his reading of Dick, in the first line of *Listen to the sirens*, the first track on Tubeway Army's eponymous album of 1978, re-issued 1979.) In the dystopian world of Dick's novel (possibly set in 1988), the "pols" (police) want a "fingerprint, voiceprint, footprint, EEG wave pattern" from the protagonist, Jason Taverner:

> … seated, he allowed terminals to be placed here and there on his head; the machine cranked out three feet of scribbled-on paper, and that was that. That was the electrocardiogram [*sic*! Checked in two separate editions of the book].

Despite having the EEG print Taverner suspects that the pols will not be able to find his information in their extensive data pool. Later when Taverner is being sought by the pols, they suggest that "we may be able to catch him with an EEG-gram projection from a copter", to get "a match of patterns". Clearly the view here is that EEGs are sufficiently individualised as to permit identification, even if recorded with leads placed "here and there" on the head.

Through its incarnation as the film *Blade Runner* (1982), probably the best known of Dick's novels is *Do androids dream of electric sheep?* (1968).[2] There may be EEG references here too, specifically in the allusions to the "Penfield mood organ", a method of "artificial brain stimulation" which features in both the first and last sections of the book. For example, Rick Deckard, squabbling with his wife, "at his console ... hesitated between dialling for a thalamic suppressant (which would abolish his mood of rage) or a thalamic stimulant (which would make him irked enough to win the argument)." Different dialling codes on the organ permit the selection of different moods, such as 888 for "the desire to watch TV, no matter what's on it" or 670 for "long deserved peace". (Music aficionados will know that this dialling trope also appears in Gary Numan's *I dream of wires* from the *Telekon* album of 1980.) As a neurologist reading this book (en route to, and in the interstices of, an international neurology conference!), I immediately thought the Penfield mood organ must be a reference to Wilder Penfield (1891–1976), whose work (with Herbert Jasper) stimulating the cortex of awake epilepsy patients undergoing surgery allowed him to map the functions of various regions of the brain.[3] The possible influence of Penfield on Philip Dick is acknowledged in a psychology textbook.[4] I do not know whether Dick ever underwent an EEG. His biographer Lawrence Sutin speculates a possible diagnosis of temporal lobe epilepsy to explain some of Dick's experiences, in particular a series of "visions and auditions" experienced in February-March 1974 which influenced his later writing.[5]

Ursula Le Guin (1929–2018) is another author categorised as within the sci-fi genre who has explored the narrative possibilities of EEG. The plot of *The lathe of heaven* (1971)[6] revolves around EEG recordings. Dr William Haber of the Oregon Oneirological Institute records EEGs during the dreams of George Orr:

> As soon as the cap was in place he switched on the EEG ... Eight of the cap's electrodes went to the EEG; inside the machine, eight pens scored a permanent record of the brain's electrical activity (20),

Somehow, Orr's dreams affect outward reality ("effective dreaming"), a faculty which Haber seeks to take control of, using his Augmentor which operates by "instigating and then reinforcing ... d-state activity" (56), for his own advancement, with catastrophic results.

In *The word for world is forest* (1976),[7] sometimes regarded as Le Guin's indictment of the Vietnam War, colonists from Earth have enslaved the peaceful Athshean people. Raj Lyubov, the colony anthropologist, has studied the Athsheans:

> He had wired countless electrodes onto countless furry green skulls and failed to make any sense at all out of the familiar patterns, the spindles and jags, the alphas and deltas and thetas, that appeared on the graph.

However,

> It was with Selver [an Athshean] as EEG subject that he had first seen with comprehension the extraordinary impulse-patterns of a brain entering a dreamstate neither sleeping nor awake.

Suffering a migraine headache, Lyubov wonders what Selver would do:

> Although knowing nothing of electricity he could not really grasp the principle of the EEG, as soon as he heard about alpha waves and when they appear ... there appeared the unmistakable alpha-squiggles on the graph recording what went on inside his small green head; and he had taught Lyubov how to turn on and off the alpha-rhythms in one half-hour lesson.

Electromyography and nerve conduction studies (EMG/NCS)

Literary accounts of EMG/NCS might be anticipated in patient accounts and fictional narratives featuring individuals with neuromuscular disorders.

In his account of the episode of Guillain-Barré syndrome (GBS) he suffered in 1981–2, the author Joseph Heller (1923–1999), best known for his 1961 novel *Catch-22*, reported two EMG examinations.[8] The first, performed at the Mount Sinai Hospital in New York, lasted less than fifteen minutes, whereas the second, performed at a rehabilitation facility, the Rusk Institute at the New York University Medical Centre, lasted more than two hours. "The worst both times ... was the needle plunged into the palm of the hand near the base of the thumb." At Rusk, all four limbs were examined as well as the face.

> None of the pain from the individual electric shocks or from the needle punctures was so intense as to make one wish to cry out. It was the repetitions of the electric shocks that rapidly wore me down, and which gradually proved more and more terrible ...

Although "[m]y F-wave responses were not too good" and "the doctor muttered to himself that there was definite facial involvement", Heller was subsequently informed that the "results of the EMG test were inconclusive, neither confirming nor eliminating Guillain-Barré".

In *Solomon's Porch: the story of Ben and Rose*, a college professor in his 50s develops a neurological illness which is labelled as GBS[9] (I have critiqued this diagnosis elsewhere[10]). It does not appear that EMG/NCS is ever performed, which may account for some of the diagnostic confusion.

Poetic rendering

Incredible as it may seem, both EEG and EMG/NCS have also been stimuli for poetry.

Daniel Hoffman's (1923–2013) poem "Brainwaves", from the collection entitled *The Center of Attention* (1974), begins "When his head has been wired with a hundred electrodes" and asks: "Is it good/For a man to be made aware that his soul/Is an electric contraption,".[11]

"The Nerve Conduction Studies" is by Simon Armitage (born 1963),[12] from which these selected lines are quoted:

> We loop conductive strips over the toes
>
> and fingers, press conductive strips and pads
> into the calves and wrists, ..
>
> ...
>
> the trace comes up on the screen and we ask
>
> for a second or third flick of the switch
> if the jolt doesn't travel the distance
> the first time.
>
> ...
>
> These tests are well known to hold true; we trust
> they prove nothing less than you dared hope for.

Acknowledgment

Adapted from: Larner AJ. "Neurological literature": neurophysiology. *Advances in Clinical Neuroscience & Rehabilitation* 2017;16(5):14–15.

References

1. Dick PK. *Flow, my tears, the policeman said.* London: Gollancz, 1974: 76,78,79,210.
2. Dick PK. *Do androids dream of electric sheep?* London: Gollancz, 1968:1–4,189–192.
3. Penfield W, Jasper H. *Epilepsy and the functional anatomy of the human brain.* Boston: Little, Brown, 1954.
4. Banyard P, Flanagan C. *OCR psychology. AS core studies and psychological investigations* (3rd edition). Hove: Psychology Press, 2013:133.

5. Sutin L. *Divine invasions. A life of Philip K. Dick.* London: Gollancz, 2006 [1989]:231–232.
6. Le Guin UK. *The lathe of heaven.* London: Gollancz, 1971.
7. Le Guin UK. *The word for world is forest.* London: Gollancz, 1976:45,80.
8. Heller J, Vogel S. *No laughing matter.* New York: Simon & Schuster, 1986:38,54–55,191–194.
9. Riley J. *Solomon's Porch: the story of Ben and Rose.* Baltimore: America House, 1999.
10. Larner AJ. GBS100: some literary and historical accounts. In: Willison HJ, Goodfellow JA (eds.). *GBS100: Celebrating a century of progress in Guillain-Barré syndrome.* Peripheral Nerve Society, 2016:20–27.
11. Hoffman D. *Beyond silence: selected shorter poems 1948–2003.* Baton Rouge: Louisiana State University Press, 2003:168.
12. Armitage S. *The universal home doctor.* London, Faber and Faber, 2002:43–44.

Neurological literature: Render's syndrome

In a previous piece published some years ago (2006), two recently published books on Asperger's syndrome and autism were reviewed.[1] The reviewer took exception to what he perceived to be the possible pathologisation of variants of human behaviour characterised by social impairments, all absorbing narrow interests, repetitive routines, speech and language peculiarities, problems of non-verbal communication, and motor clumsiness under the rubric of "Asperger-like syndrome" or "autism" related to failure of theory of mind, that is the apparent ability to attribute mental states to others.

It must be mentioned here that the evidence of Hans Asperger's involvement in the Nazi euthanasia programme, reported in 2018,[2] was not known at the time of the publication of these books or of the review. The term Asperger syndrome is no longer used in the most recent diagnostic systems.

The reviewer suggested the possibility of conceptualising a converse disorder characterised by what he chose to term "hypermentalising," the presumption of knowing others' mind states (excessive theory of mind?). Needless to say, further experience has indicated that other authors have also considered and written about this latter possibility, not least one of the 20th century's finest writers, Ursula Le Guin (1929–2018), but reaching rather different conclusions.

In a short story/novella entitled *Vaster than empires and more slow*, published in 1971, a character named Osden is initially described thus:

> Mr. Osden is really a very rare case. In fact, he's the first fully cured case of Render's Syndrome – a variety of infantile autism which was thought to be incurable. . . . The therapy was completely successful.[3]

The name Render is, by Le Guin's admission, taken from the protagonist (Charles Render) of a story by Roger Zelazny (1937–1995), initially published as *He Who Shapes* in 1964 and subsequently in 1966 as *The Dream Master*.[4] (The potential of dreams has also been explored by Le Guin, as described in a previous article.[5])

Osden is "an empath". Indeed, as a consequence of his treatment, his autistic defence has been unlearned and he has a supernormal empathic capacity, feeling the feelings of others as well as his own. Indeed Osden's faculty of "wide range bio-empathic receptivity" is not species-specific, "he could pick up emotion or sentience from anything that felt". This ability equips him to be the "Sensor" of an Extreme Survey expedition to explore a new, alien world.

I had envisaged the hypothetical hypermentaliser as having "highly developed social skills, 'team workers' who are good at motivating other people to work for them" with an "excessive interest in other people's business".[1] Osden, however, fails entirely to fit this pattern. He cannot form any human relationship, the sum of his treatment having been to "turn an autism inside out". He is surrounded by a "smog of cheap second hand emotions" and sometimes puts his head in a polythene bag (sic) in the belief that this cuts down on the empathic noise he receives from others. He is helplessly obedient to the demands of others' emotions, reactions, and moods. His colleagues find him arrogant and venomous, a spreader of discord, and one calls him "Mr No-Skin", a metaphor reflected in his physiognomy: "He looked flayed. His skin was unnaturally white and thin showing the channels of his blood". Osden reports that his original autistic defence of total withdrawal from others has been replaced by re-transmission of the negative or aggressive affects others feel towards him. The mission Commander, Haito Tomiko, thinks autism may be preferable.[3]

Zelazny's Render may perhaps have had some symptoms along the autistic spectrum: "after the death of Ruth [his wife] and of Miranda, their daughter, ... he had begun to feel detached. Perhaps he did not want to recover certain empathies; perhaps his own world was now based upon a certain rigidity of feeling" (Ref.4, p. 23). Osden, by contrast, having been "cured", cannot detach.

Another potential instance of knowing too much of others' minds is reported by Douglas Adams (1952–2001) in *The Restaurant at the End of the Universe* (1980), the second novel in his extremely popular *Hitchhiker's Guide to the Galaxy* series. The enlightened, accomplished and above all quiet Belcerebron people of Kakrafoon are punished for this behaviour by a galactic tribunal which inflicts upon them telepathy, "that most cruel of all social diseases". The consequence is that "in order to prevent themselves broadcasting every slightest thought that crosses their minds to anyone within a five mile radius, they now have to talk very loudly and continuously" about inconsequential subjects.[6]

One putative attribute of hypothetical hypermentalisers was that they were "vocative and willing to express opinions, often forcefully, however little knowledge they actually have, opinions which they can alter dramatically dependent upon the needs of the situation".[1] If humans struggle to intuit beyond their subjectivity, then hypermentalisers may assume that everyone else is a hypermentaliser and behave, like the afflicted Belcerebron people, accordingly. Whether that is deemed pathological behaviour is for others to decide.

Acknowledgment

Adapted from: Larner AJ. "Neurological literature": Render's syndrome. *Advances in Clinical Neuroscience & Rehabilitation* 2018;18 (1):21.

References

1. Larner AJ. *Asperger's syndrome and high achievement: some very remarkable people* by Ioan James; *Different like me. My book of autism heroes* by Jennifer Elder. *Adv Clin Neurosci Rehabil* 2006;6(5):36.
2. Czech H. Hans Asperger, National Socialism, and "race hygiene" in Nazi-era Vienna. *Mol Autism* 2018;9:29.
3. Le Guin UK. *The found and the lost. The collected novellas of Ursula K Le Guin.* New York: Saga Press, 2016:1–36.
4. Zelazny R. *The Dream Master.* New York: iBooks, [1966] 2001.
5. Larner AJ. "Neurological literature": neurophysiology. *Adv Clin Neurosci Rehabil* 2017;16(5):14–15.
6. Adams D. *The Hitchhiker's Guide to the Galaxy. The complete trilogy of five.* London: Pan, 2007:230.

Neurology at the movies

A number of previous articles have examined the portrayal of neurological disorders in literary texts. Novels and stories have been a potent stimulus for film adaptations, and hence it is not surprising that neurological disorders, with their dramatic possibilities ("based on a true story"), sometimes crop up in films. However, films often exercise a powerful suggestion to viewers, and hence incorrect or inauthentic portrayals of neurological disease might exert adverse effects.

This article reviews some examples of "neurology at the movies". Psychiatric disorders portrayed in film are not discussed here, examples of which have been documented.[1] The power of such films to influence public opinion is of note, for example *One Flew Over the Cuckoo's Nest* (1975), based on the novel by Ken Kesey, probably did a great disservice to the cause of ECT.

Personal film viewing experiences have been supplemented by recourse to an internet movie database (IMDb.com) and reviews from *Time Out* magazine (www.timeout.com/film).[2] Documentary films are not considered here, biographies and dramas being the genres most likely to involve portrayals of neurological disease.

Epilepsy

Epilepsy in films has been systematically (and entertainingly) examined by Baxendale.[3] Included are film versions of Dostoyevsky's novels *The Idiot* and *The Brothers Karamazov* which feature characters with epilepsy. Also noted in this review is a film version of Shakespeare's *Othello* (1965), presumably based on Othello's blackout which is labelled as epilepsy by Iago. Objections to the notion that Othello has epilepsy have been raised, including the circumstances and the prompt recovery, which suggest syncope as a more likely diagnosis.[4]

More recent films with an epilepsy connection include *The Exorcism of Emily Rose* (2005) and *Requiem* (2006), both based on a documented German source case of the early 1970s. Emily Rose believes herself to be possessed by demons and undergoes an exorcism, only to die a couple of days later. The priest conducting the exorcism is then accused of "negligent homicide" when it transpires that he suggested cessation of Emily Rose's epilepsy drugs. A courtroom drama ensues, one issue being whether this patient had epilepsy and psychosis. In *Requiem*, the protagonist is Michaela who suffers seizures and hallucinations and stops anti-epileptic drug therapy of her own volition.

Multiple sclerosis

The celebrated cellist Jacqueline du Pre (1945–1987) is perhaps one of the most high profile sufferers of MS. The biopic *Hilary & Jackie* (1998) documents her relationship with her sister, but the *Time Out* review fails to even mention Jackie's multiple sclerosis. The theme of young talent cruelly robbed by disease is also evident in the drama *Go Now* (1995), when a young soccer player develops MS. On a more positive note, in the TV drama *The West Wing*, President Bartlett (Martin Sheen) seems able to run the White House and the USA despite his MS, although he has concealed this diagnosis from the voters. The occurrence of serious neurological illness in heads of state, and whether this should be known to the electorate, has been previously reviewed.[5]

Parkinson's disease

Based on the Oliver Sacks celebrated book, *Awakenings* (1990) is an account of postencephalitic parkinsonism and the effects of levodopa. Otherwise, film accounts of PD seem few, despite its prevalence. The comedy drama *What we did on our holiday* (2006) features an elderly patient with PD.

Motor neurone disease

Despite its clinical rarity there have been a few films featuring motor neurone disease. In the US, the condition is sometimes known as Lou Gehrig's disease because the legendary New York Yankees first baseman developed this condition, as seen in *A Love Affair: the Eleanor and Lou Gehrig Story* (1978). MND is a surprising backdrop for a comedy romance in *Hugo Pool* (1997) wherein an LA pool cleaner falls in love with a young man dying with the disease. More typical of the "young life blighted by cruel disease" genre is *Jenifer* (2001).

Stroke

Biopics have occasionally featured stroke, for example *The Patricia Neal Story* (1981), about the actress, sometime wife of Roald Dahl, whose stroke-related aphasia threatened her acting career.[6] Julian Schnabel's film of *Le scaphandre et le papillon* (*The diving bell and the butterfly*, 2007), based on Jean-Dominique Bauby's account of locked-in syndrome from the inside, is perhaps one of the most compelling film accounts of neurological disease.

Coma

A study of 30 movies depicting prolonged coma found misrepresentation to be common (e.g. awakening from prolonged coma with cognition intact) ,which might impact on public perceptions of coma.[7]

Miscellaneous others

Many neurologists may never see a case of X-linked adrenoleukodystrophy unless they attend a showing of *Lorenzo's oil* (1992), documenting the Odone family attempting to develop a treatment for this rare condition which has afflicted their son. Lorenzo's oil, a 4:1 glyceryl trioleate-glyceryl trierucate combination, reduces hexacosanoic acid levels, and following clinical trial has been recommended in asymptomatic boys with normal brain MRI results.[8]

Daniel Day Lewis won an Oscar for his rendition of Christy Brown, a sufferer from cerebral palsy, in *My left foot* (1989).

Jack Nicholson portrays a writer with obsessive compulsive disorder in *As good as it gets* (1997), although an altogether more compelling rendition is given by Tony Shalhoub in the US TV serial *Monk*.

Some films featuring characters with amnesia or memory loss, some in the context of Alzheimer's disease, have already been noted.[9]

Conclusion

To paraphrase:[1] Should neurologists watch films? What has cinema ever done for neurology? Is "biopic" simply a blend word for "biographical myopic"? Although licence is integral to the art of film making, the majority of (non-documentary) filmic portrayals of neurological disease are simply dishonest. Maybe they should carry a health warning.

Acknowledgment

Adapted from: Ford SF, Larner AJ. Neurology at the movies. *Adv Clin Neurosci Rehabil* 2009;9(4):48–49.

References

1. Byrne P. Why psychiatrists should watch films (or What has cinema ever done for psychiatry?). *Advances in Psychiatric Treatment* 2009;15:286–296.
2. Pym J (ed.). *Time Out film guide* (17th edition). London: Random House, 2009.

3. Baxendale S. Epilepsy at the movies: possession to presidential assassination. *Lancet Neurol* 2003;2:764–770.
4. Larner AJ. Has Shakespeare's Iago deceived again? http://bmj.com/cgi/eletters/333/7582/1335, 2 January 2007.
5. Owen D. Diseased, demented, depressed: serious illness in Heads of State. *Q J Med* 2003;96:325–336.
6. Larner AJ. Tales of the unexpected: Roald Dahl's neurological contributions. *Adv Clin Neurosci Rehabil* 2008;8(1):22.
7. Wijdicks EF, Wijdicks CA. The portrayal of coma in contemporary motion pictures. *Neurology* 2006;66:1300–1303.
8. Moser HW, Raymond GV, Lu SE et al. Follow-up of 89 asymptomatic patients with adrenoleukodystrophy treated with Lorenzo's oil. *Arch Neurol* 2005;62:1073–1080.
9. Larner AJ. "Neurological literature": cognitive disorders. *Adv Clin Neurosci Rehabil* 2008;8(2):20.

Parkinson's disease before James Parkinson

Introduction

Every neurologist knows that James Parkinson (1755–1824) published *An Essay on the Shaking Palsy* in 1817. In this work Parkinson described six personally observed cases, although three were only seen in passing, what Professor Andrew Lees has evocatively termed "street watch methodology", an experience which may be familiar to many neurologists even today. The eponym of Parkinson's disease was promoted later in the nineteenth century (1877) by Jean-Martin Charcot.[1]

A question long asked is whether Parkinson was describing a new disease in 1817, or whether he was simply the first to crystallise the clinical gestalt which we now recognise as "Parkinson's disease" (PD).

Parkinson and his pamphlet

Like authors before and since, Parkinson attempted a review of the previous literature in his account of the shaking palsy, mentioning the works of authors dating from classical antiquity (Galen) up until the eighteenth century (e.g. Gerard van Swieten, Hieronymus David Gaubius, William Cullen). Two authors whose works seem to have been of particular significance to Parkinson were Sylvius and Boissier de Sauvages.

Franciscus Sylvius de la Boë (1614–1672) was a Dutch physician and scientist who made a distinction between "those tremors which are produced by attempts at voluntary motion, and those which occur whilst the body is at rest"; the latter he termed *Tremor coactus*. This distinction still forms an important component of clinical history taking in the assessment of tremor disorders. Galen and van Swieten had also distinguished between rest and action tremor.[2]

François Boissier de Sauvages de la Croix (1706–1767) was a French physician and botanist. His interest for Parkinson was his description of *Scerotyrbe festinans*, the phenomenon whereby "Patients, whilst wishing to walk in the ordinary mode, are forced to run". Festination or festinant gait is a reflection of the postural instability which is one of the cardinal features of PD.

Whether these authors were describing PD is not clear, since they each mentioned only one aspect of the clinical phenotype. In recent years, an account by the Hungarian physician Ferenc Pápai Páriz (1649–1716) has been identified, the *Pax corporis* of 1690, in which all four cardinal signs of PD are described.[3] Parkinson does not reference this work, and it would seem highly unlikely that he knew of it, since it was written in Hungarian.

Parkinson's disease before Parkinson?

Appeal to the historical record may help to answer the question as to whether cases conforming to Parkinson's description occurred before his pamphlet. In this context it should be remembered that "shaking palsy" might have been used in ways other than that denoted by Parkinson. For example, Parkinson's almost exact contemporary Caleb Hillier Parry (1755–1822), based in rural Bath rather than cosmopolitan and industrial London, described in 1815 the "shaking palsy" in which the "head and limbs shake, more especially on any muscular exertion", a description perhaps more suggestive of essential tremor than Parkinson's disease.[4]

The surgeon and anatomist John Hunter (1728–1793) has been suggested to have described a case of PD in his Croonian Lecture of 1776:

> "Lord L-'s hands are almost perpetually in motion, ... When he is asleep his hands etc are perfectly at rest, but when he wakes, in a little time they begin to move."[5]

The French painter Nicolas Poussin (1594–1665) was from 1650 troubled with worsening tremor. A sophisticated tremor analysis of lines in selected of his works produced between the 1620s and 1660s has concluded that they show a progressive decrease in movement velocity, which would be consistent with a diagnosis of PD.[6]

Leonardo da Vinci (1452–1519) may also have described a case of PD. In a manuscript now in Windsor Castle he wrote:

> " ... in paralytics ... who move their trembling limbs such as the head or the hands without permission of the soul; which soul with all its power cannot prevent these limbs from trembling."[5]

Calne and colleagues suggest that the reference to "paralytics" indicates a difficulty with voluntary movement[5] which might now be interpreted as hypokinesia.

Non-medical narratives

Non-medical narratives may sometimes contain descriptions of clinical disorders. There are several examples of novels which feature characters with PD, most published in recent years.[7,8] Charles Dickens (1812–1870) may have described progressive supranuclear palsy in 1857, over a century before the definitive clinical account of Steele, Richardson and Olszewski (1964).[9] Dickens may also have described Parkinson's disease in his characterisation of Frederick Dorrit in the novel *Little Dorrit* (1857). He "stooped a good deal", turned round in a "slow, stiff, stooping manner", and spoke with a "weak and quavering voice", which might be indicative of the typical posture of PD and, possibly, the hypophonic voice.[10]

William Shakespeare (1564–1616) is credited by one influential literary critic, Howard Bloom, with the "invention of the human",[11] so it is perhaps not surprising that his plays and poetry are claimed to describe various clinical disorders including paralysis, stroke, sleep disturbances, epilepsy, dementia, and the neurology of syphilis.[12] Claims for PD have also been made,[13] for example in this quote from *Troilus and Cressida* (I:ii:172–5), wherein Ulysses is describing the ageing Achilles:

> And then, forsooth, the faint defects of age
> Must be the scene of mirth; to cough and spit
> And with a palsy fumbling on his gorget,
> Shake in and out the rivet.

The gorget is a piece of armour protecting the throat.

Conclusion

There are occasional accounts dating prior to 1817, in both medical and literary sources, which are suggestive of PD. The relative paucity of these reports has been ascribed to the fact that the disease typically occurs in those aged greater than the prevailing life expectancy of earlier historical periods, and that the symptoms were not easily distinguished from "normal senescence".[5] This echoes Parkinson's own comments in 1817 to the effect that remedies were seldom sought for the symptoms and signs he was describing, which may also explain why three of his cases were seen only in passing on the street.

Acknowledgment

Adapted from: Larner AJ. Parkinson's disease before James Parkinson. *Adv Clin Neurosci Rehabil* 2014;13(7):24–25.

References

1. Parkinson J. *An Essay on the Shaking Palsy 1817.* Chichester: Wiley-Blackwell, 2010.
2. Koehler PJ, Keyser A. Tremor in Latin texts of Dutch physicians: 16th-18th centuries. *Mov Disord* 1997;12:798–806.
3. Bereczki D. The description of all four cardinal signs of Parkinson's disease in a Hungarian medical text published in 1690. *Parkinsonism Relat Disord* 2010;16:290–3.
4. Larner AJ. Neurological contributions of Caleb Hillier Parry. *Adv Clin Neurosci Rehabil* 2004;4(3):38–9.
5. Calne DB, Dubini A, Stern G. Did Leonardo describe Parkinson's disease? *N Engl J Med* 1989;320:594.
6. Haggard P, Rodgers S. The movement disorder of Nicolas Poussin. *Mov Disord* 2000;15:328–34.
7. Haan J. Protagonists with Parkinson's disease. In: Bogousslavsky J, Dieguez S (eds.). *Literary medicine: brain disease and doctors in novels, theater, and film* (Frontiers of Neurology and Neuroscience Volume 31). Basel: Karger, 2013:178–87.
8. Van der Brugger H, Widdershaven G. Being a Parkinson's patient: Immobile and unpredictably whimsical. Literature and existential analysis. *Medicine Health Care and Philosophy* 2004;7:289–301.
9. Larner AJ. Did Charles Dickens describe progressive supranuclear palsy in 1857? *Mov Disord* 2002;17:832–3.
10. Larner AJ. Charles Dickens qua neurologist. *Adv Clin Neurosci Rehabil* 2002;2(1):22.
11. Bloom H. *Shakespeare: the invention of the human.* London: Fourth Estate, 1999.
12. Fogan L. The neurology in Shakespeare. *Arch Neurol* 1989;46:922–4.
13. Stien R. Shakespeare on parkinsonism. *Mov Disord* 2005;20:768–9.

GBS100: Some literary and historical accounts

The 100th anniversary of the description of acute demyelinating neuropathy with cerebrospinal fluid *dissociation albumino-cytologique* by Gullain, Barré, and Strohl, was celebrated in 2016.

Introduction

The importance of hearing patient narratives of disease – "hearing the patient's voice" – is increasingly recognised as a complement to the technical narratives of disease produced by clinicians. As well as being of intrinsic interest, the patient perspective may broaden medical sensibility to, and perception of, the experiential aspects of disease, and rightly give the impression that clinicians are actually listening to their patients rather than simply shaping their narratives for their own purposes.

As for other neurological diseases, there are many patient accounts of GBS (see for example Box, and http://www.guillainbarresupport.org/group/the-reading-rooms/forum/topics/books-related-to-gbs), only a few of which are discussed here, alongside some fictional accounts and some possible historical cases.

Patient narratives of GBS

The American author Joseph Heller (1923–1999), most noted for his 1961 novel *Catch-22*, developed GBS in late 1981 and subsequently wrote an account of his illness, *No Laughing Matter* (1986).[1] The book consists of alternating chapters by Heller and his friend Speed Vogel, so that both patient and collateral narratives are provided, although it might be argued that Vogel is simply Heller's alter ego (p.220), since during the author's illness Vogel lived in his house, wore his clothes, forged his signature on cheques, dealt with his fan mail, and "more or less assumed his identity" (p.72).

From the Heller/Vogel account, neurological problems began with weakness (difficulty pulling open a door, removing a heavy sweater over his head), along with dysphagia (trouble swallowing a meal after the first few mouthfuls, a symptom calculated to ring alarm bells in a "prodigious eater") and cacogeusia (food tasting metallic). At the gym, simple stretching exercises proved difficult:

> ... lying supine on a mat ... Bending each leg in succession, I was supposed to wrap my arms about the shin and lift my head to touch my chin to my knee. I could not come close, on either side. (p.22)

Heller could only do 7–9 of his usual 15 push-ups. The following day, a Sunday, Heller again noted food tasted metallic, as well as chewing his food more slowly than usual, and he reflected that:

> ... something neurologically unpleasant was taking place inside me, something I could not control and could not fathom. All of my limbs felt tired. (p.19)

He spoke to his physician to report his symptoms, who diagnosed GBS over the telephone and arranged to see him, followed shortly thereafter by a neurological consult (with Dr Walter Sencer) and admission to the medical intensive care unit of the Mount Sinai Hospital in New York (Sencer published a number of articles in the *Journal of the Mount Sinai Hospital*, later the *Mount Sinai Journal of Medicine*, in the fifties and sixties but none relate to GBS). At no time did Heller report an experience of numbness or pain (p.21).

During his 22 day ICU admission he did not require ventilation, although a tracheostomy was mooted at one point, but his weakness was profound, with dysarthria, dysphagia requiring a nasogastric tube, and respiratory and cardiac monitoring. His major gripe was sleep deprivation, and then a fear of not waking from sleep, which led to low mood and psychiatric consultations. Treatment was entirely supportive, Heller's illness predating effective immunotherapies for GBS.

There was some doubt about the diagnosis because two lumbar punctures returned normal results and it was with relief (according to Heller) that a third puncture (all were reported to be painless) showed a raised protein, confirming the suspected clinical diagnosis.

Despite a weakness so profound that he could not lift his head or roll over, Heller commented that:

> I never once throughout the entire experience thought of myself as weak ... I was paralyzed, not weak. And in truth, *I* wasn't weak. My *muscles* were weak. (p.162; italics in original)

The corner was turned shortly after Christmas 1981, with gradual neurological improvement thereafter such that after three months and three days he left Mount Sinai Hospital for a rehabilitation facility (the Rusk Institute at the New York University Medical Center) until mid-May 1982.

In passing, Vogel gives an answer to the perennial question of why we refer to "Guillain-Barré syndrome" and not "Guillain-Barré-Strohl syndrome", despite the tripartite authorship of the original 1916 paper. One of Heller's friends was the novelist Mario Puzo (1920–1999), author of *The Godfather* (1969), later made into a celebrated film. Informed of Heller's diagnosis by a mutual friend, Puzo apparently blurted out:

> "My God, that's terrible!"
> "Hey Mario, you know about Guillain-Barré?"
> "No, I never heard nothing about it [*sic*]," Mario replied. "But when they name any disease after two guys, it's got to be terrible!" (44)

By extrapolation, then, perhaps naming a disease after three guys (Guillain-Barré-Strohl) rather than two would render it simply too awful to contemplate (e.g. Gerstmann-Straussler-Schenker disease?).

It was also in 1981 that Tony Benn (1925–2014), an English Labour Party politician and socialist, developed GBS, just at the time that he was campaigning (ultimately unsuccessfully) for the deputy leadership of his party. Brief notes on his illness appear in his political diaries,[2] beginning with an entry on 5th May:

> I wasn't feeling very well today. I have had this tingling in my legs and now my hands, and my face has been very hot and my skin has been rough.

After consulting a fellow Member of Parliament who was medically qualified and being reassured, Benn then consulted his general practitioner on 14th May:

> ... I reported the fact that I have got this tingling in my legs. At the moment, walking is like having on wellington boots full of water with a sponge in the feet. I don't have any feeling in my feet and my hands tingle. ... he thinks it might be some nerve condition.

By 1st June, referral to a neurologist was made, and on 4th June:

> I was taken to see Dr Clifford Rose [(1926–2012)], who examined me. I hadn't got reflexes in my legs or arms.
>
> He told me, "I think I know what this is. If this was only a medical consideration, I would recommend you came into hospital at once." I said, "Well, I'm perfectly happy to do that because I am simply incapacitated."

Benn was then in hospital from 6th-17th June, when there are no diary entries.[2] Following discharge from hospital, he noted on 24th June that "I have to rest in the afternoon, and it's still painful to walk", but there do not seem to be any other comments on possible sequelae in the abridged diary entries, other than "very tired" on 26th September, although this could have been related to his political campaigning prior to the Party Conference which started that day. Overall therefore it seems that Benn's GBS was a mild episode, with prominent sensory symptoms, unlike Heller who seems not to have had any sensory features.

An account of recovery from "Guillain-Barré disease" by an ex-patient, Lucile Marie Hoerr Charles, Ph.D., a college professor, appeared in 1961 in the journal *Psychosomatic Medicine.*[3] Her illness followed a routine smallpox vaccination (and was indeed written up and published as such[4]). She had been affected two years earlier and was paralysed for six weeks; looking back:

> It has been a tremendous experience of both body and soul; a slow, painful, miserable, uncertain, frightening business; often wonderful, and full of amusement and beauty also.

Pain was a significant factor in this illness:

> In a few days my hands became numb and, when I held them under the faucet, I could not tell the difference between hot and cold water. Soon, severe pain came. My whole body seemed to be just one cramp.

Despite making a good physical recovery,

> ... convalescence after leaving the hospital was also a dark, trying period – in some ways worse than acute illness. No more support by institutional routine, nor by the constant bustle, energy, authority and tender-loving-care of medical people who were pushing hard to make me well.

I'm sure many, if not all, neurologists have encountered GBS patients who report feeling "abandoned" after hospital discharge, despite good or excellent neurological recovery.

Fictional accounts of GBS

Paralysis and the recovery from it are subjects calculated to attract writers for their dramatic potential.

Although not perhaps amounting to a genre, a number of classic novels, primarily intended for children ("improving literature"), feature characters who develop paralysis: Katy Carr in *What Katy Did* (1872) by Susan Coolidge; Clara Sessman in *Heidi* (1880) by Johanna Spyri; Colin Craven in *The Secret Garden* (1909) by Frances Hodgson Burnett; and Pollyanna Whittier in *Pollyanna* (1913) by Eleanor H Porter.[5,6] All these novels predate the original description of GBS, but the fictional possibilities of this paralysing disorder have subsequently been exploited on occasion.

Likewise, playwrights have sometimes featured characters with paralysis, for example in *The Sacred Flame* (1928) by W Somerset Maugham (himself medically qualified), and in *Whose life is it anyway?* (1978) by Brian Clark, featuring post-traumatic paraplegia and quadriplegia respectively.

In *Solomon's Porch: the story of Ben and Rose* by Jane Riley,[7] Ben Windham, a college professor in his 50s, develops a neurological illness which is labelled Guillain-Barré syndrome. Whether the author had any experience of the disease, firsthand or otherwise, is not clear, but there are certainly elements in the description of the disease within the novel which jar for the clinical reader. The patient suffers progressive weakness over a few weeks (contrary to the blurb: "... gone to a party ... when he left, he was crippled"), but despite seeing numbers of clinicians and undergoing a lumbar puncture no clear diagnosis emerges, other than polyneuropathy, possibly related to his underlying diabetes. Despite this lack of diagnostic clarity, a referral to rehabilitation services is made, before transfer to another medical centre where the diagnosis is immediately made by a physician and confirmed by a neurologist who labels some of the previously consulted professionals "irresponsible". However, the time frame of the novel is a little difficult to follow and it may be that neurological decline has been going on for more than eight weeks, indeed the neurologist considers that this is the "slow kind" of GBS, and "considers yours chronic inflammatory demyelinating polyneuropathy" (p.67–8); so, not GBS at all! This may explain the treatment with prednisolone (p.67,81) as well as plasma exchange. The patient's wife is still, perhaps justifiably, a little baffled:

> I don't really understand the difference between GBS and CIDP. You seem to be somewhere in between the symptoms for those two. (p.88; also 206)

So, subacute demyelinating polyradiculoneuropathy (SIDP), perhaps?

When the patient weakens again, nearly 18 months later, the prednisolone still seems to be continuing (p.106), prior to more plasma exchange, IVIg, and cyclophosphamide. More perplexingly, the patient complains of loss of sensation from the chest down, suggesting a sensory level (p.41,54,85), and eventually is found to have cervical spine stenosis (p.115) requiring surgical intervention, presumably some form of decompression. Whilst the concurrence of two neurological diseases is not impossible, it is implausible. Furthermore, the patient's wife is informed by the physician shortly after the GBS diagnosis that the "leading cause of death related to GBS is suicide" (p.69), though how a paralysed patient might achieve this is not made clear.

Although accuracy or consistency is not necessarily to be anticipated in a work of fiction, one seriously worries for any GBS patient or family who might use this book as a source of information about the disease; the frontispiece disclaimer, with direction to Guillain-Barré Foundation International for information regarding the disease, is a welcome inclusion.

In *Thaw* by Monica Roe,[8] the narrating voice is that of Dane Rafferty, an 18 year-old skier recovering from GBS in a rehabilitation centre in Florida, far distant from his family and friends in Upstate New York. The action takes place over a 2–month period, with flashbacks to premorbid days and disease onset. Hence the focus is more on the recovery phase, particularly the input from a physiotherapist, Anya, and an occupational therapist (no doctor ever darkens these pages!); this is concordant with the author being a "traveling physical therapist" (according to the blurb) presumably with experience of treating GBS patients:

> Recovery from Guillain-Barré is a strange process. After you get to the totally helpless point and hang out there for a while, the whole thing begins to reverse itself. ... Trouble is, during all that time when you can't move, your joints start to tighten up, so by the time you can actually tell your muscles to move on their own, the joints may be too stiff to let it happen. (p.56)

As Dane's recovery progresses (relatively quickly), some of the techniques of neurorehabilitation are mentioned, for example the tilt table, and the patient's perspective on this:

> ... this table contraption that can be cranked from horizontal to completely vertical, bringing the person on it along like Frankenstein's monster rising from the slab. Supposedly, being upright and putting weight on your feet is good for your bones and joints even if you can't do it yourself. ... It also makes you dizzy if you do it for too long at first. (p.69–70)

Later Anya sets Dane to work with the inflatable ball ("It makes my muscles burn like hell ... but it's really been helping my balance and torso strength"; p.192), and standing using the parallel bars:

> ... the sequence of steps that we always go through to get me standing: plant both feet on the ground, as far back as possible; shift weight forward through my legs. At this point, [Anya] usually pulls my hips forward and up, giving just a little extra power to my upward push. (p.193–5)

There is something heartfelt and, one senses, personal about the battles of the physiotherapist, Anya, with her recalcitrant patient, Dane, and with patient relatives complaining about lack of recovery in their loved ones. When Dane is refusing physiotherapy Anya tells him:

> You all want to be fixed, want us to perform miracles we can't guarantee and provide answers we can't give. ... You'll still turn right around and blame us if it doesn't end up exactly the way you hoped it would. (p.207)

This lament sounds like the voice of experience, but, like the other passages quoted, is seamlessly assumed within the narrative. Most readers will probably be more concerned with whether Dane recovers fully, gets back to skiing, and makes it up with his girlfriend (who ditched him when he was paralysed, intubated and ventilated – girls surely know how to pick their moment!). But there is much to enjoy in this book if reading with neurological spectacles on.

Historical diagnoses of GBS

Appeal to the historical record may help to answer the question as to whether cases of GBS occurred before 1916. However, since CSF findings were part of the diagnostic characterisation by Guillain and his colleagues, and lumbar puncture was only performed after the 1890s, cases conforming to the original clinical and investigational description (*dissociation albumino-cytologique*) occurring before the 1916 publication would seem unlikely. Hence inferences based on clinical features are the only recourse to answer the question of historical cases.

For example, Reich suggested that the renowned American neurosurgeon Harvey Cushing (1869–1939) suffered from GBS in 1918 when an undiagnosed illness characterised (in Cushing's diaries) by symmetrical weakness, numbness, and paresthesias of the hands and feet, areflexia, bilateral facial paresis, diplopia, and fever prevented him from operating.[9]

Another, more formalised, example of this diagnostic revisionism relates to the diagnosis of Franklin Delano Roosevelt (1882–1945), 32nd President of the United States of America (1933–45), who suffered a paralytic illness in 1921 which is widely believed to have been due to poliomyelitis. Goldman and colleagues re-examined the clinical features as recorded in biographies of FDR (he never underwent lumbar puncture or neurophysiological testing as far as is known) and undertook a Bayesian (i.e. probabilistic) analysis of eight key symptoms.[10] By multiplying prior probabilities by symptom probabilities, Goldman et al. calculated that six out of the eight symptoms had posterior probabilities which favoured a diagnosis of GBS over poliomyelitis. It is an interesting analysis, which certainly attracted widespread attention when first published, but essentially inferential. The exact determination of FDRs diagnosis is never likely to be established, but Goldman et al. persist in their view.[11]

Could other previous fictional accounts of paralysis in fact be describing GBS? Any such claim would of course be entirely speculative. Since both Katy Carr and Pollyanna Whittier develop paralysis following traumatic accidents, GBS would not seem to be a likely diagnosis. Few details are given about the onset of illness in Clara Sessman and Colin Craven, but as they both subsequently recover from these illnesses it might be wondered whether they had GBS, in Colin's case sufficient to produce lower limb atrophy.

Conclusion

It seems implausible that GBS did not exist before G, B, and S took to print, thus characterising GBS as a disease entity. This same condition seems to be described, for example, in the reports by Landry (1857) and by Wardrop (1834; see also *Lancet* 1987;i:861–2). An argument has also been made for William Barnett Warrington, who presented possible cases in 1903 and 1914.[12] Thus a "100th anniversary" of GBS is in some ways a cultural construct. Clinical knowledge of GBS which has accrued over the century has sometimes transferred into the literary domain, spawning both personal and fictional (or possibly "factional") accounts of the disease, as well as attempts at retrospective diagnosis, which may inform and/or frustrate readers, depending on the perspective (lay, professional) from which they approach these documents. At best, these narratives may allow clinicians to hear the patient voice which may ultimately inform their approach to the management of sick patients.

Acknowledgment

Adapted from: Larner AJ. GBS100: some literary and historical accounts. In: Willison HJ, Goodfellow JA (eds.). *GBS100: Celebrating a century of progress in Guillain-Barré syndrome*. Peripheral Nerve Society, 2016:20–27.

References

1. Heller J, Vogel S. *No laughing matter*. New York: Simon & Schuster, 1986.
2. Benn T. *The Benn diaries. Selected, abridged and introduced by Ruth Winstone*. London: Arrow Books: 1996:514–520.
3. Charles LM. Morale in recovering from Guillain-Barré disease. Account of an ex-patient. *Psychosom Med* 1961;23:298–304.
4. Kisch AL. Guillain-Barré syndrome following smallpox vaccination; report of a case. *N Engl J Med* 1958;258:83–84.

5. Keith L. *Take up thy bed and walk: death, disability and cure in classic fiction for girls.* London: Routledge, 2001.
6. Larner AJ. Some literary accounts of possible childhood paraplegia and neurorehabilitation. *Dev Neurorehabil* 2009;12:248–252.
7. Riley J. *Solomon's Porch: the story of Ben and Rose.* Baltimore: America House, 1999.
8. Roe MM. *Thaw.* Asheville, North Carolina: Front Street, 2008
9. Reich SG. Harvey Cushing's Guillain-Barré syndrome: an historical diagnosis. *Neurosurgery* 1987;21:135–141.
10. Goldman AS, Schmalstieg EJ, Freeman DH Jr, Goldman DA, Schmalstieg FC Jr. What was the cause of Franklin Delano Roosevelt's paralytic illness? *J Med Biogr* 2003;11:232–240.
11. Goldman AS, Schmalstieg EJ, Dreyer CF, Schmalstieg FC Jr, Goldman DA. Franklin Delano Roosevelt's (FDR) (1882–1945) 1921 neurological disease revisited; the most likely diagnosis remains Guillain-Barré syndrome. *J Med Biogr* 2016;24:452–459.
12. Ziso B, Larner A. William Warrington (1869–1919): GBS before G, B, and S? *Eur J Neurol* 2016;23Suppl1:868 (abstract 32236).

Some patient accounts of GBS

Bed Number Ten by Sue Baier and Mary Zimmeth Schomaker (1986)

Nothing but time. A triumph over trauma by Judy Light Ayyildiz (2000)

Guillain-Barré Syndrome: My Worst Nightmare by Byron Comp (2004)

A Solitary Confinement by Robin Sheppard (2007)

Going Full Circle: My Fight Against Guillain Barré Syndrome by Phillip Taylor (2008)

My Wake-up Call – A Survivor of Guillain-Barré Syndrome by Jerry L Jacobson (2011)

Guillain-Barré Syndrome: My Journey Back by Shari Ka (2011)

Blue Water, White Water. A true story of survival by Robert C Samuels (2011)

Why didn't I die? by Barbra Sonnen-Hernandez (2011)

Happily Ever After: My Journey with Guillain-Barré Syndrome and How I Got My Life Back by Holly Gerlach (2012)

My GBS Story. A Life Changed by Cindy Herron (2014)

Index

www.ingramcontent.com/pod-product-compliance
Lightning Source LLC
Chambersburg PA
CBHW060412200326
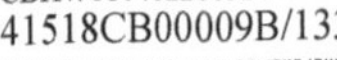